Clinical Research Transformed

Olli S. Miettinen • Johann Steurer
Albert Hofman

Clinical Research Transformed

Springer

Olli S. Miettinen
Faculty of Medicine
McGill University
Montreal, QC, Canada

and

Department of Medicine
Weill Cornell Medical College
New York, NY, USA

Johann Steurer
Horten Center for Patient-oriented
Research and Knowledge Transfer
University of Zürich
Zürich, Switzerland

Albert Hofman
Department of Epidemiology
Harvard T.H. Chan School of Public Health
Boston, MA, USA

ISBN 978-3-030-06175-3 ISBN 978-3-030-06176-0 (eBook)
https://doi.org/10.1007/978-3-030-06176-0

Library of Congress Control Number: 2019931861

This Springer imprint is published by the registered company Springer Nature Switzerland AG.
The registered company address is: Gewerbestrasse 11, 6330 Cham, Switzerland

You see things; you say 'Why?'
But I dream things that never were; and I say 'Why not?'

– George Bernard Shaw

Foreword

Central in any clinician's practice of medicine is *the need to know about hidden truths concerning patients' health*: When a patient complains about some new symptom, the doctor needs to know about the presence/absence of its possible underlying illnesses; when a patient's actual illness has been established, the doctor may need to know about the causal origin of this case of that illness; and most importantly, the doctor needs to know about the future course of the case, especially about the way this depends on the choice of treatment. To these ends, the doctor needs to possess, or have access to, the relevant segment of the *scientific knowledge-base* of clinical medicine.

While there already is an abundance of published clinical research, the evidence produced by it has not really translated into the knowledge doctors need for those insights into hidden truths about their patients' health; the research, while 'patient-oriented,' has not really been patient-*relevant.* This disappointing realization by the authors was the starting point for the development of this book.

To help remedy the wanting relevance that has plagued clinical research up to now, the authors of this book developed, and present in it, a *novel theory-framework* – of concepts and principles – for all three of the principal lines of directly practice-relevant clinical research. Thus transformed, they believe clinical research would produce the evidence-base that would provide for the development of the requisite knowledge-base for clinical medicine. The transformed research the authors expect to provide for transformation of today's clinical medicine – still essentially prescientific – into *genuinely-scientific clinical medicine.* This transformation they expect to make clinical medicine more productive and efficient, and thereby also more economical.

This book's authors did not attribute the wanting relevance of the research to any fundamental deficiencies in what clinical researchers – both medical and statistical – have customarily aimed to optimize, namely, the methodology of their studies. Rather, the authors deemed the meagre relevance of the research to have been due to failure to address what clinical doctors really need to know about, namely, the *probabilities* of the relevant-but-hidden truths about their patients' health, and in particular, these probabilities with specificity to the cases' particulars in relevant respects. Such knowing – probabilistic and maximally case-specific – about relevant-but-hidden truths concerning a patient's health the authors call *gnosis*.

While the authors thus bring this ancient term for esoteric spiritual knowing into modern use in reference to the esoteric medical knowing that is in the essence of clinical medicine, the linguistic basis for this is that the concept of gnosis in this book subsumes dia-*gnosis*, etio-*gnosis*, and pro-*gnosis*. These terms for the three species of esoteric knowing in clinical medicine strongly suggest 'gnosis' as the most apt omnibus term for them.

But at issue in this is more than a neologism for a familiar concept. For, the concept the word 'gnosis' denotes in this book actually is quite new, and in an important sense. As the authors explain, today's preeminent dictionaries of medicine do not present diagnosis and prognosis as species of clinicians' *knowing* (about the health of the patient), and etiognosis they don't even recognize as belonging in the lexicon of today's medicine. Diagnosis those dictionaries present as a 'determination' (of the nature of the patient's illness), and different from this, prognosis they present as a 'forecast' or 'prediction' (of the future course of the patient's health). (The authors' concept of clinicians' gnoses is not restricted to knowing only high-probability truths nor, even, to knowing what the highest-probability truth is, whatever be the probability.)

Recognition that central in clinical doctors' work is such *knowing* – probabilistic and case-specific, about hidden truths in their patients' health – naturally would lead to clinical researchers' concern to develop a *scientific knowledge-base* for gnoses in the authors' meaning of this term of theirs. This vision of progress was the prompting for the development of this book on the theory – concepts and principles – of truly patient-relevant '*gnostic clinical research.*'

The authors underscore that, in truly-relevant gnostic clinical research for whichever discipline of clinical medicine, a *great multiplicity of probabilities* needs to be addressed for whichever truth of gnostic concern, this on account of all the distinctions that need to be made in the gnostic profiles of the cases for a start. As a simple example of this, a set of ten diagnostic indicators, each of them addressed in terms of only two categories, already implies distinctions among 1024 different diagnostic profiles, representing subdomains of the domain of case presentations for diagnosis that is at issue. In an etiognostic study, the causal history at issue adds to this, and so do treatment and prospective time in prognostic studies.

This complexity the authors understood to mean that the distinctions need to be made in the framework of a *statistical model* for the probability in question. Thus, the core concept in this book is the generic *Gnostic Probability Function, GPF*. In diagnostic research, this is a *prevalence* function that is subject to being studied directly, while in etiognostic and prognostic research, it typically is derived through an *incidence* function. Thus, *epidemiological* concepts are central to this research, and the case-specifying particulars are represented by *statistical* variates. The *objects of study* are the parameters in the GPF that has been designed for the study. This means that the objects of study are designed in statistical terms and that the objects' design – for relevance – defines the form of the study result and dominates the study's methods' design.

The theory of gnostic clinical research the authors see, and present, as an extension of critically-developed theory of epidemiological research on the etiology/etiogenesis of illness (for population-level preventive medicine). For this reason, they characterize gnostic clinical research as *meta-epidemiological clinical research.* In this, they emphasize the need for a tenable conception of the etiogenetic study – that it is not a 'case-control study,' and even less a 'cohort study,' but a *case-referent* study aka case-*base* study.

Particularly notable about this epidemiological parentage of the theory of the transformative clinical research that this book is about, is the etiogenetic viewpoint in the synthesis of the data assembled in an intervention-prognostic study, most notably a randomized trial on a treatment. In the synthesis of the data assembled in such a trial, deployment of the epidemiological case-base approach, notably with representative sampling of the study base, provides for addressing a prognostic probability function for each of the outcome events documented in the trial. This has been a major point in the efforts of this book's senior author – *Olli S. Miettinen* – to entice truly-competent epidemiological researchers to extend their research horizon from the advancement of the knowledge-base of community medicine – epidemiology that is – to that of clinical medicine.

Centrally involved in the theory of meta-epidemiological clinical research presented in this book is *logistic regression,* which already is well ingrained in epidemiological research on the etiogenesis of illness. Its role in the theory presented in this book is so central that there no longer is any role for Cox regression (or Poisson regression, for that matter). In this statistically-unified theory of the field of gnostic clinical research, the variant of logistic regression for addressing prognostic probability functions has previously been the missing element. It could be termed *Miettinen regression.*

Now that Miettinen's previous, passing advocacies of meta-epidemiological clinical research take full expression in this book, it is relevant to take note of something expressly epidemiological in his past: For half a century already, he has played a pivotal role, the impact of which hardly can be overestimated, in the reformation of epidemiological research – in the transformation of this research from an activity of 'doctors who could count' to research in the framework of educatedness in the theory of the research, which has a foundation in statistics as well as in medicine. For his pioneering work as a 'developer and teacher' of epidemiological research, he received his first honorary doctorate well over three decades ago already. And the point of this here is that Miettinen's transformation of epidemiological research bodes well for the transformation of clinical research that he advocates in this book.

This book includes quite comprehensive a Glossary of the carefully-used terminology in it, much of which will be unfamiliar for medical academics preparing for gnostic clinical research, with very concise definitions of the terms. And it also includes a Retrospective Overview of the teachings in it, serving to retrace the main features of the train of thought in it. That Overview can serve as an alternative, actual introduction to the contents of this important but quite challenging book, for study even before its Part 1, entitled 'Introduction to Transformative Clinical Research.'

An Appendix is constituted by the written version of the lecture – very well attended – which Miettinen gave in the Nobel Forum of the Karolinska Institute (KI) in Stockholm in February 2018. This lecture was a presentation of his vision of how the transformation of clinical research – which would be transformative of clinical medicine – would best come about. It was Miettinen's expressed wish that the medical faculty of the KI would see the need for such clinical research as is advocated in this book and would incorporate the precepts in this book about that research into its curriculum of education in epidemiological research – for the needed, avant-garde, globally-oriented education of both epidemiologic and clinical academics who aim to make a career in gnostic clinical research.

While there is no doubt in our minds that the research would be of great benefit to patients everywhere, and also to various systems of clinical healthcare, we have to wait and see whether the KI will be in a position to accommodate Miettinen's educational expectations on the KI, preparatory to the Institute's role in the research itself. But it is our view that the KI and its medical faculty should feel very honored by Miettinen's high expectations on them, and we sincerely hope that they will be able to accommodate those expectations.

Professors of Epidemiology
Karolinska Institute, Solna, Sweden

Anders Ahlbom
Anders Ekbom

Preface

The societal burden of modern medicine, notably when societally sponsored, was an abiding concern of the Scottish doctor *Archibald (Archie) Cochrane* (1909–1988). This led him to devote a sabbatical year of his to thinking about the ways the costs of the U.K. National Health Service (NHS) could be reduced, and he published, in 1972, a book on the subject. In it, he explained how his 'random reflections' on the matter led him to realize that the NHS is unduly costly because it is *inefficient*, and that it is inefficient because its *doctors don't have the requisite knowledge* to choose the most effective treatments.

From those insights, Cochrane derived the idea that the care by the doctors in the NHS would become more effective and efficient, and thereby less costly, if *randomized trials* advanced the doctors' knowledge about the comparative effectiveness of the available options for treatment.

This idea of Cochrane's, through his advocacy of it in that famous little book, led to a major escalation in the conduct of those trials: Tens of thousands of them are now published each year. And this abundance of those trials, in turn, led to their 'systematic reviews' in the framework of a program (informal, international) dubbed the Cochrane Collaboration. Hundreds of such 'Cochrane reviews' are now annually deposited in the Cochrane Library (in cyberspace).

Like Cochrane, we, the authors of this book, also have devoted much thought to the state of the knowledge-base of medicine and, especially, to research intended to advance this vitally-important knowledge. And in this, alas, we've come to realize that, despite the enormous amount of 'patient-oriented' original research that already has been completed and also 'systematically reviewed' – research not only on the effects of treatments but on diagnostics too – *clinical medicine still is largely devoid of its requisite, directly patient-relevant knowledge-base*. Our explanation for the continuing lack of major progress in the development of the knowledge-base of medicine is that *the research, while patient-oriented, has not really been patient-relevant*.

Clinical trials on treatments' comparative effectiveness (and safety) have not been patient-relevant simply by virtue of the treatments in them having been randomly assigned, nor has their relevance been assured by supplementation of the randomization with 'blinding' of its result together with the rest of the trials' now-common methodology: advance specification of the 'primary' and 'secondary' outcomes (for both efficacy and safety); design of the trial's size by means of statistical 'sample size determination'; 'analyzing' the data by means of 'Cox regression' and thus quantifying the effects in terms of 'hazard ratios'; treating non-adherence to the assigned treatments as though inconsequential upon substitution of 'intention to treat' for treatment proper; adjusting for 'multiple comparisons' by means of 'Bonferroni corrections'; etc.

For a randomized trial to really be patient-relevant, it would need to contribute to the knowledge-base of doctors' treatment-related prognostications – their knowing, at the time of the choice of treatment and with specificity to the patients' various prognostic profiles at that time, about the *probabilities* (profile-conditional) of the prospective occurrence of various possible outcomes, with specificity also to the choices between the compared treatments and various periods or points of prognostic time.

Thus, for real relevance for doctors' prognostic concerns about their patients, any randomized trial, inherently focused on cases from the defined *domain* of patients' admissibility into it, needs to address suitably-designed *prognostic probability functions*, each of these having to do with the probability of the prospective occurrence of a particular type of outcome of treatment – the way this probability depends on (suitably-defined, subdomains-defining) prognostic indicators, the choice of treatment, and prognostic time, all of these jointly considered.

For *diagnoses* – doctors' knowing about the probabilities of the presence of particular ones of the possible underlying illnesses (as explanations of the patient's sickness) – relevant are not the teachings of 'clinical epidemiologists' about the 'sensitivity' and 'specificity' for the illness at issue of the various items in the diagnostic profile of the case, nor the 'likelihood ratios' of the elements in the profile contrasting the presence of the illness with its absence. For, the diagnostician is not, and should not be, concerned with those 'accuracies,' nor to move from completely unconditional 'prior odds' of the presence of the illness to its corresponding 'posterior odds' by sequential multiplications by the 'likelihood ratios.'

The true concern of diagnosticians is to know about the probability of the presence of the illness in question directly, conditionally on the patient's diagnostic profile as a whole. Thus, research truly relevant to diagnostic probability-setting is about *diagnostic probability functions*, each of them addressing, for a particular domain of case presentation, the way the probability of the presence of a particular illness is a joint function of the diagnostic indicators involved in the definition of the diagnostic profiles of cases from the domain.

Clinical research transformed to production of (empirical versions of) such *gnostic* – dia-, etio-, and prognostic – probability functions would serve to make clinical medicine truly knowledge-based, truly scientific. Such research – *such gnostic clinical research* – would be, in this way, *transformative of clinical medicine* into closer conformity with the Cochranian ends of enhanced effectiveness and efficiency and, thereby, into greater affordability.

This book is about the *theory* – concepts and principles – of thus-transformed clinical research. In this, our point of departure is our critically-formulated conception of the essence of clinical medicine (Sect. 1.1), and the closing Part VII is a retrospective overview of the text, retracing the precepts in it on clinical research transformative of clinical medicine into genuinely knowledge-based, scientific medicine.

As the presentation involves a large number important but subtle concepts, many of them novel to readers preparing for the transformed-and-transformative clinical research we advocate, that closing Part VII is followed by a Glossary of the most important terms.

We devote an Appendix to '*machine learning*' as an adjunct, or possibly even an alternative, to the transformed clinical research we envision as transforming clinical medicine – from today's largely agnostic, opinion-based medicine to scientifically learned, knowledge-based medicine.

Another Appendix outlines our vision of how the needed transformation of 'patient-oriented' clinical research – for the development of the requisite knowledge-base (gnostic) for genuinely-scientific clinical medicine – will most likely come about, namely, by the educational and research leadership role of the to-be-excellent *epidemiologic* segment of a particular, very distinguished, faculty of medicine.

Montreal, QC, Canada — Olli S. Miettinen
Zürich, Switzerland — Johann Steurer
Boston, MA, USA — Albert Hofman

Acknowledgments

About the development of this book, we owe nothing to colleagues upholding the existing orthodox conceptions of *medicine's interface with science*. To wit, this book's development was not tethered to the major premise about this interface in the already century-old but still highly-influential 'Flexner report' on medical education, nor to the counterpart of this underpinning the recent yet already very widespread Evidence-Based Medicine (EBM) movement, championed by 'clinical epidemiologists.' For, we take serious exception to the Flexnerian notion that medicine is scientific by virtue of the 'scientific way of thinking' students of medicine purportedly learn from scientists working in the laboratories of medicine, and just as unrealistic we take to be the EBM notion that each practitioner of clinical medicine can, and should, critically follow all of the relevant literature on clinical research, and on this basis continually update their knowledge relevant to their practice – in disregard of what clinical-scientific experts say.

As this book thus is, essentially, a research-cultural orphan, our heroes to here acknowledge are not so much colleagues sharing in the genesis of the teachings we present as the adoptive parents of them. A near-final version of the manuscript of this book we shared with the epidemiology professors *Anders Ahlbom* and *Anders Ekbom* of the Karolinska Institute (in Stockholm). We are very grateful to them for their ready acceptance of our eminently heterodox precepts on the vitally-important field of clinical research, and their expression of this in a Foreword for this book.

In the various technical aspects of the development of the manuscript – mainly the various intricacies of Microsoft's Word but also the implementation of statistical computing – we were fortunate to have the very expert collaboration of our colleague Jakob Martin Burgstaller in Zurich. For this, we owe a debt of gratitude to him.

With particularly great appreciation, we acknowledge the financial support of the Helmut Horten Foundation, through its funding of the Horten Center for Patient-Oriented Research and Knowledge Transfer of the Department of Medicine, Faculty of Medicine, University of Zurich. This Center's overall mission, explicit in its name, was the contextual impetus for the development of this book (on clinical research that is not only patient-oriented but maximally patient-relevant). And this

Center also was the financial basis of its director's – Steurer's – work on this book project.

The senior author of this book – Miettinen – wishes to acknowledge, also, an important contribution specific to his work in the development of this book. While already an emeritus professor and thus free from routine academic duties, his concentration on this mission could have been distracted from by the various non-academic duties that normally are unavoidable. But there was no such distraction, even. His wife, Judith Seidman, even though still holding a high office in the country's capital, saw to that.

Contents

Part I
Introduction to Transformative Clinical Research

Chapter 1
The Essence of Clinical Medicine

Contents

Abstract In this book – introduction to the kind of clinical research that would produce the (still-missing) scientific knowledge-base for clinical medicine (cf. Preface) – the point of departure naturally is the essence of the work of clinical doctors as distinct from that of all other professionals involved in clinical healthcare. Distinctive of the work of doctors in clinical healthcare is the central role in it of the pursuit and attainment of firsthand insights into hidden truths about the health of their clients. Such esoteric insights, ones of probabilistic ad-hoc knowing – *gnosis*: dia-, etio-, and/or prognosis – result from bringing general medical knowledge – *gnostic clinical knowledge* – to bear on the available facts on their clients. While thus distinct from other, 'paramedical' professions of clinical healthcare, clinical medicine also is distinct from the other species of (the genus) medicine: from community medicine – from epidemiology, that is.

Keywords Definition · Medicine · Clinical medicine · Community medicine · Epidemiology · Diagnosis · Etiognosis · Prognosis · Gnosis · Science

1.1 Prevailing Conceptions of Clinical Medicine

Critical thinking about clinical research at large necessarily is predicated on a tenable conception of *medicine* at large, and then of that which distinguishes *clinical* medicine within medicine-not-otherwise-specified.

O. S. Miettinen et al., *Clinical Research Transformed*,
https://doi.org/10.1007/978-3-030-06176-0_1

The pursuit of a tenable conception of medicine, and of clinical medicine within it, naturally begins with the definitions of these concepts in *dictionaries* of medicine; and as the mission in this is to achieve tenable conceptions of them, the dictionary definitions are to be read as counselled by Francis Bacon [1]: "Read not to contradict, nor to believe, but to weigh and consider."

The dictionary to first consult might well be *Stedman's* [2], which in its Preface is characterized as "the most up-to-date authority on medical language." In this dictionary, *medicine* is defined as:

> The art of preventing or curing disease; the sciences concerned with disease in all its relations.

And for *clinical* medicine the definition in this dictionary is:

> The study and practice of medicine in relation to care of patients; the art of medicine as distinguished from laboratory science.

These definitions might be juxtaposed with their counterparts in *Dorland's* [3], which in its Preface is characterized as "the outstanding authoritative guide to the language and usage in medicine and related health care fields," this in response to the demand for "agreed-upon body of terminology for the fruitful interchange of ideas." According to this authority, *medicine* is:

> The art and science of the diagnosis and treatment of disease and the maintenance of health;

and *clinical* medicine is:

> The study of disease by direct examination of the living patient.

Rather than simply believing these (discordant, less-than-clear) definitions, weighing and considering them (à la Bacon, above) obviously is called for; and this inescapably leads to the (surprising and disappointing) conclusion that *the concept of clinical medicine remains devoid of even an agreed-upon definition of its essence, to say nothing about a definition that is not only agreed-upon but also tenable*. But in what follows, we present, for the reader to weigh and consider, a conception of clinical medicine very different from those above [4], the one we regard as tenable.

1.2 The Knowledge-Based Essence of Clinical Medicine

1.2.1 Teaching as the Essence of Clinical Medicine

In the practice of clinical medicine, doctors provide professional healthcare to their clients, patients and others (who, different from patients, are not suffering from and complaining about sickness [4]); and so also do various 'paramedical' professionals collaborating with clinical doctors – nurses, psychologists, nutritionists, social workers, etc. The work of all of these professionals is 'clinical' in the etymological meaning of this adjective, which derives from the Greek word for bed. Clinical healthcare is provided directly – commonly 'at the bedside' – to its recipient, not indirectly, as is the case with consultants' inputs and laboratory 'studies,' for example.

The essence of clinical doctors' professional work – "in relation to the care of patients" and other clients – is not "preventing or curing disease." After all, rarely is a clinician able to prevent or cure a case of a disease or other illness, even in modern medicine. Instead, the essence of clinical doctors' work is that which actually is the etymological meaning/denotation of the very word *'doctor,' which is Latin for 'teacher.'* Disease (L. *morbus*) is but one species of ill-health/illness [4], the others being defect (L. *vitium*) and injury (Gr. *trauma).*

The *essential function of clinical doctors*, we say, is to teach their clients about their health, including about the means by which it could be changed for the better. Decisions about treatments are, in principle at least, prerogatives of doctors' suitably-informed clients rather than in the purview of doctors themselves [4]; and more to the same effect, rarely are the chosen treatments carried out by the doctors who teach about them. Treatments, notably when medicational, are generally executed by the clients of doctors.

To wit, *'doctoring'* would more appropriately mean teaching than treatment, by a doctor.

1.2.2 Gnoses as the Basis of Clinicians' Teachings

Teaching a person about their own health presupposes knowing about this – and, specifically, on a level deeper than the available facts relevant to this. As the basis of the teaching, a clinical doctor consulted by a client needs to know what facts are relevant to ascertain in the context of the type of case-presentation that is at issue; and in particular, the doctor commonly needs to know the meaning of the ascertained set of facts – the thus-established 'profile' of the case – in respect to relevant *hidden truths* about the client's health.

One species of such deeper professional **knowing** in clinical medicine is, we say, *diagnosis*: knowing about whether a hidden case of a particular type of illness is present. Another species of it is *prognosis*: knowing about whether a particular type of health outcome will emerge or prevail in the future. And a third species of this knowing is *etiognosis*: knowing about the causal origin – etiology/etiogenesis – of an existing case of illness – or sickness not due to illness – in respect to whether a particular antecedent of the case was causal to it. Diagnosis, etiognosis and prognosis are the three species of clinical doctors' case-specific *esoteric* knowing, the three species of the genus **gnosis** at the core of clinical medicine [4].

The proposition that knowing – of this esoteric, gnostic kind – is in the essence of clinical medicine (as the basis of doctors' teachings) is, remarkably, a novel one: Stedman's [2] defines diagnosis not as a species of knowing but in process terms – as "The determination of the nature of a disease, injury, or congenital defect." Prognosis it defines as "A forecast of the probable course and/or outcome of a disease." Dorland's [3], in turn, defines diagnosis as "1. the determination of the nature of a case of disease. 2. the art of distinguishing one disease from another"; and prognosis it defines as "a forecast as to the probable outcome of an attack of disease; the prospect as to recovery from a disease as indicated by the nature and symptoms of the case." Etiognosis is not defined in either one of those dictionaries.

1.2.3 Knowledge as the Basis of Clinicians' Gnoses

While, as a matter of logic and a professional-ethical imperative, clinical doctors' teachings are based on their gnostic insights into their clients' health, these insights doctors gain by bringing *relevant knowledge* – general (abstract; i.e., placeless and timeless) medical knowledge – to bear on the available facts on the case in question. Depending on what the gnosis is about, the relevant general knowledge is either diagnostic, etiognostic, or prognostic. Thus, fundamental to whichever discipline/'specialty' of clinical medicine – a 'learned profession' as it is – is knowledge in the particular meaning of the *gnostic clinical knowledge* that is relevant to practice in this discipline of clinical medicine. (A doctor practicing a particular discipline of medicine could reasonably be viewed as a medical specialist if there were, also, generalists of medicine; but there are no generalists of modern medicine – just as there are no generalists of professional sports, say.)

The set of available facts constituting the ad-hoc input into a clinician's gnosis – the *gnostic profile* of the case – generally underdetermines the (hidden) truth that the gnosis is about. Therefore, contrary to the implications of the definitions of diagnosis and prognosis in eminent dictionaries of medicine (above), the general medical knowledge relevant to diagnosis cannot generally be categorical so as to provide for "determination" of whether a particular illness is present; and for prognosis it cannot generally be categorical so as to provide for a "forecast" about the client's future health. In general, the medical knowledge underpinning gnoses in clinical medicine – and secondary to this the (gnosis-based) teachings of clinical doctors – needs to provide for *probabilistic* knowing about the clients' health; it needs to address *gnostic probabilities*.

1.3 The Needs for Knowledge Expanded by Science

Prior to the advent of medical science, the case-specific facts ascertained by doctors toward diagnosis derived almost exclusively from the history and physical examination of the patient; and as for prognosis, the remedies to improve the prospective course of the patient's health were very few.

Thus, in late seventeenth century, the 'British Hippocrates,' Thomas Sydenham, "began the treatment of virtually every disease by opening a vein with a lancet. In America, purging, blistering …, sweating through the use of heat and steam, and especially bleeding … also became the common medical therapies for almost all ills and were considered 'best practices'" [5, p. 16].

In the first medical school in America, as of its founding in 1765, the leading clinician was the 'American Sydenham,' Benjamin Rush. "As late as 1796, Rush still believed that 'there was but one fever in the world … and one disease,' the 'morbid excitement induced by capillary tension,' that responded best to the remedy of bloodletting and purging" [5, p. 23].

The advent of (laboratory-based) medical research has, as is well known, led to major expansion of what clinicians need to know, in lieu of the few, grand conjectures of Sydenham and Rush. For, consequent to research in pathology, doctors now need to think – and know – about *a multitude of actual somatic anomalies* – illnesses [4] – potentially underlying sickness – symptoms and/or overt signs [4]. And besides, on the basis of laboratory-level medical research in various 'basic sciences of medicine' there has been, and continues to be, *extensive and multifarious development of novel products and processes* for (potential) use in clinical medicine. In the face of these two lines of science-based innovation in what needs to be thought – and known – about, the requisite knowledge-base of modern medicine is vastly more complex than the conjectures that sustained the practices of Sydenham and Rush.

In these terms, the science-based expansion in doctors' needs for knowledge has to do with the *gnostic implications* of the medical products and processes that have become available for them through development inspired by knowledge from medical science. Thus, different from doctors prior to the advent of medical science, modern doctors (in some disciplines of clinical medicine) need to know, for instance, about the prognostic implications of (the processes of) thrombolysis, some of these processes (of treatment) involving the use of SK (streptokinase), some others the use of TPA (tissue plasminogen activator), etc. But they *need not know* the scientific basis for the development of such options for the treatment of thrombosis, nor even the structures of the thrombolytic agents.

1.4 Agnostic Medicine versus Pseudomedicine

With a discipline of clinical medicine viewed as a knowledge-based profession, one in which the relevant knowledge unique to doctors enables them to achieve (esoteric) knowing about their clients' health in terms of diagnostic and other gnostic probabilities (Sect. 1.2.3), the question arises: What about cases in which the knowledge relevant for the gnosis at issue remains non-existent or otherwise unfamiliar to the doctor dealing with the case? Does such a case fall outside the domain of clinical medicine, for the particular doctor at least?

Practice of clinical medicine we regard as *knowledge-based, genuine medicine* as long as the probability-setting in its gnoses is based on cognizance of the prevailing state of the needed gnostic knowledge – however wanting this knowledge may be. Immaterial to this is, we hold, whether the practitioner is a graduate of an accredited school of medicine and licensed to engage in the practice in question.

Practice without this cognizance, if free of pretenses of it, still is medicine rather than pseudo-medicine; it is medicine without full competence in it.

On the other hand, practice in essential ignorance about or disregard of the prevailing state of the relevant gnostic knowledge, while nevertheless affecting the possession and deployment of this knowledge, is practice devoid of the essence of clinical medicine (outlined above); it is *pseudomedicine, quackery* [4]. (According to Stedman's, quackery is unlicensed practice of medicine, while Dorland's defines it as "the fraudulent misrepresentation of one's ability and experience in the diagnosis and treatment of diseases or of the effects to be achieved by the treatment offered.")

1.5 Clinical Medicine as a Species of Medicine

According to *Stedman's* [2], clinical medicine is "the art of medicine [not otherwise specified] as distinguished from laboratory science" (Sect. 1.1) – which implies that all of medicine is constituted by the art of clinical medicine, and that this art is to be distinguished from medical science, all of which is laboratory-based science. We take exception to this, to both of these implications.

To us, clinical medicine is not a unitary art/discipline but the aggregate of the existing multitude of its constituent disciplines. And to us, clinical medicine is a species of the genus medicine, the essence of medicine – clinical and other – being doctors' gnosis-based teaching of their clients (or proxies of these) about the clients' own health (Sects. 1.2.1, 1.2.2, and 1.2.3). The specific difference that characterizes the clinical species of medicine has to do with the nature of clinical doctors' clients: *clinicians' clients are individuals, cared for individually* (rather than collectively, as a population).

That specific difference in our definition of clinical medicine implies its counterpart for another species of medicine: *community medicine*, in which a doctor cares for a single client, the population of a community of individuals collectively (rather than its members individually). We take *'epidemiology'* to be a synonym of that term for this neighbor of clinical medicine in the genus medicine [4]. At variance with this, Stedman's [2] defines community medicine as "the study of health and disease in a defined community; the practice of m. [medicine] in such a setting." In Dorland's [3], community medicine is left undefined.

A notable but non-definitional difference between clinical medicine and community medicine has to do with their respective purposes: clinical medicine is preventive (prophylactic) as well as therapeutic-cum-palliative, and rehabilitative besides, while community medicine is solely preventive.

References

1. Bacon F (1999) On studies. In: Vickers B (ed) Francis Bacon. The essays or counsels civil and moral. Oxford University Press, Oxford
2. Stedman's medical dictionary, illustrated in color, 28th edn. Williams & Wilkins, Philadelphia (2013)
3. Dorland's illustrated medical dictionary, 32nd ed. Elsevier Saunders, Philadelphia (2012)
4. Miettinen OS (2015) Medicine as a scholarly field: an introduction. Springer, Cham
5. Abrams JE (2013) Revolutionary medicine. The founding fathers and mothers in sickness and health. New York University Press, New York

Chapter 2
The Essence of Clinical Research

Contents

Abstract Critical conception of the distinguishing essence of clinical *medicine* within clinical healthcare at large, and also as a species of medicine at large (Chap. 1, above), provides for correspondingly-critical conception of clinical *research* within medical research at large. From the understanding that medicine is not a science flows, first, the understanding that clinical research is extrinsic to (clinical) medicine, with intended service to (clinical) medicine the distinguishing essence of it within research at large; and second, that the service of medical research to medicine proper is of two fundamentally different kinds. With only one of these – *gnostic clinical research* – serving to provide for *scientific medicine*, reasonably construed.

Keywords Definition · Medical research · Clinical research · Patient-oriented research · Clinical epidemiology · Evidence-based medicine · Basic clinical research · Gnostic clinical research · Scientific medicine · Medical science

2.1 Prevailing Conceptions of Clinical Research

In a book on *clinical research*, Stephen Glasser discusses the various ways in which this subject has been defined, which leads to his conclusion about their "validity" and to a definition of his own [1]:

> So, there is a wide range of definitions of clinical research, some valid, some not. I have chosen to adopt a 'middle of the road' definition that encompasses the term 'patient-

O. S. Miettinen et al., *Clinical Research Transformed*,
https://doi.org/10.1007/978-3-030-06176-0_2

> oriented research,' which is defined as research conducted with human subjects (or on material of human origin) for which the investigator directly interacts with the human subjects at some point during the study.

And very notably, the U.S. National Institutes of Health defines clinical research [2] as:

> Research on human subjects, that is:
>
> 1. Patient-oriented research. Research conducted on human subjects (or on material of human origin such as tissues, ...) for which an investigator (or colleague) directly interacts with human subjects. It includes (a) mechanisms of human disease, (b) therapeutic interventions, (c) clinical trials, or (d) development of new technologies.
> 2. Epidemiological and behavioral studies.
> 3. Outcomes research and health services research.

We, however, hold that the *definition of this class of research should specify* either the *object* of the research in question – the counterpart of the genome and/or inheritance in the case of defining genetics – or the *aim* of the research – the counterpart of understanding the functioning of the human body in the case of physiology (in the modern meaning of this term, different from the term's denotation in Nobel Prize for "Physiology or Medicine"; Sect. 3.2.1). This is to say that, in our view, this class of research is not productively defined by anything that has to do with the means used in studying its object or pursuing its aim. For, the means should not be preordained by the definition of the research but should be adopted ad hoc, with a view to optimization of the learning from the piece of research in question.

2.2 The Practice-Serving Essence of Medical Research

As medicine is not a science (or a set of sciences; Chap. 1, above), *medical research is not an aspect of medicine* (while research is immanent in and central to all empirical sciences). The common tenet that medicine is a science in addition to being an art is but a (profound) misunderstanding (Sect. 1.1).

Even though medicine is not a science, aspects of it are objects of inquiry in certain disciplines with no inherent relation to medicine, scholarly disciplines such as the sociology and economics. But actual *service to medicine* – to the health-related concerns intrinsic to it – is the very raison d'être and essential purpose of another major class of medicine-related research. Now, only research intended to serve the concerns intrinsic to (the practice of) medicine – applied research in this meaning of the term – can reasonably be taken to be *medical research* (clinical or epidemiological; Sect. 1.5). Hence, clinical research is to be construed as research (medical) intended to serve the concerns intrinsic to (the practice of) clinical medicine – research for the advancement of clinical medicine.

Thus construed, all of clinical research is 'applied' – applications-motivated – research rather than 'pure'/'basic' research, driven by interests of the investigators.

The raison d'être of clinical research is the *utility* of the attained knowledge, not anyone's interest in the knowledge.

2.3 The Fundamental Duality in Medical Research

In broadest terms, medical research makes two types of contribution to medicine (the practice of it). One of these two types of contribution characterizes each of the *'basic sciences of medicine,'* despite the basic (rather than applied) orientation of them. Specifically, research in each of these sciences has the potential of leading to discoveries that, through the intermediary of suitable and successful 'development,' result in novel products and processes for use in medicine – most notably novel tests for diagnostic (or prognostic) purposes and novel agents for use in treatments (prophylactic, therapeutic, or palliative). These sciences are, in this sense, basic to clinical medicine, but they serve (just as unwittingly) community medicine (epidemiology) as well, most eminently through the development of vaccines for community-level preventive medicine. This justifies the (routine) omission of the specification 'clinical' in the term 'basic medical sciences' in the context of viewing them as 'basic' to clinical medicine.

Knowledge from those 'basic sciences of medicine' does not constitute the *knowledge-base of the practice of medicine,* notably the knowledge-base of the estimation of diagnostic and other *gnostic probabilities,* which is in the essence of clinical medicine (Sect. 1.2.3). Nor are these probabilities addressed even in post-graduate medical education. And so, competence – expertise – in the estimation of gnostic probabilities has been presumed to be attainable only post-educationally, from extensive personal experience in clinical practice. Recently, however, it has become widely understood that the genuine source of this knowledge is constituted by diagnostic and other *gnostic clinical research.*

Awareness of the pivotal importance of gnostic clinical research for the practice of clinical medicine, together with the doctrine that each clinical practitioner needs to personally and critically follow the progress of this research, was at the root of the genesis of *'clinical epidemiology'* as 'a new basic science' that future clinicians need to study (Sect. 6.1) – as the basis for practicing *'evidence-based medicine.'* But by no means is 'clinical epidemiology' a science, and even less 'a new basic science' of clinical medicine. And the idea of each practitioner personally and critically (*sic*) following gnostic clinical research is altogether untenable as to its premises of the requisite time-availability and competence.

The point of all this in the present context is that scientific advancement of clinical medicine requires not only research on the laboratory level – in the 'basic sciences of medicine' – but also on the clinical level; that the research in those sciences needs to be supplemented by *gnostic clinical research* – as the source of the knowledge-base of clinical doctors' gnoses about the health of their patients and other clients (Sect. 1.2).

2.4 Medical Science vis-à-vis Scientific Medicine

Medicine has, as is well known, a long history prior to the advent of science of any kind, and prior to the advent of medical research in particular. Medicine therefore has a long history of having been founded on beliefs devoid of foundation in science. Most eminent among these was belief in the Hippocratic-and-Galenic doctrine about imbalances among the four bodily 'humors' as constituting the essence of various illnesses. This doctrine implied the need to direct treatments to restoration of the humors' balance, and the presumedly effective means to this end was bloodletting, commonly practiced even by leading doctors till quite recently (Sect. 1.3).

This doctrine, underpinning 'humoral medicine,' was overturned by Rudolf Virchow's 'cellular pathology' and, especially, by the novel understanding that various communicable diseases are 'caused' by (tissue invasion of) microbial agents. That 'revolutionary' understanding was brought about, very famously, in the late nineteenth century, by *the laboratory-level research of Louis Pasteur and Robert Koch*; and it was of *enormous practical consequence in medicine*, as it soon led to very effective preventive treatments, by vaccinations directed to various communicable diseases. Even though these 'causal' understandings involved some conceptual errors [3, 5], their impact on thought in medicine at large has subsequently been both extensive and profound.

The discoveries of the microbial basis of various communicable diseases, by the research of Pasteur and Koch, were not tantamount to these giants of medical science having discovered, in their laboratories, the means of preventing these diseases: required for the prevention was the subsequent *development* of the agents – vaccines – for use in these interventions and also of the knowledge-base of using them for the prevention and control of epidemics of these diseases in the practice of (community) medicine. Thus, the laboratory-level research was not tantamount to inauguration of *scientific medicine*, not even in respect to the prevention of some communicable diseases. And even at present, the already-abundant availability of, notably, diagnostic tests and therapeutic agents, developed on the basis of laboratory-level discoveries, is commonly the basis for agnostic medicine (Sect. 1.4), or even medical malpractice, rather than for something justifiably called scientific medicine.

Thus, a tenable conception of the sense in which an action in medicine (which is not science; Chap. 1) is scientific cannot be that something in it has its origin in science. An action in medicine is not scientific if it violates the imperatives of logic, which are inviolable in science itself and, by extension, in all extra-scientific actions aptly characterized as scientific. And an action in medicine, however logical and even knowledge-based, is not scientific if its knowledge-base does not derive from science, from medical research (Sects. 2.2 and 2.3), that is. Put in the affirmative, *medicine is scientific to the extent that its theoretical framework is rational – logical – and its knowledge-base in this framework derives from (medical) science* [3].

Given that essential to clinical medicine are the gnoses in it (Sect. 1.2.2), clinical medicine is scientific not on the basis of any insights from the 'basic sciences of medicine' but on the grounds of the *rational theory-framework of the gnoses* in it together with (gnostic) *clinical research as the basis of the gnoses* – of the gnostic probabilities constituting the foundation of the doctoring of the clients (Sect. 1.2.2).

2.5 Gnostic Research versus Gnosis Proper

Gnostic clinical research is science in the process meaning of 'science'; for any gnostic clinical study is an inquiry into a scientific object of study – the magnitude of a particular type of gnostic probability in a given domain of client presentation in the abstract (Sect. 1.2.3), specifically into the way in which this probability depends on a particular set of gnostic indicators, in the case of prognosis commonly together with prognostic time and the choice of prospective treatment. Assembly of gnosis-relevant facts naturally is involved, eminently, in the execution of a piece of gnostic clinical research.

Facts on a set of gnostic indicators are ascertained, also, in the pursuit of gnosis in the practice of clinical medicine; and this fact-finding is commonly referred as 'investigation' or 'study.' But this fact-finding is not done for the purpose of advancing scientific knowledge; rather, the gnostic fact-finding in the practice of clinical medicine is done so as to be more specific about the type of case that is at hand – preparatory to bringing correspondingly-specific general clinical knowledge (gnostic) to bear on the gnostic probability-setting in the individual case (in suitably 'individualized,' 'personalized' medicine).

This process of gnosis-oriented fact-finding and the facts' translation into gnoses in the practice of clinical medicine can be, and ideally is, scientific; *but it is not science*. It is scientific to the extent it is an element in *scientific medicine*, which to us is medicine with a logical theoretical framework and a knowledge-base from science (Sect. 2.4, above).

2.6 Clinical Research as a Species of Medical Research

As clinical medicine is a species of the genus medicine (Sect. 1.5), a consequence of this is that clinical research is a species of medical research, the other species of this research being community-medicine research, commonly termed *epidemiological research*. And just as we define clinical research as research aimed at advancement of the practice of clinical medicine (Sect. 2.2), epidemiological research is, to us, research aimed at advancement of the practice of community medicine.

In both clinical and epidemiological research, we hold, an important segment is conducted in the *laboratories* of 'basic medical sciences' (Sect. 2.3).

References

1. Glasser SP (ed) (2008) Essentials of clinical research. Springer, Dordrecht, pp 3–4
2. Clinical Research. In: Glossary of NIH terms. Retrieved August 11, 2016 from http://grants.nih.gov/grants/glossary.htm#ClinicalResearch
3. Miettinen OS (2015) Medicine as a scholarly field: an introduction. Springer, Cham
4. Abrams JE (2013) Revolutionary medicine. The founding fathers and mothers in sickness and health. New York University Press, NewYork
5. Carter KC (2003) The rise of causal concepts of disease. Case studies. Ashgate Publishing Company, Burlington

Chapter 3
Clinical Research and Clinical Medicine at Present

Contents

Abstract The doctrinal underpinnings of both 'basic' and gnostic clinical research are, at present, in suboptimal alignment with their respective reasons for being (in the advancement of clinical medicine). Medical academics representing the sciences (biological) that are viewed as 'basic' to medicine commonly mistake the discoveries from their research to be 'translatable' into the requisite knowledge-base of (the practice of) clinical medicine. And those whose research – of statistical type – actually should serve the development of this directly practice-serving knowledge (gnostic) fail in this, on account of the theoretical framework of the research remaining seriously misguided or otherwise underdeveloped. Clinical medicine itself, in consequence, remains out of alignment with what would reasonably be expected in this Information Age.

Keywords Basic clinical research · Translational research · Translational medicine · Diagnostic research · Etiognostic research · Prognostic research · Screening research · Published research, thesis research · Status quo of clinical medicine

O. S. Miettinen et al., *Clinical Research Transformed*,
https://doi.org/10.1007/978-3-030-06176-0_3

3.1 Prevailing Ideas about Clinical Research

3.1.1 Ideas about 'Basic' Clinical Research

Clinical research can be said to have begun with the scientific work of the chemist *Louis Pasteur* and, separately, that of the physician *Robert Koch*. Their research was of enormous consequence to medicine, to community medicine in particular. For, it famously was the basis for rapid development of practicable-and-effective vaccines for the prevention and control of common major epidemics of various communicable diseases. (Cf. Sect. 2.3.)

That research by Pasteur and Koch in the late nineteenth century – while inaugurating laboratory-level medical science with special reference to medical microbiology and focused on this particular one of the 'basic sciences of medicine' – quickly became the basis of *grand ideas about laboratory-based medical research* at large, as described in a grand epos on the history of medicine [1]. So, by the close of that century already, so explains that grand epos (p. 251), "the physician found himself at last free from the quicksands of dogmatism and metaphysics, armed with solid scientific principles [*sic!*], endowed with a large armamentarium of instruments and drugs." (Those "solid scientific principles" are not delineated in that epos.)

Those ideas have endured ever since. They are crystallized in that epos in a very notable maxim about laboratory-level medical research (p. 254): "[Modern medicine] is "made in laboratories, just as in the nineteenth century it was made in hospitals and in the Middle Age in libraries."

That idea about laboratories as the sole locus of medical research has recently given rise to the concepts of *'translational medical research'* and *'translational medicine*,' with the difference, if any, still quite ill-defined. The European Society of Translational Medicine, we're told [2], "defines TM as an interdisciplinary branch of the biomedical field supported by three pillars: benchside, bedside, and community." And attached to this 'definition' is the explication that, "Accordingly, TM is a highly interdisciplinary field, the principal goal of which is to coalesce assets of various natures to promote enhancements in prevention, diagnosis, and therapies."

The impression from this is that those two terms denote, quite interchangeably, a very grand concept founded on laboratory-level medical research. This concept appears to represent an *attempted fusion of inherently very distinct concepts*. In this (con)fusion, lost is not only the practice proper versus practice-advancing research duality (Chap. 1 vs. Chap. 2) but also of the purpose-based duality constituted by the aim in laboratory-level ('benchside') clinical research (à la Pasteur and Koch) to provide for the development of novel tools for clinical practice and the counterpart of this aim on the clinical ('bedside') level, namely to advance the knowledge-base of clinical medicine (Sect. 2.3).

While these grand ideas – dubious if not obviously untenable – now surround and animate laboratory-level clinical research, there also are, at present and quite independently of these, ideas specific to *clinical-level research* for advancement of the knowledge-base of clinical medicine. These ideas are differentiated according to what species of clinical gnosis is at issue. They are addressed in the Sections that follow.

3.1.2 Ideas about Diagnostic Research

The status quo of the theory of diagnosis and diagnostic research comes to focus in an *eminent book on diagnostic research* [2], in its introductory chapter already. Said in it is (p. 1) that

> Diagnostic evaluation is the first crucial medical intervention in an episode of illness ...

and (p. 2) that

> diagnosis covers not only test accuracy but also the basis for prognosis and appropriate treatment choice, ...

And about the concept of test (diagnostic) is said (p. 3) this:

> Diagnostic testing can be seen as the collection of additional information intended to (further) clarify the character and prognosis of the patient's condition and can include patients' characteristics, symptoms and signs, history and physical examination items, or additional tests using laboratory or other technical facilities.

So, in this eminent book on diagnostic research, diagnosis is not seen to be a species of doctors' esoteric knowing about their clients' health (cf. Sect. 1.2.2) but, curiously, as an "evaluation," which is construed as constituting an "intervention." This obfuscation is compounded by the statement that "diagnosis covers ... test accuracy." And quite odd is the notion – common in the circles of 'clinical epidemiology' (Sect. 6.1) – that the entirety of fact-finding for the diagnostic profile of a case (e.g., ascertainment of the patient's age) is diagnostic "testing," characterized by its particular "accuracy" for the diagnosis in question.

With this *utter confusion* about the relevant elementary concepts of medicine, this eminent book is about that *"test accuracy"* – with 'sensitivity' etc. the measures of this – instead of being about research on diagnostic probabilities, specific to various diagnostic profiles defining subdomains of defined domains of diagnostic challenges.

With this level of development of the general theory of diagnosis as the foundation for diagnostic research, the orientational *ideas about the nature of diagnostic studies are seriously misguided,* such as these (p. 1):

> the most important designs are the cross-sectional study (to determine the accuracy and added discriminatory value of diagnostic procedures) and the randomized controlled trial (to evaluate the clinical impact of [additional] testing).

Without parsing the particulars and misguidedness of statements like these here, we simply refer to Part IV of this book of ours, which is devoted the theory of diagnostic research. For, it is only in the light of the concepts and principles there that those ideas about diagnostic research – commonly held at present – can be critically understood.

Eminently illustrative of the prevailing culture surrounding and permeating diagnostic research is the succession of two very major studies intended to advance the knowledge-base of *diagnosis about pulmonary embolism* [3, 4]: they did not address that which is the diagnostic concern to know about, namely the profile-conditional probabilities of the presence of this disease in at least one relevant domain (of type of case presentation).

3.1.3 Ideas about Etiognostic Research

Research for the knowledge-base of etiognosis in the practice of clinical medicine has remained practically non-existent, in contrast to diagnostic research (in the misguided meaning outlined in Sect. 3.1.2, above). This hardly is surprising, given that *even the very term 'etiognosis' remains a neologism* (Sect. 1.2.2), different from the familiarity of the terms 'diagnosis' and 'prognosis' – though with the common conceptions of these two gnoses remaining malformed (Sects. 1.2.2 and 3.1.2, above).

The relative inattention to etiognosis in clinical medicine has, arguably at least, its origin in *Robert Koch's definition of tuberculosis* as the somatic anomaly that is caused (*sic*) – rather than characterized – by the presence of mycobacteria (which he discovered) in the affected tissue(s). This was a *conceptual mistake*: He should have conceptualized this illness as mycobacteriosis and termed it accordingly – with the aprioristic understanding that this anomaly (somatic) is caused by (effective) exposure to the agent (mycobacterium) together with susceptibility to its pathogenetic effects [5]. (Contemporary definitions of tuberculosis, and of other microbial diseases likewise, perpetuate Koch's conceptual error. However, this error has not spread to the definitions of illnesses with non-microbial agents in their essence, illnesses such as trichinosis and asbestosis.)

This inattention to the concept of etiognosis and its consequent neglect of etiognostic research for clinical medicine is lamentable, given that etiognostic challenges commonly parallel or immediately follow diagnostic ones. Thus, when a patient complains about a particular symptom, the doctor's challenge is not inherently diagnostic (about the possible presence of particular illnesses as causes of the symptom); for parallel with this can be the etiognostic challenge – to know about possible non-illness causation of the symptom, most notably by the use of some particular medication(s). And when the presence of a particular illness already is a given (per attained rule-in diagnosis about it), the challenge may be to achieve gnosis about its causal origin – iatrogenic etiology/etiogenesis in particular – with a view to prevention of recurrence of the illness.

Different from clinical research, etiology/etiogenesis of illness has been a *central concern in epidemiological research*, in the development of the knowledge-base for community medicine, for the population-level preventive medicine that is the essential concern in this non-clinical species/branch of medicine (Sect. 1.5). Nevertheless, the principles of etiogenetic research remain poorly developed, even on the most elementary level.

Emblematic about the underdevelopment of the theory of etiogenetic research is the still-persistent notion that an etiogenetic study can be of either one of two possible types. These two types – 'designs' – used to be termed the prospective study and the retrospective study, respectively, but are now termed the *cohort study* and the *case-control study*, respectively. The flaw of logic in this duality is revealed by the current terminology already: cohort is a type of population (Sect. 5.2.2), and its logical alternative is dynamic population (Sect. 5.2.1), while 'case-control' isn't any type of population.

The *singular essence* of etiogenetic study can be – and needs to be – deduced from the very concept of etiology/etiogenesis, and this is of neither one of those two types [6]. It is addressed in Sects. 7.4.4 and 15.6 here, with special reference to the development of the knowledge-base for etiognosis in clinical medicine.

3.1.4 Ideas about Prognostic Research

Like the concept of diagnosis and that of etiognosis, *the common conception of prognosis still is an underdeveloped one*: it remains commonplace to hold that an illness – or the patient's condition more broadly – has a prognosis; and when prognosis is understood to be a mental entity of doctors, it is construed as a "forecast" (Sect. 1.2.2), implying essential certainty, rather than probabilistic knowing – knowing about probability, however low.

Besides and in particular, *it remains commonplace to not subsume case-specific knowing about treatment effects under prognosis*. In consequence of this, *studies of the effects of treatments, very notably, do not address treatment-conditional prognostic probabilities*, even though this would be a very useful and practicable purpose of those studies. An eminent example of this lack of focus on the advancement of the knowledge-base of prognosis is the Women's Health Initiative trial [7]. A major reason for this failure in treatment trials may well be lack of mastery of the theory of achieving the truly pragmatic, prognostic focus in treatment trials. The relevant theory is addressed in Sect. 7.4.5 and Chaps. 20 and 21 here.

3.1.5 Ideas about Screening Research

The medical *concept of screening*, according to Stedman's Medical Dictionary [8] is this:

> Examination of a group of usually asymptomatic people to detect those with a high probability of having a given disease, typically by means of an inexpensive diagnostic test.

Rephrased in a more scholarly way – which does not allow such qualities as "usually," "typically," and "inexpensive," nor such loose and otherwise untenable elements as "high probability" – this definition is:

> Application of a diagnostic test to asymptomatic people as the first phase in an attempt to detect latent cases of the presence of a given illness.

The concept of test in this definition is the ordinary one of clinical medicine, not the one of 'clinical epidemiologists' that encompasses all of the fact-finding for a diagnostic profile of a case (Sect. 3.1.2).

Screening in this common definition of the concept – which refers to (a population of) "people" rather an individual – is an activity in *community medicine*. It is 'mass screening' of a population rather than something in clinical medicine. Those with a positive result of the screening test (as defined for the purpose) are referred to care in *clinical medicine*. The clinical care resulting from the referrals may involve replication of that initial test; but regardless, this test's positive result is supposed to be followed up by the application of further tests/diagnostics toward possible early (pre-symptomatic, 'pre-clinical') rule-in diagnosis about the illness in question, this as a predicate for early, and thereby presumedly more effective, treatment.

Such sreening-and-referral (in community medicine) serves its purpose – epidemiological, of reducing overt-case morbidity and/or mortality from the illness (Sect. 5.3) – on its *two clinical premises*: that the referral resulting from a positive result of the screening-test (in community medicine) indeed prompts the pursuit of rule-in diagnosis about the illness (in clinical medicine); and that such early (pre-clinical) detection of the illness indeed is followed by early treatment (in clinical medicine) that is more effective – more commonly curative – than treatment once the illness already is overtly manifest, in symptoms and/or clinical signs. It follows that *screening research is clinical research*, both diagnostic and interventive, intervention-prognostic.

The purpose of here taking up screening research separately from both diagnostic and intervention-prognostic research is merely to caution clinical researchers about the prevailing culture of screening research for community medicine. In this culture, 'mass' screening is treated as a community-level intervention (*sic!*). Predicated on this, the community-level morbidly/mortality implications are studied by means of clinical-type trials with arbitrarily-set design parameters, trials which seriously mislead both the inputs to public policies about the screening in question as well as perceptions of the effectiveness of early treatments relative to late ones [9]. The prime example of this confused culture now is the recent trial on CT screening for lung cancer [10], on which the U.S. National Institutes of Health spent 300 million dollars. (CT imaging of the chest and competent reading of the images scarcely qualifies as "an inexpensive diagnostic test"; cf. above.)

3.1.6 Ideas about the Impact of Clinical Research

Quite telling about the prevailing sense of purpose in clinical research is the conception and quantification of a study's merit in terms of the *'impact factor'* of the journal in which its report is published. This measure quantifies the frequency with which articles published in that journal have recently been cited in the medical literature at large.

In this context it is worth noting the frequency of citations of *Gregor Mendel's article on genetics,* seminal to the entire field of genetics. Even though he sent copies of his article – published in the *Proceedings of the Brno Natural Science Society* – to a number of leading scientists, it "was cited only four times between 1866 and 1900 – virtually disappearing from scientific literature" [11, p. 54].

3.2 Clinical Research Proper at Present

3.2.1 Research Leading to Nobel Prize

One indication of the prevailing state of clinical research are the accomplishments that have recently been celebrated by the awarding of the Nobel Prize for "Physiology or Medicine" to the researchers involved. Since 2000, the thus-celebrated contributions to "physiology" – which at the time when these prizes were introduced (in 1900) meant natural philosophy relevant to medicine [12], but in this context now presumably means laboratory-level, 'biomedical' sciences – or directly to "medicine," have practically all been in the nature of *biological "discoveries*." To wit:

2000, "for their discoveries concerning signal transduction in the nervous system" (Arvid Carlsson, Paul Greengard, Eric R. Kandel)
2001, "for their discoveries of key regulators of the cell cycle" (Leland H. Hartwell, R. Timothy Hunt, Paul M. Nurse)
2002, "for their discoveries concerning genetic regulation of organ development and programmed cell death" (Sydney Brenner, H. Robert Horvitz, John E. Sulston)
2003, "for their discoveries concerning magnetic resonance imaging" (Paul Christian Lauterbur, Peter Mansfield)
2004, "for their discoveries of odorant receptors and the organization of the olfactory system" (Richard Axel, Linda B. Buck)
2005, "for their discovery of the bacterium Helicobacter pylori and its role in gastritis and peptic ulcer disease" (Barry Marshall, John Robin Warren)
2006, "for their discovery of RNA interference - gene silencing by double-stranded RNA" (Andrew Z. Fire, Craig Mello)
2007, "for their discoveries of principles for introducing specific gene modifications in mice by the use of embryonic stem cells" (Mario Capecchi, Martin Evans, Oliver Smithies)
2008, "for his discovery of human papilloma viruses causing cervical cancer" (Harald zur Hausen); "for their discovery of human immunodeficiency virus" (Françoise Barré-Sinoussi, Luc Montagnier)
2009, "for the discovery of how chromosomes are protected by telomeres and the enzyme telomerase" (Elizabeth Blackburn, Carol W. Greider, Jack Szostak)
2010, "for the development of in vitro fertilization" (Robert Edwards)

2011, "for their discoveries concerning the activation of innate immunity" (Bruce Beutler, Jules Hoffmann); "for his discovery of the dendritic cell and its role in adaptive immunity" (Ralph M. Steinman)
2012: "for the discovery that mature cells can be reprogrammed to become pluripotent" (John Gurdon, Shin'ya Yamanaka)
2013, "for their discoveries of machinery regulating vesicle traffic, a major transport system in our cells," (James Rothman, Randy Schekman, Thomas Südhof)
2014, "for their discoveries of cells that constitute a positioning system in the brain" (John O'Keeffe, May-Britt Moser, Edvard Moser)
2015, "for their discoveries concerning a novel therapy against infections caused by roundworm parasites" (William C. Campbell, Satoshi Ōmura); "for her discoveries concerning a novel therapy against Malaria" (Tu Youyou)
2016, "for his discoveries of mechanisms for autophagy" (Yoshinori Ohsumi)
2017, "for their discoveries of molecular mechanisms controlling the circadian rhythm" (Jeffrey C. Hall, Michael Rosbash, Michael W. Young)
2018, "for their discovery of cancer therapy by inhibition of negative immune regulation" (James P Allison and Tasuko Honjo)

The point of note here is that *none of these prizes was for gnostic clinical research* – which does not produce discoveries but, in the appropriate theoretical framework (logical), serves to produce gnostic knowledge (Sect. 1.2.3) and, thus, to provide for scientific medicine (Sect. 2.4).

Peter Medawar – this exceptionally illustrious Nobel laureate in "physiology or medicine" ("for discovery of acquired immunological tolerance") – has written, inter alia, about the academic status of 'applied' science relative to its 'pure' counterpart, from the historical perspective. He explains [13] that *'pure science'* used to mean science in which knowledge is derived deductively from self-evident 'first principles,' and that it has historically been deemed to be superior to any empirical science. The term 'pure science,' he explains, now denotes empirical science devoid of any purpose of application of the knowledge acquired. He – this eminent representative of 'basic medical research' – notes, lugubriously, that "the idea of the superiority of pure over applied science has remained, and with the dire equation *Useless = Good*"; and elsewhere he makes this point even more explicitly: "one of the most damaging forms of snobbism in science is that which draws a class distinction between pure and applied science" [14]. Common synonyms of 'pure science' now are 'basic science' and 'fundamental science' [15]. Hence, 'basic medical science'actually is a contradiction in terms.

This system of values in academia is, to an extent, inimical to all of medical research, which we take to be, by definition, 'applied' – purposive – research (Sect. 2.2). And to the extent that this still is the case, it is even more so in respect to gnostic clinical research, which we think of as 'quintessentially applied' medical research [5, p. 7].

Quite apart from the (lamentable) system of values in medical (and other) academia, a sufficient reason for the absence Nobel Prizes for gnostic clinical research can be taken to be the thus-far-attained quality of this research – reflecting its underpinnings in the poorly-developed general theory of medicine itself (Chap. 1), and its consequent *underdevelopment of the theory of gnostic clinical research* (Chap. 2 and Sect. 3.1, above), which this book endeavors to rectify (cf. Preface).

Perhaps there will some day be a *Nobel Prize for a faculty of medicine, celebrating its having pioneered a world-wide program of faculty-wide programs of gnostic clinical research* in medical academia, each of the faculty-specific component programs led by the faculty's department cultivating (the theory of medicine and) the theory and practice of gnostic clinical research: The prime candidate for this honor we take to be the very faculty that provides these awards, as we make plain in Appendix 2.

3.2.2 Research Published in Medical Journals

Particularly telling about the goings-on in clinical research at present are recent reports on it, most notably reports published in the preeminent journal of the preeminent discipline of clinical medicine – in *Annals of Internal Medicine*, that is. This journal's mission is, inter alia, to "advance standards in the conduct and reporting of medical research," and its 2015 "Impact Factor is 16.440 – the highest of any specialty journal in the Thompson Reuters' General and Internal Medicine category ..." [16].

In the second half of 2016, the titles and keywords of the first 15 original-research reports in this journal were these:

1. Anglemyer A *et alii*. Suicide rates and methods in active duty military personnel, 2005–2011: a cohort study. *Ann Intern Med* 2016; 165: 167–174.

   Keywords: suicide, prevention, military personnel, firearm-specific suicide, retrospective cohort study.
2. Bernard CL *et alii*. Cost-effectiveness of HIV preexposure prophylaxis for people who inject drugs in the United States. *Ann Intern Med* 2016; 165:10–19.

   Keywords: HIV, prophylaxis, intravenous drug abuse, cost-effectiveness.
3. Coffin PO *et alii*. Nonrandomized intervention study of naloxone coprescription for primary care patients receiving long-term opioid therapy for pain. *Ann Intern Med* 2016; 165: 245–252.

   Keywords: overdose, opioid analgesics, effect of implementing naloxone prescription, nonrandomized intervention study.
4. Cusi K *et alii*. Long-term pioglitazone treatment for patients with nonalcoholic steatohepatitis and prediabetes or type 2 diabetes mellitus: a randomized trial. *Ann Intern Med* 2016; 165: 305–315.

   Keywords: metabolic defects, nonalcoholic steatohepatitis, prediabetes, type 2 diabetes mellitus, efficacy, safety, pioglitazone treatment, randomized trial.
5. Dahlén T *et alii*. Cardiovascular events associated with use of tyrosine kinase inhibitors in chronic myeloid leukemia: a population-based cohort study. *Ann Intern Med* 2016; 165: 161–166.

Keywords: tyrosine kinase inhibitors (TKIs), long-term toxicity, vascular events, retrospective cohort study, population-based registries.

6. Edgren G *et alii*. Transmission of neurodegenerative disorders through blood transfusion: a cohort study. *Ann Intern Med* 2016; 165: 316–324.

   Keywords: neurodegenerative disorders, transfusion, transmission of diseases, retrospective cohort study.

7. Greenwood JP *et alii*. Prognostic value of cardiovascular magnetic resonance and single-photon emission computed tomography in suspected coronary heart disease: long-term follow-up of a prospective, diagnostic accuracy cohort study. *Ann Intern Med* 2016; 165: 1–9.

   Keywords: cardiovascular magnetic resonance, single-photon emission computed tomography, coronary heart disease, major adverse cardiovascular events, observational study.

8. Joynt KE *et alii*. Public reporting of mortality rates for hospitalized Medicare patients and trends in mortality for reported conditions. *Ann Intern Med* 2016; 165: 153–160.

   Keywords: quality improvement tool, public reporting of mortality rates, administrative data.

9. Lachs MS *et alii*. The prevalence of resident-to-resident elder mistreatment in nursing homes. *Ann Intern Med* 2016; 165: 229–236.

   Keywords: resident-to-resident elder mistreatment, physical injury, psychological injury, observational study.

10. Mafi JN *et alii*. Comparing use of low-value health care services among U.S. advanced practice clinicians and physicians. *Ann Intern Med* 2016; 165: 237–244.

    Keywords: nurse practitioners, physician assistants, low-value services, primary care.

11. Mark DB *et alii*. Economic outcomes with anatomical versus functional diagnostic testing for coronary artery disease. *Ann Intern Med* 2016; 165: 94–102.

    Keywords: imaging, evaluation of chest pain, coronary heart disease, economic study.

12. Park GE *et alii*. Control of an outbreak of middle east respiratory syndrome in a tertiary hospital in Korea. *Ann Intern Med* 2016; 165: 87–93.

    Keywords: respiratory syndrome, control measures, effectiveness of control measures.

13. Ranasinghe I *et alii*. Long-term risk for device-related complications and reoperations after implantable cardioverter-defibrillator implantation: an observational cohort study. *Ann Intern Med* 2016; 165: 20–29.

    Keywords: nonfatal outcomes, implantable cardioverter-defibrillator, reoperation, hospitalization, observational cohort study, incidence of ICD-related complications.

14. Walensky RP *et alii*. The anticipated clinical and economic effects of 90–90-90 in South Africa. *Ann Intern Med* 2016; 165: 325–333.

    Keywords: HIV/AIDS, treatment aims, virologic suppression, clinical value, economic value.

15. Wang C *et alii*. Comparative effectiveness of Tai Chi versus physical therapy for knee osteoarthritis: a randomized trial. *Ann Intern Med* 2016; 165: 77–86.
    Keywords: pain, disability, knee osteoarthritis, Tai Chi, randomized trial.

Some points of note on this set of reports are these:

- None of those 15 studies had to do with 'basic' medical research (cf. Sect. 3.2.1, above), and none of them addressed gnostic probabilities (cf. Sect. 2.3).
- One of those 15 studies addressed "diagnostic accuracy" in lieu of diagnostic probabilities (cf. Sect. 3.1.2).
- Several of those 15 studies addressed effects of intervention without addressing intervention-conditional prognostic probabilities (cf. Sect. 3.1.4).
- Several of those 15 studies were, in the report's title, specified in terms of the generic type of study that was at issue – whether a "Nonrandomized intervention study," "A randomized trial," "A population-based cohort study," "A cohort study," a "Long-term follow-up of a prospective, diagnostic accuracy cohort study," "An observational cohort study," or "A randomized trial" again.

Notable implications of those notes are these:

1. Internists – and ipso facto doctors in whichever discipline of clinical medicine – seemingly do not follow reports on 'basic' medical research (cf. Sects. 2.3 and 3.1.1).
2. Even though research on gnostic probabilities is essential for scientific clinical medicine (Sects. 2.2, 2.3, and 2.4), reports on this (quintessentially applied) genre of clinical research appear to be absent from the leading journal for the preeminent discipline of clinical medicine.
3. Even in a journal of this stature, and one with the express mission to also "advance standards in the conduct and reporting of medical research," the reports on original studies, in their titles already, reflect substantial underdevelopment of relevant standards and its consequent *confusion about even the core concepts* (manifest in inept and variable terms denoting them).

3.2.3 Research Providing for a Doctorate

As modern medical academia takes medicine to be a science as well as an art (Sect. 1.1), *students of medicine in the undergraduate stage already (and more so subsequently, especially as clinical fellows) are encouraged if not actually expected to engage in medical research* – to some extent. The prime example of this is, that a piece of semi-autonomous (supervised) research, without any further studies in medicine, can lead to a *Doctoral degree in medicine*. This is the culture outside the U.S. and Canada, while in these two countries undergraduate medical education as such leads to the MD (Medical Doctor) degree as the highest degree in medicine – a professional, non-academic degree. In Europe and elsewhere, *regardless of the topic of the thesis, such a Doctorate is taken to signify particularly high level of qualification for the practice of one's particular discipline of medicine and also for various leadership positions in medicine and medical agencies.*

Given the importance accorded, in Europe for example, to such a Doctorate in medicine, and the ease with which it can be acquired, it is unsurprising that it is commonly sought in the countries in which this is the culture. Thus, to take the example of the faculty of one of us (JS), in the University of Zurich in the years 2010–2015 inclusive, while there were a total of 1109 graduations in medicine – with the Master of Medicine degree – the number of theses in medicine – leading to the Doctor Medicinae degree – was almost as large, 1024.

The topics of these thesis projects are instructive to review. In 2015, in the first 10 approved theses for a Doctorate in medicine, the topics were these:

1. The Omnicarbon® Monoleaflet Aortic Valve. A Long-Term, Multicenter, Single-Country Study.
2. Acquired Vorinostat Resistance Shows Partial Cross-Resistance to 'Second-Generation' HDAC Inhibitors and Correlates with Loss of Histone Acetylation and Apoptosis but not with Altered HDAC and HAT Activities.
3. Ausgeatmetes Stickstoffmonoxid, ein Marker zur Unterscheidung von Subgruppen bei Kindern mit respiratorischen Symptomen im Vorschulalter. (Exhaled Nitric Oxide: Marker for Identification of Subgroups of Preschool Children with Respiratory Symptoms.)
4. 10 Jahre Altersschätzung an Lebenden (1994–2004) am Institut für Rechtsmedizin der Universität Zürich-Irchel. (Ten Years of Age Estimation in Living People (1194–2004) at the Institute for Forensic Medicine at the University of Zurich Irchel.)
5. Cardiac Image Fusion from Stand-Alone SPECT and CT: First Clinical Experience.
6. 17-alpha-Hydroxylase/17,20-Lyase Defizienz und Intersexualität. (17-alpha-Hydroxylase/17,20-Lyase Deficiency and Intersexuality.)
7. Moderne Koronarchirurgie am schlagenden Herzen. (Modern Coronary Surgery on Beating Hearts.)
8. Kann eine relevante Hämolyse beim Neugeborenen anhand des Carboxyhämoglobins in der kapillären Blutprobe frühzeitig erkannt werden? (Can Relevant Hemolysis in Newborns be Identified Early by Measuring Carboxyhemoglobin in Capillary Blood?)
9. Retrospektive Untersuchungen zur Morbidität bei Blutspendern mit positivem direkten Antiglobulintest (DAT). (Retrospective Investigations of Morbidity in Blood Donors with Positive Direct Anti-globulin Test.)
10. Facemasks and Aerosol Delivery In Vivo.

Such is the variety in these topics of research that *it is not possible to discern any leit motif in it*; and in particular, there clearly was no focus on directly practice-serving research as the basis for the progression from the MD-equivalent degree to the highest available degree in medicine. The thesis work typically takes some 6 months to complete, and no course work is associated with it. But in the faculty of medicine that awards Nobel Prizes in "Physiology or Medicine" (Sect. 3.2.1), the attainment of a Doctorate in medicine is much more demanding, typically requiring 4 years of thesis work (supervised) and also course work related to the topic of the thesis.

This variation in types of Doctorate in medicine – following a Master's degree in this professional field (which is not a science; Sect. 1.1) – is puzzling also in its lack of the 'harmonization' that the 'Bologna process' is supposed to have brought to higher education in Europe. And: the different Doctorates arguably are not in (the professional field of) medicine but in (the academic field of) medical research – in the context of very underdeveloped conception of the general essence of the research and of the requisite educational preparation for it.

3.3 Clinical Medicine at Present

The impact in the advancement of clinical medicine that has thus far been accomplished by clinical research is very clear in its overall gestalt: The laboratory-level branch of clinical research has led to enormous extension in the contents of the general toolkit of clinical medicine, but the 'patient'-level counterpart of this research has almost totally failed to provide the scientific knowledge-base for doctors' gnostic probability-setting, leaving clinical doctors quite unprepared for their essential function – teaching their clients about their health (Sect. 1.2.1).

Illustrative of the present state of clinical medicine – as for its relation to clinical research – are the gnoses in the case of an *adult presenting with chest pain* as the chief complaint (about sickness) and having *myocardial infarction* as the underlying illness:

1. *Diagnosis*. The pursuit of diagnosis in a case of an adult presenting with chest pain as the chief complaint initially focuses on the possibility of MI as the underlying illness. Toward diagnosis about MI in such a case, the doctor first takes the patient's 'history' and performs a 'physical examination,' both of these in a routine way and with no reference to science. Such fact-finding (s)he may supplement with diagnostic testing developed on the basis of medical science, electrocardiography first and then perhaps also a cardiac enzyme ('troponin') determination. With the diagnostic profile of the case thus established, the doctor needs to translate this into diagnosis about the presence of MI, into the probability of this. In the earliest, most critical stages of the course of the patient's illness, the already-established profile of the case is not pathognomonic – conclusive – about the presence/absence of MI, and hence the diagnosis about this can only be probabilistic. But*: in clinical medicine at present, there is no scientific knowledge-base for such (profile-specific) probability-setting* – even for this critically-important, very common diagnosis.
2. *Etiognosis*. If the diagnostic profile has led to (practical) rule-in diagnosis about MI, an element in the profile can be a positive history about recent use of a potentially thrombogenic medication (hormonal, say). Especially in the context of

such a history in a case of non-fatal MI – implying possibly iatrogenic (physician-induced) origin of the case and thus a possible means to prevent its recurrence – the doctor is concerned to know about the probability of such etiogenesis of the case of MI. To this end (s)he ascertains the etiognostic profile of the case, with special reference to the relevant particulars of the medication's use in the potentially etiogenetic segment of the past (recent) and to the modifiers of its thrombogenic potential (incl. the amount of the medication's earlier use). But again: *in clinical medicine at present, there is no scientific knowledge-base for such (profile-specific) probability-setting* – even for this critically-important, quite common etiognosis.

3. *Prognosis about the effects of therapy.* Given a rule-in diagnosis about MI, notably early in the course of the episode, the doctor's attention turns, urgently, to prognoses, ones that have critical bearing on the choice among the options for treatment (therapeutic) of the case. Among the options now are thrombolytic treatments with either SK or TPA as the therapeutic agent (cf. Sect. 1.3), resulting from successful development – 'drug development' – founded on (promising) results of laboratory-level, 'basic' medical research. For each of those two medications, the process of its development was, centrally, a matter of 'pre-marketing' patient-level clinical research. This research was constituted by clinical trials in the routine three phases – Phase I, Phase II, and Phase III – of this research; and evidence from the Phase III research satisfied the regulatory agency (the FDA in the U.S.) about the drug's efficacy (in some of the cases), whereby the agency permitted the drug to be marketed for doctors' use for thrombolysis. But for these medications' actual, suitably-informed use for thrombolysis, needed is suitable 'post-marketing' patient-level clinical research on treatments with each of those drugs – research that addresses the degree of the treatment's efficacy and safety specific to the relevant particulars of both the case and the treatment. Such research would address the probabilities of the various possible outcomes of (the course of) MI conditional on the choice of the treatment and the prognostic profile of the case. But again: *such suitably-specified prognostic probabilities, centrally relevant to decisions about therapeutic treatment, are not addressed in clinical trials at present* – not even in post-marketing trials addressing treatments aimed at prevention of fatal outcomes in cases of MI.
4. *Subsequent prognosis about the effects of prophylaxis.* At the completion of the course of a case of MI, if the patient survived, the doctor's concern turns to prognosis of a different kind: now the concern is to know about the probability of recurrence of the illness (MI), with specificity to various periods of prospective time, the choice of treatment (aimed at prevention or delay of the recurrence), and the prognostic profile of the case. In this, the main concern is to know about the way in which the time-specific prognostic probabilities depend on the choice of the treatment (preventive/prophylactic), given the prognostic profile of the case. But again: *such suitably-specified prognostic probabilities, centrally relevant to decisions about prophylactic treatment, are not addressed in clinical trials at present* – not even in post-marketing trials addressing treatments in cases of status post MI.

References

1. Marti-Ibanez F (ed) (1962) The epic of medicine. Clarkson N. Potter, Inc./Publisher, New York
2. Knottnerus JA, Buntinx F (eds) (2008) The evidence base of clinical diagnosis: theory and methods of diagnostic research. BMJ Books, London
5. Miettinen OS (2015) Medicine as a scholarly field: an introduction. Springer, Cham
3. PIOPED Investigators (1990) Value of the ventilation/perfusion scan in acute pulmonary embolism. Results of the Prospective Investigation of Pulmonary Embolism Diagnosis (PIOPED). JAMA 263:2753–2759
4. Stein PD, Fowler SE, Goodman LR, *et alii* for the PIOPED II Investigators. (2006) Multidetector computed tomography for acute pulmonary embolism. N Engl J Med 354:2317–2327
6. Miettinen OS, Karp I (2012) Epidemiological research: an introduction. Springer, Dordrecht
7. The Women's Health Initiative steering committee (2004) Effects of conjugated equine estrogen in postmenopausal women with hysterectomy. The Women's Health Initiative randomized controlled trial. JAMA 291:1701–1712
8. Stedman's medical dictionary, illustrated in color. 28th edn. Williams & Wilkins, Philadelphia (2013)
9. Miettinen OS (2015) Screening' for breast cancer: misguided research misleading public policies. Epidemiol Methods 4:3–10
10. The National Lung Screening Trial research team (2013) Results of initial low-dose computed tomographic screening for lung cancer. N Engl J Med 368:1980–1991
11. Mukherjee S (2016) The gene. Intimate history. Scribner, New York
12. Wootton D (2015) The invention of science. A new history of the scientific revolution. Harper, New York
13. Medawar P (1982) Pluto's republic. Oxford University Press, Oxford, p 15
14. Medawar P (1979) Advice to a young scientist. Harper & Row, Publishers, New York, p 45
15. Flexner A, Dijkgraaf R (2017) The usefulness of useless knowledge. Princeton Press, Princeton
16. Annals of Internal Medicine. Retrieved March 17, 2017 from https://www.acponline.org/system/files/documents/products_services/journals/branded-annals-press-release.DFP

Chapter 4
Clinical Research Transformative of Clinical Medicine

Contents

Abstract While developments founded on knowledge (biological) derived from laboratory-level clinical research have made clinical medicine well-endowed with products and processes for (selective) deployment by doctors, they naturally haven't transformed the essence of clinical medicine. And gnostic clinical research, such as it has been, has largely failed to provide the requisite knowledge (clinical) for scientific practice of clinical medicine (Sect. 3.3, above). The basis for this failure has not been paucity of gnostic clinical research but the nature of the ideas that now underpin this research (Sect. 3.1). We here present an introduction to an *alternative way of thinking about the requisite knowledge-base of clinical medicine*, one that would serve as the foundation for education in and practice of *gnostic clinical research transformative of practices in clinical medicine,* by providing for its becoming scientifically knowledge-based.

Keywords Diagnostic tests' properties · Diagnostic probabilities · Diagnostic probability functions · Etiognostic probability functions · Prognostic probability functions · Education for gnostic clinical research · CLINICAL Scholars programs · MD-PhD programs · Clinical research transformed · Clinical medicine transformed

O. S. Miettinen et al., *Clinical Research Transformed*,
https://doi.org/10.1007/978-3-030-06176-0_4

4.1 Transformative Ideas about Gnostic Clinical Research

Specific to *diagnostic research*, the transformative idea advocated in this book is an alternative to the *prevailing doctrine* that this research is to address the 'properties' – result distributions – of diagnostic tests, and also of diagnostic indicators more generally, in both the presence and the absence of the illness targeted for diagnosis (Sect. 3.1.2). The corresponding *transformative idea* is, fundamentally, that diagnostic research is to address, directly, that which diagnoses are about, namely the probabilities of the presence of the illness in question conditional on the various possible diagnostic profiles of the cases. This means, more specifically, that the research is to address the diagnostic probabilities for the illnesses at issue as joint functions of sets of diagnostic indicators, these for defined domains of case presentation for diagnosis; it is to address such *diagnostic probability functions*, DPFs.

This transformative idea about diagnostic research is paradigmatic for the other species gnostic clinical research as well – etiognostic and prognostic in addition to diagnostic – with particularly notable importance for the development of the scientific knowledge-base for decisions about treatments of choice conditionally on the prognostic profiles of patients (Sect. 3.3).

The overall idea is, simply, this: *Directly practice-serving – gnostic – clinical research would address gnostic probability functions* specific to defined domains of doctors' need to know about (profile-specific) gnostic probabilities.

4.2 Education for Transformative Clinical Research

4.2.1 The Focus on Gnostic Clinical Research

Transformative of clinical medicine would *not* be some innovative idea fundamental to thinking about, and hence to education in, *laboratory-level clinical research*. One reason for this is that clinical research on the laboratory level is *not* being misled by prevailing lead ideas about it (Sect. 3.1.1). And an added reason for this is that successful research in the 'basic sciences of medicine' is not firmly founded on any general education in these sciences. Notable in this regard is how Peter Medawar – this particularly illustrious scholar on this species of medical research (cf. Sect. 3.2.1) – viewed the relevance of serious education in a 'basic science of medicine': "very many scientists (I certainly among them) do not learn new skills or master new disciplines until the pressure is upon them to do so; thereupon they can be mastered pretty quickly .... My own career as a serious medical scientist began with devising a means of measuring the intensity of the reaction that a mouse or a man mounts against a graft transplanted upon it from some other mouse or some other man" [1].

Very different from what Medawar says about education for consequential medical research (biological) on the laboratory level, *gnostic clinical research* – addressing gnostic probability functions (Sect. 4.1, above) – is *statistical research* and therefore requires education, suitably focused, in statistics, inter alia. And the need for education in gnostic clinical research is accentuated by the need to supplant the prevailing doctrines about it (Sect. 3.1) by the theory – concepts and principles – of the research that would be transformative of the practices in clinical medicine (into those of genuinely scientific medicine).

4.2.2 The Individual Aims of the Education

The student setting out to seriously prepare for gnostic clinical research is not someone preparing for practice in one of the disciplines that jointly constitute the field of clinical medicine. Thus, at issue here is not educational preparation for research that leads to a Doctorate in medicine as a (purported) merit for a career in the practice of clinical medicine (Sect. 3.2.3).

The aims of seriously preparing for this species of clinical research are not confined to concerns to achieve competence in the *research* to advance the knowledge-base of clinical medicine; an aim closely related to this can be the more subjective one to achieve proficiency in *teaching* the scientific knowledge-base – including lack thereof – for gnoses in a particular discipline of clinical medicine. This aim, too, is a major one, given that such teaching should be an eminent feature of the education provided by schools/faculties of medicine.

The epitome of the deserving recipient of the education at issue here is a graduate student of medicine aiming to become a professor of his/her discipline of clinical medicine.

4.2.3 The Main Modules of the Education

From the foregoing it is, in many ways, evident that the very first module in educational preparation for gnostic clinical research is to address the *general theory – concepts and principles – of clinical medicine*. This module, however, is not a Part unto itself in this book, given that it is the sole subject of a recent other book [2]. In the present book, the general theory of clinical medicine is covered only in terms of ad-hoc fragments of it, as has been the case in these orientational Chapters already. The various concepts are reviewed, in terms of succinct definitions, in this book's Glossary.

As any student concerned with 'patient'-level clinical research well knows, this research is closely related to epidemiological research, and Part II here therefore focuses on the *theory of epidemiology and epidemiological research*, specifically insofar as it is expressly relevant as background for gnostic clinical research. A gnosis-serving clinical researcher generally expects – and indeed should expect – to be self-sufficient in these matters. For, in successful gnostic clinical research, all of the relevant elements of educatedness are integrated in a single mind, that of the Principal Investigator.

Just as well-known is the statistical nature of the research at issue here. The *statistics relevant to gnostic clinical research* should also be mastered by the PI of any piece of the research, rather than the PI delegating this aspect of the study to a collaborating 'biostatistician.' For, the poor development of the objects of this research at present stems, in part, from the prevailing culture of not integrating, in the mind of the PI, 'study design' in substantive medical terms with the statistical 'data analysis' that follows the collection of the study data. In mathematical sciences such as physics and astronomy, the scientist masters the relevant mathematics and does not presume it to be delegatable to a 'physicomathematician' or 'astromathematician.' Given the need to integrate the relevant statistics with the subject-matter issues in the mind of the PI, Part III of this book is devoted to the essentials of the relevant statistics in gnostic clinical research.

Then come, naturally, the principal Parts (IV through VI) devoted, respectively, to the *theory of diagnostic, etiognostic, and prognostic research* (gnostic; cf. Sect. 3.2).

4.2.4 Informal Programs of the Education

As formal programs of the PhD-level education focusing on gnostic clinical research are not yet available, needed now is self-education, informally, without it resulting in a PhD-equivalent certification of readiness for independent conduct of such research.

This education, we suggest, would center on study of *two books*: first the recent book on the general theory of medicine [2] and then this book on the theory specific to gnostic clinical research – addressing the generic objects of this research consonant with the essence of the species of gnosis at issue and then, subordinate to this, the design of the objects and methods of these studies.

As this self-education would commonly be quite challenging, *it would be good to form a group of similarly-oriented students* of these two books, meeting periodically to discuss pre-specified segments of these books. Routine participation, in the readings and discussions, of a senior epidemiological researcher and a theoretical statistician in *tutoring* roles would be very desirable and helpful, and so also would be the participation of a senior clinical scholar.

4.2.5 *Formal Programs of the Education*

The education at issue here is more ambitious and, hence, on a higher level of scholarship than are the (non-degree) Clinical Scholars programs that that have been, and still are, sponsored by the Robert Wood Johnson Foundation. And the MD-PhD programs of education that have become quite common in the U.S. and Canada lack the focus of the education at issue here.

A formal program of education in gnostic clinical research would lead to a *PhD-equivalent degree in medicine or medical research*. The need for such programs is quite obvious to us, but leaders of medical academia remain in need of persuasion about this. And the requisite development of the faculty for the programs also is challenging in the early stages of these programs.

Such a program of education, we dare say, needs to be founded on the percepts in this book. And we envision it to be centred on the *epidemiological* (rather than clinical) segment of a particular, very distinguished faculty of medicine (App. 2).

4.3 Clinical Medicine Transformed by Clinical Research

Once suitably gnosis-oriented clinical research – on gnostic probability functions (Sect. 4.1) – has produced the requisite knowledge-base for practices related to, say, myocardial infarction, the agnosticism unavoidable at present (Sect. 3.3) will be a matter of history (of largely agnostic but nevertheless genuine medicine; Sect. 1.4). For the practice of medicine (scientific; Sect. 2.4) transformed by such research, *scientific knowledge relevant to the gnoses of doctors' concern will not only exist; it will be accessible to doctors right when they need it, from cyberspace where it is codified.*

Codified in the (readily-accessible) source for *diagnosis* in the context of a given type of case presentation will be not only the relevant DPF (diagnostic probability function) for at least some of the illnesses that reasonably could be the doctor's concern but also the complete differential-diagnostic set implied by the presentation. Besides, the source (in cyberspace) will guide the process of the facts-ascertainment to the gnostic profile, in the first stage for diagnoses prior to any diagnostic testings in laboratories. And if the first-stage, pre-test probability for the illness targeted for diagnosis is not extreme enough for the purpose – either practically ruling in or ruling out this possibility – the source will specify the testing (perhaps a set of tests) whose result(s), when added to the diagnostic profile, could make it sufficiently conclusive, in terms of the testing resulting in such a pathognomonic post-test profile.

As illustrated by that innovation in diagnosis, the here-advocated gnostic clinical research will be *transformative of all three of the species of clinical doctors' gnoses* and, thus, the entire knowledge-base of clinicans' doctoring – teaching their clients about their health (Sect. 1.2), including how it could be preserved or changed for the better.

Sapere aude! – Dare to know! – was Immanuel Kant's (adopted) mantra for Enlightenment. We dare to know that such transformation of clinical research as we advocate in this book would bring about a *major improvement in the quality* and a *substantial reduction in the costs* of what has become the "vast industry" around the "sovereign profession[s]" of clinical medicine, in the U.S. in particular [3]. This knowing – vision – is our counterpart of the very influential idea of *Archie Cochrane* [4] that, in the framework of the National Health Service of the U.K., major inefficiency and its consequent major costs result from the doctors' lack of knowledge about the effectiveness of the various options for treatment – idea that translated into his highly-influential advocacy of research on the comparative effectiveness of treatments (by means of randomized trials; cf. Preface).

References

1. Medawar P (1979) Advise to a young scientist. Harper & Bow, Publishers, New York, pp 16–19
2. Miettinen OS (2015) Medicine as a scholarly field: an introduction. Springer, New York
3. Starr P (1982) The social transformation of American medicine. The rise of a sovereign profession and the making of a vast industry. Basic Books, New York
4. Cochrane AL (1972) Effectiveness and efficiency. Random reflections on health services. The Nuffield Provincial Hospital Trust, London

Part II
Epidemiological Preliminaries of Gnostic Clinical Research

Chapter 5
Core Concepts of Epidemiology and Epidemiological Research

Contents

Abstract Preparatory to gnostic clinical research is, quite importantly, familiarity with and secure internalization of certain core concepts of epidemiology and of research for the advancement of its practice. These concepts, like their counterparts in clinical medicine, are, still, less than satisfactory in their general stage of development. They, too, therefore need to be approached with the critical mind-set that is a prerequisite for learning and internalizing the general theory of clinical medicine (by self-study of a recent book; Sect. 4.2.2) and, subordinate to this, the general theory of gnostic clinical research that provides the knowledge-base for genuinely scientific medicine (cf. Sect. 3.3). We provide here a *critical introduction to the core concepts of epidemiology and epidemiological research*, ones that are preparatory to study specific to gnostic clinical research.

Keywords Definition · Epidemiology · Types of population · Morbidity · Mortality · Rate of prevalence · Rates of incidence · Epidemiological research · Basic epidemiological research · Gnostic epidemiological research

O. S. Miettinen et al., *Clinical Research Transformed*,
https://doi.org/10.1007/978-3-030-06176-0_5

5.1 The Essence of Epidemiology and Epidemiological Research

In the early 1960s, when one of us (OM) was a student of epidemiology and public health, there was an article on the "scope and methods of epidemiology" in the *American Journal of Public Health* [1], accompanied by an Editorial on it [2]. Several Letters to the Editor followed, including one introducing "epidemiologology" – the study of epidemiology [3]. The confusion about the essence of epidemiology wasn't resolved (and became the subject of OM's thesis for the Master of Public Health degree).

At present, still, authoritative definitions of epidemiology are rather variable. According to *Stedman's Medical Dictionary* [4], epidemiology is:

> The study of the distribution and determinants of health-related states or events in specified populations, and the application of this study to control of health problems.

The definition by the *World Health Organization* [5] is essentially the same as this. According to these two authorities, thus, epidemiology has, oddly, two proximate genera, ones that even in themselves are rather odd: one of these is *study*, the other is *the application of this study*. (Study of the determinants of population health – constitutional, environmental, and behavioral – definitely aren't objects of epidemiological study, only morbidity's relation to them is.)

According to some other notable sources, epidemiology is a *science*. Thus, *MacMahon et alii* noted that "Epidemiology is widely recognized as the basic science of preventive medicine" [6]. And accordingly, one of the Institutes in the *U.S. National Institutes of Health* [7] defines epidemiology this way:

> Epidemiology is the branch of medical science that investigates all the factors that determine the presence or absence of diseases and disorders.

Yet another conception of the proximate genus of epidemiology is, at present, that epidemiology is a *method*. Thus, according to the *Centers for Disease Control and Prevention* of the U.S [8],

> Epidemiology is the method used to find the causes of health outcomes and diseases in populations.

There indeed has been a good deal of preoccupation with 'the epidemiological method' as an essential feature of epidemiology (cf. above).

The *International Epidemiological Association*, in the first, 1983 edition of its dictionary [9], gave the very same definition of epidemiology as was quoted from *Stedman's* above. But according to the sixth, 2014 edition [10], epidemiology is:

> The study of the occurrence and distribution of health-related events, states, and processes in specified populations, including the study of the determinants influencing such processes, and the application of this knowledge to control relevant health problems.

This definition still lacks the logical structure of the definition of the concept of a thing: specified by a thing's logical definition is the thing's proximate genus and its specific difference within this genus [11].

To us, epidemiology is a species in the genus medicine: *to us, epidemiology is community medicine* [11–13]. In epidemiology, different from clinical medicine, the doctors' clients are populations, served as such, collectively (rather than their members individually; Sect. 1.5).

5.2 Epidemiological Concepts of Population

5.2.1 Open, Dynamic Population

The population that is the client of an epidemiologist – the population of a community, such as that of a municipality, a province of a country, or a country as a whole – is generally constituted by the residents of the jurisdiction in question. Alternatively, the population served by an epidemiologist is that of the workers in a particular trade in a given jurisdiction, the students in the schools in a given jurisdiction, the participants in a particular health-insurance scheme or, for a hospital epidemiologist, the patients in a (set of) hospital(s), etc.

Membership in such a population is defined by the state of being alive and also otherwise representing the *membership-defining state of being*, such as residency in the jurisdiction in question. Any such state of being is transient, and the population in question therefore is '*open*' – for exit from it. In consequence of its openness for exit, such a population generally has turnover of membership; it generally is '*dynamic*' in this sense [12, 13]. A population thus defined is eternal in its existence; but the size of it may decline to zero and remain at this level, even forever. (The patient population – open, dynamic – of a hospital declines to zero when the hospital is closed, and it remains zero until the hospital reopens, if ever.)

This concept of dynamic population as the general nature of the client populations of practitioners of epidemiology – of community medicine (Sect. 5.1, above) – is of central importance for clinical *studies on the etiology/etiogenesis of illness* (and of sickness without its causation in illness), addressed in Part V of this book. For, in such studies (etiognostic) the documented occurrence of cases of the illness at issue takes place in some 'catchment population' for them: people who are alive and also otherwise represent the domain of of the study, and are under 'surveillance' for the occurrence of cases of the illness at issue. Apart from being alive, members of such a population – when actually members of it – are characterized by the 'were-would' state of: were a case of the event at issue to occur, it would be 'caught' by the study's scheme of case identification.

5.2.2 Closed, Cohort-Type Population

The alternative to an open population is, as a matter of logic, a closed population – a population that is *closed for exit*: once a member, always a member (regardless of survival). The membership in a closed population – a *cohort* (L. *cohors,* 'inclosure') – is defined by experiencing the *membership-defining event.*

So, everyone who ever was (or will be) awarded the Nobel Prize in Physiology or Medicine has been (or will be), as of this event, a member of this (distinguished) cohort and will forever remain a member of it. Likewise, everyone who in 1948 was enrolled into the (famous) *Framingham Heart Study* [14] – this appellation is a misnomer for the aggregate of studies exploiting the database assembled on this cohort – became, by this enrolment event, a member of this cohort-type population and will forever remain a member of this cohort, this *source population* for a multitude of mainly etiogenetic studies (involving dynamic study populations; Sect. 5.2.1, above). And the persons enrolled into the actual *study population* of a prognostic study – a *clinical trial,* say – constitute, per this event, a cohort, membership in which is not terminated by death nor by any other basis for discontinuation of the follow-up.

Rates of survival are a topic in respect to cohorts only. While the members of open/dynamic populations are, by definition, alive throughout their membership in the population in question (Sect. 5.2.2, above), the members of a cohort are, by definition, alive at the time of the membership-defining event but may not be alive at a later point in their membership in the cohort. An eminent example of cohorts are *'birth cohorts'* addressed in demographic life tables.

5.2.3 Other Ideas About Types of Population

Subsequent to the introduction of the concepts of open/dynamic and closed/cohort-type population into epidemiology [15], some other ideas about the types of population have come to the fore.

In the *IEA dictionary* of epidemiology [10], the definitions of the principal types of population are as muddled as these: an open population is "A study population that is allowed to gain and lose members"; a dynamic population is "A population that gains and loses members"; a closed population is "A population that gains no new members and loses members only to death"; and a cohort is "any designated group of persons who are followed or traced over a period of time." No rationale for this typology is apparent, nor is any given in its source.

As will become clear in Part V and Part VI, *it is important to retain the concept of open/dynamic population totally separate from – as the logical alternative of – that of closed/cohort-type population, as set forth in Sects. 5.2.1 and 5.2.2 above.* The neologism 'dynamic cohort' must be understood to be a contradiction in terms.

5.3 The Concepts of Morbidity and Mortality

In *clinical medicine*, doctors are concerned with the health of their individual clients, serving them as individuals (rather than collectively, as a population; Sect. 1.5). The concern is principally about cases of an entity that is commonly termed disease, as has been evident from many quotes in the foregoing. To us, however, disease is only one species of a lager entity of concern in clinical medicine, namely *illness*, which subsumes *defect* and *injury* in addition to *disease* (Sect. 1.2.1).

In *community medicine* – in *epidemiology*, that is – doctors care for their client populations, collectively (Sect. 1.5). On the population level, illness acquires an 'emergent' new quality, and so does death. A population is characterized by its *morbidity* from the illness at issue and its *mortality* from the cause of death at issue.

Morbidity and mortality are, in medicine, concepts specific to community medicine, to epidemiology. They are the *frequency* of occurrence, respectively, of the illness in question and the cause-specific death in question in the cared-for population [11–13], thought of with specificity to a particular point in or period of calendar time. *Morbidity and mortality are what epidemiology is all about.*

Despite its central role in epidemiology, the (epidemiological) concept of morbidity remains entirely unfamiliar to the editors of the *IEA dictionary of epidemiology* [10]. They say that in one of the term's denotations (in epidemiology), morbidity is:

> Any departure, subjective or objective, from a state of physiological or psychological well-being;

and that in another meaning, morbidity is defined by the units in which it "could be measured":

> (a) Persons who were well.
> (b) The illnesses (periods or spells of illness) that these persons experienced.
> (c) The duration (days, weeks, etc.) of these illnesses

Given the utterly central concern for morbidity in epidemiology, these conceptions of the essence of it – by the IEA, no less – are particularly telling about the prevailing state of the theory of medicine specific to community medicine.

5.4 The Concept of Rate of Occurrence

The *frequency* with which a particular illness, or death from a particular cause, occurs in a particular segment of the population served by an epidemiologist, is quantified in terms of a suitable *rate* of this.

An epidemiological rate of occurrence results from a *division*: the *number of cases* (of the entity at issue) is divided by *the amount of opportunity* for their occurrence. The cases counted for a rate of morbidity in epidemiological practice generally are the ones that are routinely detected – rule-in diagnosed – in clinical practices; and the amount of opportunity for the cases' occurrence is specified by the epidemiologist according to what is seen to be both relevant and practicable. The inputs into the calculation of rates of morbidity are generally derived from case registries together with population registries. Rates of mortality, too, are based on primary data from clinical practices (specific to causes of death), and the inputs to rate calculation are numbers from death registries together with population registries.

If the amount of opportunity is quantified in terms of the number of instances in which a case could have occurred, then the rate (resulting from this calculation) is a pure number, a *proportion*. But if the opportunity space is an amount of population-time, the rate is the *number of cases per unit amount of population-time* (analogous to speed, as the distance per unit of time).

The *IEA dictionary of epidemiology* [10] says that "In epidemiology, ..., a rate is an expression of the frequency with which an event [*sic*] occurs in a defined population, usually in a specified period of time"; and it goes on to say – about this purportedly singular type of rate in epidemiology – that:

> The components of a rate are the numerator, the denominator, the specified time in which events occur, and usually a multiplier, a power of 10, that converts the rate from an awkward fraction or decimal to a whole number.

According to the IEA, thus, (the purportedly singular type of) rate in epidemiology has an amount of population-time as its referent; but this rate is not presented as the number of cases per unit amount of population-time. Instead, the numerator and denominator inputs to the calculation remain "components" of the result of it, along with some others – and the result of the calculation is a pure, whole number, rather than a dimensioned quantity. (Cf. above.)

The authors of the IEA dictionary declare that rates never are of the form of proportions, so that, for example, the term *prevalence rate* is to be avoided. To them, a rate inherently expresses "a change in time." To us this is but quixotic rebellion against the English language, in which the word 'rate' has many meanings and the term 'prevalence rate' is well-established not only in general but also in epidemiology.

5.5 Types of Rate

5.5.1 *Rates of Prevalence versus Rates of Incidence*

In epidemiological rates of occurrence there is the overarching, well-known duality constituted by rates of prevalence and rates of incidence, even though the IEA dictionary says that the term 'prevalence rate' is to be avoided (Sect. 5.4, above).

Prevalence of an illness has to do with the illness prevailing in the population at issue, and thus with an illness that in individual cases prevails over an appreciable period of time – a chronic condition such as autism, obesity, diabetes, multiple sclerosis, and Alzheimer's disease. It has to do with (sustained) *states* of ill-health, not (episodic) events of ill-health. Thus, a *rate of prevalence* quantifies the frequency of occurrence – presence – of a state of health (or a state merely related to health) in a population, the frequency with which the state prevails among the members of a particular population at a particular time; it is the *proportion* of the people in whom the illness prevails at the time.

The epidemiological concept of *incidence*, very distinct from that of prevalence, has to do with *events* of health (or merely related to health). Incidence is the frequency with which the event in question occurs in a particular population, in a segment of the population's course over time. It is quantified in terms of *rates of incidence*, typically in reference to overt cases of it (diagnosed in clinical practices). Rates of incidence, alone, characterize illnesses that are *acute* in the meaning of short duration – illnesses such as measles, stroke, and hip fracture. They are, from the epidemiological vantage, thought of as being of no notable duration. They thus are treated as though instantaneous, akin to sudden cardiac death from ventricular fibrillation.

Some illnesses are thought of in terms of both prevalence and incidence. This is natural for chronic illnesses with acute and discernible (rather than insidious) onset, such as status post stroke (different from adult-onset diabetes, say). And for chronic illnesses without such an onset (a particular type of cancer, say), 'incidence' actually has to do with the event of its (first rule-in) diagnosis.

The *IEA dictionary of epidemiology* [10] does not make the state versus event distinction in the entities of health (or merely related to health) that are at issue in the concepts of prevalence and incidence, respectively.

Under *Prevalence* that dictionary describes (in its usual, quite undisciplined manner) the way in which a rate of prevalence is calculated; and this it closes with the statement that "It is a proportion, not a rate" – thus expressing an elementary truism and following this with a gross falsehood. As we noted in Sect. 5.4, the concept of proportion-type rate is very well-established in the English language in general and, consistent with this, in the English-language jargon of epidemiology.

And under *Incidence* that dictionary of epidemiology presents the falsehood that it is "The number of instances of illness commencing, or of persons falling ill, during a given period in a specified population." This is to say that the numerator input into the calculation of a rate of incidence is, in itself, incidence. This is like saying that the distance covered by driving for whatever amount of time is, as such, the speed of the driving.

5.5.2 Proportion-Type Rates of Prevalence/Incidence

An epidemiologist contemplating the health of newborns in his/her client community thinks, among other topics, about the (rates of) the prevalence of (the state of) being stillborn at birth, and the incidence of (the event of) neonatal death. For both of these two rates, the opportunity space (Sect. 5.4) generally is a given number of instances in a *series of person-moments*, of babies at birth – some number N of successive births for that prevalence rate and some other, somewhat smaller number N′ for that incidence rate.

If in a series of N births, some number s were stillbirths, then the rate of prevalence for stillbirth in that series was the proportion s/N. And if of a series of N′ live births, some number d were followed by death in the neonatal period (within 28 days), then the rate of incidence of neonatal death – the neonatal mortality rate – in that series was the result of the d/N′ division.

Both of these rates, one of prevalence and the other of incidence, are of the proportion type, expressed as a (pure) number in the range from 0 to 1 or, equivalently, from 0% to 100%. And so also is, for example, the *case-fatality rate of a cancer:* the proportion of persons with a (rule-in) diagnosed case of the cancer in question that have died or will die from that disease. This rate may be conditional on not succumbing to another cause of death.

In a rather different vein, an epidemiologist may contemplate the prevalence of a particular state of health in some particular segment of his/her client population – for example, the prevalence of Alzheimer's disease in people 80–89 years of age. In respect to such a rate of prevalence there is no naturally-arising series of person-moments to think about. But the epidemiologist nevertheless contemplates a series of this type, from that segment of the client population (open/dynamic; Sect. 5.2.1) – *a representative series (finite) of the infinite number of person-moments constituting the population-time at issue.*

To say it once more, the IEA dictionary of epidemiology [10] declares that proportions like those are not rates of occurrence, thus rebelling against the English language. (Cf. Sect. 5.5.1, above.)

5.5.3 Density-Type Rates of Incidence

Epidemiologists' quantification of the incidence of an event of health in their cared-for populations is, typically, akin to demographers' quantification of mortality – the incidence of death – in human populations.

In demographic quantification of mortality, the focus is on an open (dynamic) population (Sect. 5.2.1) over a particular span of calendar time. With P the average size of such a population in the period from time t_1 to time t_2, the amount of population-time accrued by that population in that period is $P(t_2 - t_1)$. And if the number of deaths in that aggregate of population-time was d, then the incidence density in that population in that period of time was d/PT, where PT is the amount of population-time constituting the opportunity-space for death to occur (Sect. 5.4). Such a rate of death demographers call force of mortality.

In epidemiology, in reference to both morbidity and mortality, such a rate of incidence in the cared-for population (dynamic) is termed *incidence density* [13, 15, 16]. It is the rate in an aggregate of population-time – the number of the events in question per a unit amount of population-time (e.g., 30 per 100,000 person-years).

In the *IEA-sponsored dictionary of epidemiology* [10], said under "Incidence density" is this (in lieu of something like the paragraph above): "The average person-time incidence rate. Sometimes used to describe the hazard."

5.5.4 Rates of Cumulative Incidence

When a cohort of people (Sect. 5.2.2), such as the famous Framingham cohort [14], moves over time – measured for its individual members as of their respective entries into the cohort – the surviving portion of it declines in size, ultimately to zero. This is to say that, over time, any cohort experiences *cumulative incidence* of death, the rate of which ultimately reaches 100%.

The *case-fatality rate* of a cancer is of this form, but with a notable difference: in a cohort of persons with a (rule-in) diagnosis of the cancer, the rate of cumulative incidence of death from that cancer increases over the cohort time till it reaches its asymptote, a certain level less than 100%. This level is the cancer's case-fatality rate in one meaning of this term. In another meaning of the term, case-fatality rate is conditional on not succumbing to some other – 'competing' – cause of death.

Cumulative incidence-rate at a given point T = t in cohort time – this subtype of proportion-type rates of incidence in epidemiology – reflects the event's incidence-density specific to particular points in cohort time: it is the complement of (i.e., 1 minus) the exponential of the negative of the integral of the (time-specific) incidence density from T = 0 to that point T = t in cohort time [15, 16].

In the *IEA dictionary of epidemiology* [10], 'cumulative incidence' [i.e., the term] is said to be a synonym of "incidence proportion," such as "the proportion of childbirth labors that end with cesarean delivery." But the proportion of cesarean deliveries among all deliveries is not a rate of cumulative incidence. In truth, cumulative incidence-rate is a special species of proportion-type incidence-rate, quite different from the incidence proportion addressed in Sect. 5.5.2. Those simple rates are not thought of as resulting from incidence density of it operating over a defined span of cohort time; they are not calculated on this basis – to achieve conditionality on not succumbing to some 'competing' cause of death (and to remove the influence of losses to follow-up).

5.6 Prevailing Conceptions of Epidemiological Research

As we showed in Sect. 5.1, epidemiology is, at present, commonly seen to be a field of 'study' or, actually, a science, the essence of which is its characteristic type of research. The object of epidemiological research is commonly taken to be the causal origin – etiology/etiogenesis – of illness, and this is studied, on the population level, by means of the methods peculiar to epidemiological research. As we noted, epidemiology was, in 1962 already, "widely recognized as the basic science of preventive medicine" [6], and there still is broadly-based agreement about this, in epidemiological academia most notably.

We, however, define epidemiology not as a study or a science but as a species/branch of (the practice of) medicine, as community medicine (Sects. 1.5 and 5.1); and we therefore have a different conception of the essence of epidemiological research, outlined in Sect. 5.7 below.

5.7 The Purposive Essence of Epidemiological Research

5.7.1 'Basic' Epidemiological Research

In Sect. 2.2 we defined *clinical research* in terms of its purposive essence – as research for the advancement of clinical medicine. From this we deduced the proposition that a major species of clinical research is 'basic' clinical research, generally conducted on the laboratory level (Sect. 2.3). This species of clinical research has been enormously successful in the advancement of clinical medicine – by leading to the development of novel products and processes for deployment in clinical medicine (in addition to novel entities of somatic anomaly/illness).

Epidemiological research we define analogously with our definition of clinical research – as research for the advancement of epidemiology, of community-level preventive medicine. And analogously with our conception of 'basic' clinical research as a species of clinical research, one major species of epidemiological research we take to be 'basic' epidemiological research. Like 'basic' clinical research, *'basic' epidemiological research* has been enormously productive – most notably as the basis for the development of vaccines.

5.7.2 Gnostic Epidemiological Research

In the practice of epidemiology – of community medicine, that is (Sect. 5.1) – the doctor pursues diagnoses about the levels of morbidity from various illnesses in the community and about etiognostic explanations of these levels – with a view to decisions about preventive actions on the community level (education, regulation, and/or service).

For those diagnoses about morbidity levels in the community, the doctor has the ad-hoc input of the population's diagnostic profile – the population's distribution by various health-relevant characteristics (demographic, economic, etc.). It remains for the doctor to know about the morbidity levels in the various strata of the population. The general source for this knowing – these community diagnoses – in principle is *diagnostic epidemiological research*. This research addresses the rate of morbidity from the illness at issue, specific to various strata of populations, by addressing the rate as joint function – acausal, descriptive – of the diagnostic indicators considered. Acausal determinants of the level of a morbidity, such as age and gender, are commonly termed *risk factors*; but they actually are *risk indicators* without being risk factors [12].

A community doctor's etiognostic concern in regard to a particular morbidity is to know what proportion the rate is attributable, causally, to the population's pattern of histories in respect to a particular risk factor – the deviation of this pattern from some particular reference pattern (counterfactual). To this end the epidemiologist needs the added ad-hoc input of what that pattern of histories in the population actually is; and *etiognostic epidemiologic al research* is, ideally at least, the source of the knowledge (or mere evidence) for estimating the corresponding etiogenetic proportion/fraction, the one that the etiognosis is about.

References

1. Terris M (1962) The scope and methods of epidemiology. Am J Public Health 52:1371–1376
2. Payne AMM (1962) The scope and methods of epidemiology. Editorial. Am J Public Health 52:1502–1504
3. Stallones RA (1963) Epidemi(olog)^{2}y. Letter to the editor. Am J Public Health 53:1696–1700
4. Stedman's medical dictionary, illustrated in color, 28th edn. Williams &Wilkins, Philadelphia (2013)
5. WHO; definition of epidemiology. Retrieved August 11, 2016 from http://www.who.int/topics/epidemiology/en
6. MacMahon B, Pugh TF, Ipsen J (1962) Epidemiologic methods. Little, Brown and Company, Boston, p vii
7. National Institute of Deafness and Other Communication Disorders; definition of epidemiology. Retrieved August 11, 2016 from http://www.nidcd.nih.gov/health/statistics/Pages/epidemiology.aspx
8. CDC; definition of epidemiology. Retrieved August 11, 2016 from http://www.cdc.gov/EXCITE/epidemiology.html
9. Last J (ed) (1983) A dictionary of epidemiology. A handbook sponsored by the I.E.A. Oxford University Press, New York
10. Porta M (Editor), Hernan M, dos Santos Silva I, Last JM (Associate Editors). Buron A (Assistant Editor) (2014) A dictionary of epidemiology. A handbook sponsored by the IEA, 6th edn. Oxford University Press, New York
11. Miettinen OS (2015) Medicine as a scholarly field: an introduction. Springer, Cham
12. Miettinen OS (2011) Epidemiological research: terms and concepts. Springer, Dordrecht
13. Miettinen OS (2015) Important concepts in epidemiology. In: Olsen J, Greene N, Saracci R, Trichopoulos D (eds) Teaching epidemiology. A guide for teachers of epidemiology, public health, and clinical medicine, 4th edn. Oxford University Press, Oxford
14. Dawber TR, Meadors GF, Moore FE Jr (1951) Epidemiological approaches to heart disease. Am J Public Health 41:279–286
15. Miettinen OS (1985) Theoretical epidemiology. principles of occurrence research in medicine. Wiley, New York
16. Miettinen OS (1976) Estimability and estimation in case-referent studies. Am J Epidemiol 103:226–235

Chapter 6
The Epidemiological Interface of Gnostic Clinical Research

Contents

Abstract Alvan Feinstein and David Sackett pioneered the now-common tenet that active following and critical evaluation of reports from directly practice-relevant clinical research are integral parts of modern practice of clinical medicine. For this conception of the relation of clinical practice to clinical research – quite questionable – together with their conception of the essence of epidemiology – mistaken – Feinstein and Sackett adopted the term *'clinical epidemiology'* – a contradiction in terms. Feinstein was very hesitant about accepting this term – exogenous to him – for the statistical-type clinical research he was concerned with (and called clinimetrics); and he didn't attempt to define the concept. We here, apart from describing the genesis of and thinking about this contemporary version of 'clinical epidemiology,' outline the actual nature of the interface of gnostic clinical research with epidemiology, which implies that *gnostic clinical research is neither epidemiology nor epidemiological research* – but: *meta-epidemiological clinical research.*

Keywords Clinical epidemiology · Alvan Feinstein · David Sackett · Practice-relevant clinical research · Evidence-based medicine · Meta-epidemiological clinical research · Theory of medicine · Theory of gnostic clinical research · Education for clinical research · Epidemiological-clinical collaboration in clinical research

O. S. Miettinen et al., *Clinical Research Transformed*,
https://doi.org/10.1007/978-3-030-06176-0_6

6.1 The Concept of 'Clinical Epidemiology'

The *IEA dictionary of epidemiology* in its second, 1988 edition [1], different from the first, 1983 edition, had the 'Clinical epidemiology' entry. Under it were reviewed then-existing definitions of the concept, including one by Sackett [2]:

> The application, by a physician who provides direct patient care, of epidemiologic and biometric methods to the study of diagnostic and therapeutic processes in order to effect an improvement in health.

The disquisition about 'clinical epidemiology' under that entry in that dictionary was closed with this observation: "The existence of the above and other subtly different definitions suggests that this branch of epidemiology remains inchoate."

The then Editor of that dictionary, in that same year (1988), published an article [3] with this in-medias-res opening: "I seek here to make two points: first, that 'clinical epidemiology' is an oxymoron [here meaning not an oxymoronic figure of speech but a contradiction in terms]; second, that the uncritical enthusiasm with which this activity is being embraced in many medical schools constitutes a danger to health." And in 2011, a book critical about the (variously-defined) concept of 'clinical epidemiology' and, especially, about the ideas espoused under that rubric, was published, by one of us [4].

Nevertheless, the 2015 edition of that 'official' dictionary of epidemiology [5], under new editorship, still has the 'Clinical epidemiology' entry. Now the content is this:

> The application of epidemiological knowledge, reasoning, and methods to study clinical issues and improve clinical care. 'Clinical' should not be restricted to 'medical.' 'Medical epidemiology' is a complementary and commonly used term. Research often addresses etiological, mechanistic, therapeutic, and prognostic medical issues, is conducted in clinical settings, and is led by clinicians, and has patients as study subjects. While clinical epidemiology uses epidemiological principles mostly to aid decision-making involving sick individuals, the wider context is also commonly considered [refs.].

The 'clinical epidemiology' term with its contemporary denotation was launched in earnest in 1985, by the publication of a *textbook by Alvan Feinstein* [6]. The lengthy Prologue of this book was largely devoted to its author's lucubrations in the development of the book's title, the principal candidate for which had been "The Architecture of Clinical Research." In the end, this became the book's subtitle, with "Clinical Epidemiology" the lead title. *The concept of 'clinical epidemiology' Feinstein left undefined.*

Somewhat less cryptic would have been another one of Feinstein's candidate titles for the book: "Quantification of Diagnosis, Prognosis, and Therapy." But:

> [The name Quantification of Diagnosis, Prognosis, and Therapy] was rejected because it had at least four disadvantages: it was too long; it did not indicate the full scope of the contents; it would erroneously suggest a mathematical rather than clinical emphasis; and the word *Quantitative* might scare away many readers to whom the book was intended.

As for what that seminal book actually was about, more telling than any of the titles that Feinstein considered was this passage in his Prologue of the book:

> future clinicians are taught ... very little about how to evaluate the published evidence on which medical practice depends. This book is intended not only to help fill that gap in medical education, but also to help guide clinicians who actually engage in research.

So, Feinstein's seminal book on 'clinical epidemiology' was *mainly directed to future practitioners* of clinical medicine rather than to students preparing for careers in clinical research (which is the orientation here). It was, for them, an *introduction to clinical research*, with a view to their future needs as practitioners of clinical medicine.

As is evident from the quotes above, both of the two fathers of the contemporary concept of 'clinical epidemiology' – Sackett [2] and Feinstein [6] – addressed, under that rubric, research for the advancement of the knowledge-base of clinical medicine. And the justification for their use of that term for this research presumably was their recognition that needed in this research is the application of ideas of epidemiology. The puzzling 'clinical-epidemiology' term for this research [3] evidently arose from *the category error of taking the application of epidemiological ideas to be epidemiology.* (Application of scientific knowledge is not science; application of evidence from research is not research; and application of the ideas of epidemiology is not epidemiology.)

As also is evident from the quotes above, both Sackett and Feinstein had the idea that 'clinical epidemiology' is *a dimension of the practice of clinical medicine*: the lead idea was that practitioners of clinical medicine read published reports of clinical research, critically, and then apply the resulting learning to "effect an improvement in health" [2]; that they "evaluate the published evidence on which medical practice depends" [6]. According to Sackett [2], 'clinical epidemiology' bears on the practice of clinical medicine through studies of "diagnostic and therapeutic processes" and, hence, in these two aspects of practice; and for Feinstein [6], the counterpart of these two was the triad "diagnosis, prognosis, and therapy."

Neither one of those authorities on research-guided clinical medicine viewed the relevant research as the source of practice-relevant *knowledge*, for gnostic probability-setting (cf. Sect. 1.2). For, this conception of the mission in directly practice-relevant clinical research (Chap. 2) was not yet available as the lodestar for charting the theory of directly practice-relevant clinical research for either one of those two pioneers of modern 'clinical epidemiology' and the ideas about clinical research under this (odd) rubric.

It thus is to be understood that 'clinical epidemiology' in the contemporary meaning of this term was mainly introduced as a presumedly essential dimension of modern *practice* of clinical medicine, the dimension in which clinicians deploy evidence from reports on clinical research as a (scientific) guide to their practices, and not as a discipline of conducting research relevant for advancement of the scientific knowledge-base of clinical practice. It thus formed the ideological basis for the launching of the *'evidence-based medicine'* [8] movement – the core tenet of which is the idea that clinicians should not rely on experts' guidance but should, instead, personally follow the relevant research (comprehensively yet critically).

This idea about scientific practice of clinical medicine we deem to be very *unrealistic*.

6.2 The Concept of Meta-epidemiological Clinical Research

Different from Sackett and Feinstein, and from their already numerous devotees and followers under the banner of 'clinical epidemiology,' our thinking about clinical research does not begin with casual a-priori ideas about this research, notably the ideas that the relevant research addresses "diagnosis and treatment" [2] or "diagnosis, prognosis, and treatment" [6], and is groups-oriented numerical – and by this criterion 'epidemiological' – research. (Cf. Sect. 6.1, above.)

As a matter of principles of the general theory of medicine [7], our thinking about clinical research begins with our critical thinking about the essence of clinical medicine and, subordinate to this, about the essence of clinical research (Chaps. 1 and 2). From the concepts of these we deduce the essence of *the requisite knowledge-base of clinical medicine*: that it is about *gnostic probabilities* in defined domains of case presentation (Sect. 1.2); and in (logical) consequence of this, we take directly practice-relevant clinical research to be about those probabilities (Sect.2.3), for the advancement of the practice of genuinely scientific clinical medicine (Sect. 2.4).

Then, as an elementary matter of applied statistics, we take it that *probabilities are studied by studying rates*; and as a matter of the general theory of medicine [7] again, we understand that the concepts of rate of occurrence are germane to practice in the *epidemiological* branch of medicine (Sects. 1.5 and 5.1). The concepts of rate of occurrence in medicine therefore are germane (and intrinsic) to the theory of the epidemiological branch of medicine and, secondary to this, to the theory – concepts and principles – of population-level (gnostic) epidemiological research (Sect. 5.7.2). They therefore need to be learned for the study of probabilities (gnostic) for clinical medicine; and they need to be learned correctly, despite the confusion about them that now prevails (Sects. 5.4 and 5.5).

This is to say that, in our view, understanding the essence of directly practice-relevant clinical research begins with the realization that the theory of this research necessarily incorporates, importantly, some elements of the theory of epidemiology and epidemiological research, critically developed. But the conduct of epidemiological-type research for the purposes of clinical medicine involves the deployment of the theory of epidemiological research in domains that are extrinsic to epidemiology and epidemiological research. *The research at issue here therefore is not epidemiological research, and much less is it epidemiology – 'clinical epidemiology.'*

As gnostic clinical research, on account of its extra-epidemiological purpose, is not epidemiological, and as it nevertheless is dependent on the theory of epidemiology and epidemiological research, we think of, and describe, it as *meta-epidemiological clinical research* [7].

6.3 Epidemiological Preparation for Clinical Research

As gnostic clinical research is, in its form, an extension of population-level, statistical-type (rather than laboratory-level, biological-type) epidemiological research (Sect. 6.2, above), preparation for this species of clinical research (Sect. 2.3) involves study of the theory of population-level epidemiological research. The core *concepts* of population-level epidemiological research – together with the terms denoting them – were addressed in Chap. 5 above, with focus on critically-adopted, tenable versions of these.

Those concepts are here supplemented by just as critically-adopted core *principles* of that branch of epidemiological research, with focus on research on the causal origin – *etiology/etiogenesis* – of illnesses (or of the level of morbidity from them). For this is what population-level epidemiological research characteristically is about, with the aim of developing the scientific knowledge-base for population-level preventive medicine (which is the essence of epidemiological practice). Correct understanding of the theory of this research is relevant not only for etiognostic clinical research but also for prognostic clinical research [9].

In its traditional conception, an etiologic/etiognostic study was taken to inherently be – and in its still-common misunderstanding it can be – of the form of what now is called a *case-control study*. In such a study, a group of persons with the illness in question is compared with a similar group of persons without that illness, in respect to their respective distributions in terms of histories regarding the causal factor at issue. Much confusion has plagued the selection of the control group to make it truly 'comparable' to the case group in such a study, and this confusion still continues. In point of fact, this problem will never be solved, as the case-control conception of an etiogenetic study is logically untenable.

The requisite essence of an etiogenetic study needs to be deduced (by analytic logic) from the essence of etiogenetic/etiognostic – outcome-explanatory – causation, which is distinct from prognostic – outcome-changing – causation [10]: If antecedent A is causal (etiogenetic) to (event-type) outcome O, this means that in a population of people with a positive histories for either A or to its alternative (in the causal contrast), the incidence density of O is higher among those with A – *ceteris paribus* (i.e., all else being equal). Hence, needed for an etiogenetic study is a defined study population-time constituted by that associated with the index history (A present) together with that associated with the reference history (alternative present). For quantification of the relative sizes of the index and reference incidence densities of O in this *study base* – which is the *referent* of the study result – needed is identification of the complete series of cases of O occurring in this population-time together with a fair sample (finite) of the person-moments in it (infinite in number), both of these series documented in relevant regards. The data on these two series are synthesized into the study result for the outcome's incidence-density ratio in its referent [11], the study base [9] – conditional on the ceteris paribus factors (potential confounders). This *case-base* or *case-referent* study is the logical alternative to the traditional case-control study (above).

Such is, still, the understanding of these matters that the IEA dictionary of epidemiology [5] presents the term 'case-referent study' as a synonym of 'case-control study,' and 'case-base study' as "a variant of the case-control study in which the controls are drawn from the same study base as the cases regardless of their disease status [refs.]."

And the confusion is compounded further by the presumed existence of the so-called *cohort study* as an alternative to the case-control study. That dictionary [5] gives "concurrent, follow-up, incidence, longitudinal, panel, [and] prospective study" as synonyms of the term; and it gives as the concept's definition this: "The analytic [etiologic] epidemiological study in which subsets of a defined population can be identified who are, have been, or in the future may be exposed or not exposed – or exposed in different degrees – to a factor or factors hypothesized to influence the occurrence of a driven disease [refs.]."

In the face of this (manifest) confusion it should be understood that the *study population* in the logically-constructed etiologic (etiogenetic, etiognostic) study – the case-base or case-referent study – inherently is a dynamic one, inseparably imbedded ('nested') in the study's *source population,* which can be either dynamic or of the cohort type. The source population may be defined directly, or indirectly as the 'catchment population' of the cases (given the definition of case identification).

6.4 Meta-epidemiological Preparation for Clinical Research

Upon having gained a tenable understanding not only of the core concepts of epidemiology and epidemiological research (Chap. 5) but also of the principal – etiologic/etiogenetic – species of population-level epidemiological research (Sect. 6.3, above), strictly epidemiological preparation for gnostic clinical research is essentially complete.

The relevance of this epidemiological preparation for clinical research may be seen to be limited to only one species of gnostic clinical research, and the least important species of it at that – namely *etiognostic* clinical research. But in point of fact, understanding the case-base or case-referent structure of the logically-constructed etiogenetic study (Sect. 6.3, above) has its main relevance in the most important species of gnostic clinical research: in *prognostic* clinical research, including, very notably, in intervention-prognostic trials [9]. This we explain in the statistical Sect. 7.4.5 and more thoroughly in the Chapter on deriving prognostic probability functions from clinical-trial data (Chap. 20).

While understanding the correctly-construed etiogenetic study – the study that is so central in epidemiological research – is critically relevant for understanding etiognostic and prognostic clinical research, a very different and rather peripheral type of epidemiological study is preparatory to understanding *diagnostic* clinical research. This epidemiological study is not a causal one but acausal, purely descriptive: it is a study addressing the way the prevalence of a particular illness (chronic) depends (descriptively) on some determinants of it, in a particular domain of people. Study of such a *prevalence function* is directly paradigmatic for studying a *diagnostic probability function* designed (as to its form) for a particular domain of case presentation for diagnosis.

All in all, thus, critical understanding of epidemiological research (on rates) constitutes critically-important preparation for critical understanding of research on *probabilities – gnostic probability functions* – for the scientific knowledge-base of clinical medicine.

6.5 Epidemiological-Clinical Collaboration in Clinical Research

As gnostic clinical research is meta-epidemiological in its theoretical underpinnings (Sect. 6.2) while clinical in its substance and relevance, it needs to be collaborative between the epidemiologic and clinical segments of medical academia.

Gnostic clinical research as collaboration between epidemiologic and clinical academia is truly productive only when both of the parties in this collaboration have had suitable *educational preparation* for this research. In this, the beginning is education of both epidemiologic and clinical academics in the theory of this meta-epidemiological research – along the precepts presented in this book. And needed to this end is the development of such a program of education by the epidemiologic segment of a leading faculty of medicine. Most fitting for this role we take to be the medical faculty of the Karolinska Institute, as is argued in Appendix 2 of this book.

References

1. Last JM (ed) (1988) A dictionary of epidemiology. A handbook sponsored by the IEA, 2nd edn. Oxford University Press, New York
2. Sackett DL (1969) Clinical epidemiology. Am J Epidemiol 89:125–128
3. Last J (1988) What is "clinical epidemiology"? J Public Health Policy 9:159–163
4. Miettinen OS (2011) Up from clinical epidemiology & EBM. Springer, Dordrecht
5. Porta M (Editor), Greenland S, Hernan M, dos Santos Silva I, Last JM (Associate Editors), Buron A (Assistant Editor) (2014) A dictionary of epidemiology. A handbook sponsored by the IEA, 6th edn. Oxford University Press, Oxford
6. Feinstein AR (1985) Clinical epidemiology. The architecture of clinical research. W. B. Saunders Company, Philadelphia
7. Miettinen OS (2015) Medicine as a scholarly field: an introduction. Springer, Cham
8. Guyatt G, Cairns J, Churchill D *et alii* (1992) A new approach to teaching the practice of medicine. JAMA 268:2420–2425
9. Miettinen OS (2004) Epidemiology: Quo vadis? Eur J Epidemiol 19:713–718
10. Miettinen OS (2010) Etiologic study vis-à-vis intervention study. Eur J Epidemiol 23:671–678
11. Miettinen OS (1976) Estimability and estimation in case-referent studies. Eur J Epidemiol 103:226–2235

Part III
Statistical Preliminaries of Gnostic Clinical Research

Chapter 7
The Logistic Regression Model

Contents

Abstract Among the statistical preliminaries of education in the theory of gnostic clinical research, centrally important are, first, the precursors of logistic regression, culminating in the emergence of the *General Linear Model;* and then the generalization of this to the *Generalized Linear Model,* with *logistic regression model* a special case of this. Against this backdrop we address the *ubiquitous applicability of logistic regression as the statistical framework for gnostic clinical research,* not merely as an option but as *the only appropriate statistical-model framework for this research.*

Keywords Statistical models in general · 'Data analysis' as synthesis · The regression model · Regression toward the mean · The general linear model · The generalized linear model · The logistic regression model · The model for diagnostic probability · The model for etiognostic probability · The model for prognostic probability

O. S. Miettinen et al., *Clinical Research Transformed*,
https://doi.org/10.1007/978-3-030-06176-0_7

7.1 The Precursors of the General Linear Model

7.1.1 *The Shared Essence of the Precursors*

In books and teachings of statistics, eminent topics have been – and still are – the three closely related ones of: '*Analysis of variance*,' '*Analysis of covariance*,' and '*Regression analysis*.'

In all three of these topics, the statistical model addresses a *random variate* whose distribution, conditional on some non-random variate(s), is *Gaussian* – 'normal,' 'bell-shaped' – with a particular mean and a particular variance, variance being the average of a variate's squared deviations from the mean. These two 'parameters,' mean and variance, fully specify any particular Gaussian distribution.

In the essence of all three of these models is the feature that the value of the random variate's mean depends, potentially at least, on some determinant(s) of this value, represented by the *non-random variate(s)* in the model; but the random variate's variance is (assumed to be) independent of the determinant(s) of the value of the mean, this feature of the model being termed the 'homoscedasticity' assumption.

7.1.2 *The Analysis of Variance Model*

In the 'analysis of variance model,' the random variate at issue – Gaussian – has a mean whose value depends on a *nominal-scale determinant*, a nominal scale being characterized by discrete categories without any natural order among them. The names of the (nominal) categories, some N in number, could be Category 1, Category 2, … , Category N. The term for the model is a misnomer. For, at issue is not analysis but *synthesis* of data, and the synthesis is not directed to learning about the variance of the random variate; it *focuses on the mean*, the relation of the mean to the (nominal-scale) determinant of it.

A simple example of these models might address the mean of systemic blood-pressure – defined as the weighted average of the diastolic and systolic pressures with weights 2/3 and 1/3, respectively – in relation to ethnicity, represented by three categories. An 'analysis-of-variance' model would define a random variate (Y) as representing the numerical value of the pressure (statistical variates inherently being numerical) and having a Gaussian distribution with means M_1, M_2, and M_3 in those ethnicity categories 1, 2, and 3, respectively, with the variance of the distribution invariant among them. The random variate (Y) is the '*dependent*' variate in the meaning that the value of its mean depends on ethnicity; and the ethnicity categories are represented in terms of suitably-defined '*independent*' – non-random – variates (Xs).

The form of the 'analysis-of-variance' *model* in this simple example is:

$$M = B_0 + B_1 X_1 + B_2 X_2,$$

where M is the mean of Y and the two independent variates are indicators of two particular ones of the three ethnic categories. One possibility in this framework is to take X_1 and X_2 to be indicators of Category 2 and Category 3, respectively – an *indicator variate* being one that takes on the value 1 for the category it indicates, 0 otherwise.

In terms of this model, B_0 is the value of M when $X_1 = X_2 = 0$, that is, for Category 1 (i.e., $B_0 = M_1$); and for Category 2 and Category 3 the values of M are represented by $B_0 + B_1$ and $B_0 + B_2$, respectively (i.e., $M_2 = B_0 + B_1$, and $M_3 = B_0 + B_2$). Thus, the difference between M_1 and M_2 is represented by B_1; B_2 represents the difference between M_1 and M_3; and the difference between M_2 and M_3 is the difference between B_1 and B_2.

In this 'analysis-of-variance' framework *it is feasible to accommodate, jointly, whatever number of nominal-scale determinants* of the magnitude of the mean of the dependent variate. A simple example of this is the addition of the two categories of gender for consideration jointly with the three categories of ethnicity. These two determinants jointly imply a *single nominal-scale determinant* with six categories (as each of the three categories of ethnicity is split into two subcategories based on gender).

When involved in the definition of the independent variates is only a single determinant, the model is said to be for *'one-way analysis of variance'*; with two determinants the corresponding term (naturally) is *'two-way analysis of variance';* etc.

A limiting – 'degenerate' – case of 'analysis of variance' models for the mean of a Gaussian variate is, naturally, of the form of $M = B$, involving no indicators for distinguishing among *subdomains of the referent domain* of the distribution, say adults not otherwise specified.

7.1.3 *The Analysis of Covariance Model*

Continuing with the simple example above, suppose age is introduced as a determinant for consideration jointly with ethnicity or, for that matter, jointly with ethnicity and gender.

As age is not a nominal-scale characteristic but a *quantitative* one, its incorporation into the model – in terms of a continuous independent variate (X_i) representing the *numerical* value of age – is not analogous to adding gender to ethnicity (Sect. 7.1.2, above). In simplest terms, only a single term ($B_i X_i$) needs to be added to the model, despite the fact that innumerable levels of age are at issue.

A *model* incorporating one or more indicator variates (à la 'analysis of variance' model; Sect. 7.1.2, above) and, in addition, one or more quantitative ones, is termed an 'analysis of covariance' model. This too is a double misnomer (just as 'analysis of variance' is), as at issue is not analysis but synthesis of data (cf. Sect.7.1.2, above) and the synthesis is not directed to any covariance but, again, to the mean of the dependent variate, to its dependence on the set of independent variates (cf. Sect. 7.1.2, above).

Covariance in this context, just as in 'analysis of variance,' has to do with covariation of pairs of the independent variates: for any given pair of variates, it is the average of the product of their respective deviations from their means, the covariance of X_i and X_j being the average of $(X_i - M_i)(X_j - M_j)$, M_i and M_j being the respective means. The concern for covariation of the independent variates is no greater when quantitative independent variates are involved jointly with indicator variates, relative to involvement of indicator variates alone. And in particular, the absence of such covariation – correlation – is not an assumption in either type of model, that of 'analysis of variance' or that of 'analysis of covariance.' The essential novelty here is, merely, that involved is a quantitative determinant in addition to one (or more) whose scale is nominal. The separate determinant/independent variates can no longer be represented in terms of a single nominal-scale variate.

7.1.4 The Regression Analysis Model

Particularly notable among the three precursors of the General Linear Model is the 'regression analysis' model or, more simply, the 'regression' model.

In the original meaning of this term, at issue was, literally, a regression. Thus, for example, the mean of peoples' heights in any given category of their parents' height shows *'regression toward the mean'*: the offspring of tall people, while they also tend to be tall, are on the average less tall than their parents; and the offspring of persons of less-than-average height, while they also tend to be of less than the average height, are on the average taller than their parents [1]. In this phrasing of the phenomenon, no provision is made for secular trend in the heights of people (adults).

A different example of 'regression toward the mean' is the *replication-distribution* of the measurement result on a physiologic 'parameter' such as the mean blood pressure considered in Sects. 7.1.2 and 7.1.3 above. The mean of the values from repeat measurements at any given level of the result of the first measurement tends to show 'regression toward the mean': where the first result of the measurement deviates to a given extent from the mean in a particular direction, the mean of the repeat readings tends to deviate in the same direction but to a lesser extent.

This latter example is illustrated and explained by Fig. 7.1. In it, the Y and X axes address the second and first readings, respectively; the possible values of the data points are represented by an ellipse centered on the identity line; and the X-conditional distributions of Y are represented by vertical lines across the ellipse. Midpoints of those lines across the range of Y (under the ellipse) illustrate the regression toward the mean – the logical necessity of this in repeat measurements in the context of irreproducibility of ('errors' in) these.

The generic *model* in these examples is $M = B_0 + B_1X$, where M is, as in 'analysis of variance' and 'analysis of covariance,' the mean of the Gaussian dependent variate and X is a quantitative independent variate. This is, in today's statistical

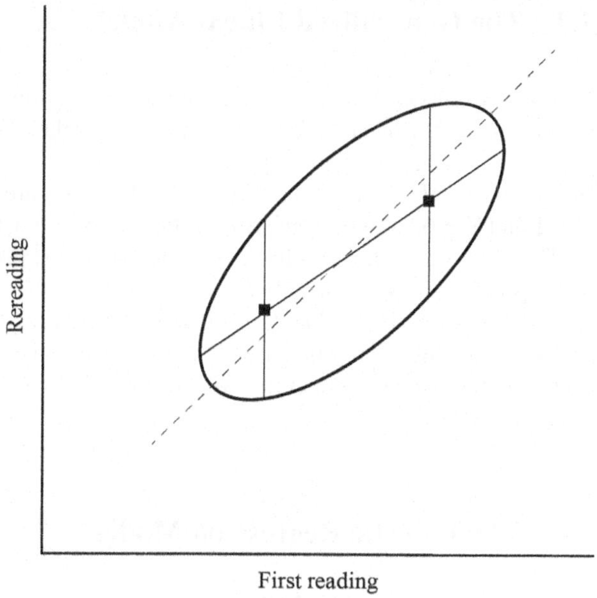

Fig. 7.1 Distribution of rereadings conditionally on first readings: 'regression toward the mean'

jargon, the model specific to *'simple regression.'* With more than one X, the model is said to be one of *multiple regression.*

7.2 The General Linear Model

An important generalization of the three models addressed in Sects. 7.1.2, 7.1.3, and 7.1.4 above, is the General Linear Model. It, too, addresses the mean of a Gaussian dependent variate Y (random), formulating this dependent parameter, *M*, as a compound of the form B_0 + sum (over i = 1, 2, …) of terms B_iX_i; but it places no constraints on the distributions (non-random) of those independent variates X_1 etc. This generalization across those three precursors of it is the *meaning of 'general'* in the term 'general linear model' in statistics.

The *meaning of 'linear'* in the appellation of this model has nothing to do with straight lines; it refers to the mathematical concept of *'linear compound'*: given quantities Q_1, Q_2, etc., a linear compound of these is the sum $C_1Q_1 + C_2Q_2 + \ldots$, where C_1 etc. are the 'coefficients' that define a particular linear compound of the set of quantities constituted by the Qs.

So, the 'general linear model' is linear in the sense that *the dependent parameter, M, is formulated as a linear compound of the independent parameters B_0, B_1, etc.*, the coefficients in this linear compound being 1, X_1, etc. The model is, in this way, 'linear in the parameters.'

7.3 The Generalized Linear Model

One or both of two further generalizations are incorporated into any given case of the Generalized Linear Model. One of these is relaxation of the constraint that the dependent variate be Gaussian in its distribution; it can have, most notably, the *Bernoulli distribution*, in which the possible values are only the two constituted by Y = 1 and Y = 0, taking place with probabilities *P* and 1 – *P*, respectively.

The other generalization has to do with the mean (*M*) of the dependent variate's distribution: the linear formulation need not be given to *M* as such; it can be given to a *transform of M*, so that *M* itself is formulated as the *inverse transform* of the linear compound – as nonlinear in this sense. Our concern focuses on the generalized linear model in the particular meaning of the *logistic* regression model, addressed in Sect. 7.4 below.

7.4 The Logistic Regression Model

7.4.1 The Essence of the Model

The 'logistic regression' model is a particular – very important – example of the generalized linear model.

In this model, the dependent variate has the Bernoulli distribution (Sect. 7.3, above); and the linear-compound formulation is given to the *'logit' transformation* of the mean (*M* = *P*) of this distribution, to log [*P* / (1 – *P*)]:

$$\log\left[P/(1-P)\right] = B_0 + B_1\mathrm{X}_1 + B_2\mathrm{X}_2 + \ldots$$

This generalized linear model is tantamount to a nonlinear formulation of the probability of Y = 1:

$$P = 1/\left[1+\exp(-\mathrm{L})\right],$$

where L is the linear compound in the model for the logit of *P* (above) and 'exp' refers to 'exponential,' meaning 'antilog of' (i.e., *e* – the base of natural logarithms – to the power of what follows).

7.4.2 The Central Relevance of the Model

In educational preparation for a stellar career as a scholar advancing – and teaching – the knowledge-base (gnostic) of a particular discipline of clinical medicine, the need is to learn the relevant topics in the education well, meaning correctly and securely. The development of this foundation for the career requires, inter alia, focus on the relevant, without the distraction of accumulating less-than-secure knowledge on non-essential topics.

In this spirit, in the statistical preliminaries of studying the theory of gnostic clinical research – which is to address *gnostic probability functions* (Sect. 4.1) – the focus needs to be on the statistical fundamentals of this research. And in this, the focus needs to be on the *logistic regression model*, as this model is *centrally relevant in all three of the species of gnostic clinical research*, leaving no need for the deployment of other types of statistical model in this research.

That proposition about logistic regression in gnostic clinical research is substantiated in Sects. 7.4.3, 7.4.4, and 7.4.5 below – and it is explicated further in the Chapters addressing the three species of this research.

7.4.3 The Model in Diagnostic Research

Concerning the theory of diagnostic research, a highly influential article was published in 1959 [2]. In it, the point of departure was the premise that, while the concern in diagnosis is to know the probability that a particular illness is present, knowledge relevant to diagnosis necessarily is of the form that is the reverse of this – that diagnosis-relevant knowledge is about the probability of the patient's "symptom complex" conditionally on the presence and absence of the illness in question. On the basis of knowledge of this type, so went the theorizing, diagnostic probabilities need to be derived by means of *Bayes' Theorem*. These ideas have been central in the diagnostic thinking of 'clinical epidemiologists' (Sects. 3.1.2 and 6.1); but they are seriously mistaken (Chap. 13).

A very different concern in clinical research has been the development of ways to summarize the elements in a diagnostic profile in terms of a score summarizing this multi-dimensional information in terms of a single number, a diagnostic score. This involves the concern to develop suitable weighting of the items of information in the profile, expressed numerically as realizations of statistical variates (Xs), and the available statistical means to this end used to be only the *'Fisher discriminant function.'*

Then, in the late 1960s, *logistic regression* was introduced into medical research. The linear compound in it is a discriminant, having, like the Fisher discriminant, relative weightings for the realizations of the statistical variates (Xs) that are involved in the scoring and are subject to statistical optimization. But an *important novelty* in the logistic framework for discriminant scoring was that it provided for translating the realizations of the (statistically-optimized) scoring function to their corresponding values of probabilities for the two possibilities (realizations of the Bernoulli Y) addressed in the discrimination (Sect. 7.4.1).

Logistic regression, unquestionably, provides *the appropriate statistical-model framework for research on diagnostic probability functions* (Part IV in this book).

7.4.4 The Model in Etiognostic Research

The deployment of logistic regression is well-established in epidemiological research on the etiology/etiogenesis of illness, even if 'Cox regression' also is commonly, though unjustifiably, used.

In an etiologic/etiogenetic study for etiognosis about a health event, the study base is the aggregate of population-time of the study population's – open, dynamic – course over time documented for the study (Sect. 6.3). For the incidence density (ID) of the event whose etiogenesis is at issue, a suitable model is 'log-linear':

$$\log(\mathrm{ID}') = B_0 + B_1 \mathrm{X}_1 + B_2 \mathrm{X}_2 + \ldots,$$

where ID′ is the numerical value of ID (i.e., ID multiplied by the unit amount of population-time). This model represents the causal relation of the ID to history of the etiogenetic factor at issue insofar as, apart from the terms representing the etiogenetic history, all relevant *extraneous determinants* of the ID's level are suitably represented by the (confounder) terms in this model.

Let us consider the simple case in which the etiogenetic history at issue is represented by X_1 alone – with $\mathrm{X}_1 = 1$ and $\mathrm{X}_1 = 0$ representing *positive (index) history* and *negative (reference) history*, respectively. In this (simple) case, the effect at issue is represented by

$$\log(\mathrm{ID}' | \mathrm{X}_1 = 1) - \log(\mathrm{ID}' | \mathrm{X}_1 = 0) = B_1,$$

and this means that the causal incidence-density ratio (*IDR*) contrasting the index and reference histories is:

$$IDR = \exp(B_1).$$

Causal *IDR* is what an etiognostic study is all about, as it implies the *etiognostic probability* as (IDR – 1) / IDR in the case of the index history (and 0 in the case of the reference history).

More generally, the *IDR* is the exponential of the sum of all the terms in the linear compound in which the contrast indicator (here X_1) is involved, with the value of this indicator set to indicate the index history (by its realization 1).

The database (in its statistical form) produced in an etiognostic study involves data on two series: the *case series* (in which Y = 1) and the *base series* (in which Y = 0). These derive from the population-time of the study base (Sects. 6.3 and 15.6). Logistic discrimination between these two series with the linear compound of the log-linear model for the ID (above) addresses *quasi-IDs*, in which the population-time (denominator) inputs to IDs are replaced by the corresponding numbers of person-moments in the base series. But the result of the fitting of this logistic model provides a result for the actual *IDR* (above), as the sizes of the base series from the index and reference segments of study population-time are (stochastically) proportional to those two amounts of population-time conditionally on the confounder variates in the model.

7.4.5 The Model in Prognostic Research

As logistic regression is the natural theoretical framework for diagnostic research, inherently addressing diagnostic probabilities through proportion-type rates (of prevalence), this species of regression is, just as naturally, the appropriate framework for addressing prognostic probabilities through *proportion-type rates of incidence, so long as the time horizon of the prognoses is very short* (Sect. 5.5.2). Different from diagnostic research, the linear compound in the model needs to provide for causal interpretability of the difference in probabilities (prognostic) from the treatment-conditional functions. This may require suitably inclusive and accurate representation of the prognostic indicators in the model (for control of confounding).

When the prognostic time-horizon is long enough so that deaths from extraneous causes and/or losses to follow-up can occur, matters become more complicated. In this common situation in prognostic studies, the now-common theoretical framework is 'Cox regression.' But, regarding the event at issue in the population-time of the study cohort's follow-up, the Cox model – of 'proportional hazards' – addresses only its incidence-density ratio, modelled to be constant over prognostic/cohort time. The result of this model's fitting to study data does not, as such, translate into rates of cumulative incidence and, thereby, into prognostic probability functions.

The statistical framework for prognostic research that does provide for studying prognostic probability functions – and involves logistic regression – has been introduced by one of us [3, 4]. At the core of it is, as it were, an etiogenetic study – of a particular type – concerning the event's occurrence in the study base. Like any etiogenetic study, this semblance of it centers on the *series of cases* of the event in question identified as having occurred in the study base, here formed by the study cohort's follow-up for the event. This series is documented in respect to the events' timings on the scale of prognostic time together with the persons' prognostic profiles (at 'baseline,' time zero) and the type of treatment adopted (at baseline, for prospective implementation). (Documentation of the events' timings is not a feature of Cox regression; it is irrelevant on account of the model's 'proportional hazards' assumption, according to which the event's incidence-density ratio is constant over prognostic time.)

In this semblance of an etiogenetic study, the *base series* – a sample of the person-moments, infinite in number, constituting the study base – has the special feature of being selected as a *representative sample of the population-time of the study base*. This series is, naturally, documented analogously with the counterpart of this for the case series. (In Cox regression, the study base is probed at the times of the cases' occurrence, in terms of addressing the time-specific 'risk sets' in it, constituted by the person-moments in the cohort's cross-sections at those times, all of these.)

While these two series provide for addressing, in the usual manner of etiogenetic studies (Sect. 7.4.4, above), the incidence-density ratio (*IDR*) of the outcome-event's occurrence, contrasting two histories regarding the choice of the treatment at baseline, *the selection of the base series as a representative sample provides for proceeding from the IDR function to the actual incidence-density functions*, treatment-specific, for the range of prognostic time at issue – and, hence, for studying the corresponding cumulative-incidence functions, which is tantamount to studying prognostic probability functions.

In all of this, the need is to understand, first, the essence of the logistic function for this semblance on an etiogenetic study. The dependent parameter in it is the logit of the probability of a person-moment in the union of the case and base series being, conditionally on the Xs in the linear compound, a member of the case series (in which $Y = 1$). Hence, the linear compound in the logistic model/function represents the *logarithm of the quasi-rate* – the number of cases divided the number of probes of the population-time – specific to whatever realization of the Xs in the linear compound.

In consequence of this implication of the logistic model/function of the case-base data, together with the special nature of the base sample here, the incidence-density in the study base is:

$$\mathrm{ID} = (\mathrm{b} / \mathrm{B}) \exp(\mathrm{L}),$$

where b is the size of the base series, representative of the study base (cf. above); B is the size of the study base, the amount of population-time constituting it; and L is the linear compound in the logistic model deployed [3]. The index and reference ID functions are the versions of this function when evaluated at the treatment indicator's respective values (1 and 0) for these.

Given the result for each of the treatment-specific ID functions, the corresponding results for *cumulative incidence*, and thereby for cumulative prognostic probabilities – specific not only to prognosticate time and treatment but also to the prognostic indicators at T_0 can be derived from the integral of each of the ID functions of time from zero time to the end of the risk period at issue (Sect. 5.5.4). More on this in Sect. 20.2.3.

References

1. Stigler SM (2016) The seven pillars of statistical wisdom. Harvard University Press, Cambridge, MA
2. Ledley RS, Lusted LB (1959) Reasoning foundations of medical diagnosis. Science 130:9–21
3. Miettinen OS (2004) Epidemiology: quo vadis? Eur J Epidemiol 19:713–718
4. Miettinen OS (2010) Etiologic study vis-à-vis intervention study. Eur J Epidemiol 25:671–675

Chapter 8
Statistics from the Model's Fitting to Gnostic Data

Contents

Abstract Given the logistic model/function constituting the overall object of a gnostic clinical study, 'analysis' (synthesis) of the study data is, in essence, a computer-based fitting of that model to the data, using a suitable software system. The fitting produces the *overall result* of the study in terms of empirical values of the parameters in the model; and it produces *inferential statistics* related to these 'point estimates.' This result is excessively discriminating among the case profiles when the data are, as usual, rather sparse and multiple parameters are involved in the object function (for discrimination among them). There thus commonly is the need to correct for this bias with suitable '*shrinkage*' of the initial result of the fitting.

Keywords Object of study · Result of study · Shrinkage of the result · Statistics from the data · 'Point estimate' · 'Internal estimate' · 'Confidence interval' · 'Standard error' · Test statistic · P-value

8.1 The Study Result from the Model's Fitting

The *objects design* for a study to advance the knowledge-base of clinical medicine specifies the *form of the gnostic probability function,* for a specified *domain*, the function that the study is to address by producing empirical content of that form, from that domain. That design specifies (the form of) a linear compound of a set of parameters in a logistic-regression model (Chap. 7, above). Implicit in this is the

O. S. Miettinen et al., *Clinical Research Transformed*,
https://doi.org/10.1007/978-3-030-06176-0_8

principle that *the objects design is to be carried all the way to the statistical form of the regression model/function (logistic) to be studied.*

The study result is obtained by fitting – by the use of a suitable computer-software system – the designed model/function (logistic) to the data assembled in the execution of the methods design of the study. The output of the model's fitting goes well beyond the empirical content of the designed function's form. *The result of the study is constituted solely by the empirical – fitted – values of the object parameters in the model* (distinct from the parameters associated with confounder variates, if any).

In this way, the objects design determines what the result from the model's fitting to the data is to be taken to be; and in particular, *the fitting of the designed function should not be used for second thoughts on the design of the object function* – by deleting from the model terms in the light of the 'inferential statistics' accompanying the parameters' fitted values. Quite another matter is the possibility of producing a second-stage result by applying 'shrinkage' to the result initially obtained (Sect. 8.3, below).

8.2 The Statistics from the Model's Fitting

8.2.1 Point Estimates

The concept of statistic is, in theoretical statistics, that of a function of data. And consistent with this, in the context of 'data analysis' – this common term is a misnomer for synthesis of data – *a statistic is a number derived from the data* (e.g., the mean of a set of the realizations of a variate).

The first-order statistics derived by fitting a logistic-regression model to a body of data are, naturally, the result-defining values – the 'maximum likelihood estimates' – of the parameters in the designed model. In statistical jargon these values are termed *'point estimates.'* A 'point estimate' is, in theoretical statistics, a data-based realization of an 'estimator' – the function (of data) that is definitional to it. (A likelihood function is, by its maximization, the basis of those 'estimates' in logistic-regression 'analysis' of data.)

From the vantage of empirical science, which is the context here, *these values are not actual estimates of the parameters' values.* They are, simply, the parameters' empirical values from the particular study at issue, results of measurement in this sense. Much more than these empirical values go into those parameters' *actual estimation* – not by data but *by scientists*, who consider the results from the study on the function as just one of the inputs to their judgements in the estimation. The first-order input other than the study result per se to actual estimation is the *genesis of the result*, bearing on judgements about *bias*.

8.2.2 *Inferential Statistics*

One class of inputs to scientists' estimation – ultimately judgemental – of the values of a set of parameters (of Nature) addressed in logistic-regression 'analysis' (synthesis) of a set of data has to do with the *precisions* of these values; that is, with their *reproducibility* in hypothetical replications of the study in all relevant regards (of which time and place are not part), including the study's degree of informativeness (per its size, i.a.). The *precision* of a parameter's empirical value is addressed in terms of the 'inferential statistics' that statistical software-systems on logistic regression routinely derive from the data, associating them with the parameters' empirical values.

Preeminent among these precision-quantifying statistics is the *'standard error'* (SE) of a parameters' empirical value. It is the empirical value of the 'standard deviation' of its replication-distribution – of the square root of its variance (which is the mean of the values' squared deviations from their mean). A parameter's empirical value together with its SE are commonly used to derive a *'confidence interval'* for, or an *'interval estimate'* of, the parameter's actual value (theoretical). Most common is the 95% interval, derived as the 'point estimate' plus and minus 1.96 times its SE. The *concept of a 95% 'confidence interval'* is this: the statistic is so derived that, in hypothetical replications of the study (infinite in number), 95% of them contain the parameter's true value – conditionally on full validity of the study. (The term thus is a misnomer for the statistic; Sect. 19.2.5.)

Another one of these statistics is the *'P-value,'* having to do with testing a 'null hypothesis' about the parameter's value, which in the context of a regression parameter B_i generally is that $B_i = 0$. In the IEA dictionary of epidemiology [1] P-value is defined as:

> The probability that a test statistic would be as extreme as observed or more extreme if the test hypothesis were true.

Our definition of P-value [2] is different from that ordinary one, and analogous with the definition of confidence interval (above). To us it thus is a statistic *designed to behave in a particular way in hypothetical replications of the study*: Conditionally on the *'null hypothesis'* (here $B_i = 0$) its distribution is uniform in the 0–1 range, so that Pr $(P < \alpha) = \alpha$ for any α in this range; and so derived that, in addition, its distribution on the *'alternative hypothesis'* (here $B_i > 0$ or $B_i < 0$) is shifted to the left in this range, so that Pr $(P < \alpha) > \alpha$.

In logistic regression, the P-value for a particular parameter's empirical value is based on this value together with its SE, on the *'test statistic'* derived as that value divided by its SE. This statistic ('Wald statistic') is taken to have, on the 'null hypothesis,' the Gaussian replication distribution with mean 0 and variance 1. The test statistic's value corresponds to a particular *cumulative probability* of that distribution, and this is taken to be the P-value (one-sided) if the hypothesis ('alternative') is $B_i < 0$; and if the hypothesis is $B_i > 0$, then the P-value is the complement of this cumulative probability. The two-sided P-value is derived as the smaller one of the one-sided P-values multiplied by 2 – insofar as it is taken to be reasonable to entertain the two-sided 'alternative hypothesis' of $B_i \neq 0$.

8.3 'Shrinkage' of the Study Result

The logistic probability function derived from the data in a gnostic clinical study is prone to exaggerate the discriminative implications of the linear compound in it: relatively high values of that compound – discriminant score – tend to translate into probability values with a positive bias; and conversely, relatively low values of it tend to translate into probability values with a negative bias. These biases tend to be manifest in a replication of the study: with the new empirical values for the parameters, the sets of X-values that in the context of the original result translated into relatively high, or relatively low, values of the probability would in this replication of the study translate into values closer to the typical. They would show *'regression toward the mean'* (cf. Sect. 7.1.4).

The extent of this special type of bias inherent in a multi-parameter linear compound from *'multiple regression'* is most pronounced when the number of parameters in the model is largest in relation to the amount of 'information' in the body of data to which the model is fitted; and by the same token, it declines with increasing information, ultimately vanishing. The information can be quantified as NP(1 − P), where N is the size of the study series an P is the proportion of 'cases' (Y = 1) in it. As a reasonable 'rule of thumb,' the bias is *negligible* if the number of the object parameters is less than 10% of the amount of information in the data.

Insofar as the intent is to provide for the study result's application as such, rather than to merely make a contribution to the aggregate of results on the set of parameters being studied, the result from the model's initial fitting to the study data requires correction for its 'overparametrization bias,' if this isn't negligible (per the criterion above). This correction is a matter of suitable *'shrinkage'* of the linear compound's discriminativeness.

Perhaps the most obvious means of accomplishing this shrinkage is the *'leave one out'* method. With one of the data-points left out, the model is fitted to the remaining N – 1 of them, and the resulting values for the parameters are coupled with the set of X-values in the left-out data-point. The result of this is a pair of data for the left-out instance: the realization of the value of Y and the value L = l of the logistic compound L. The corresponding pairs of data are produced for all the other data-points as well, left out one at a time. Then, a logistic model involving $B'_0 + B'_1 l$ is fitted to these data. The result implies the needed shrinkage, the replacement of the initial linear compound L by $L^* = B'_0 + B'_1 L$. (In this, $B'_0 > 0$, $B'_1 < 1$).

References

1. Porta M (Editor), Greenland S, Hernan M, dos Santos Silva I, Last JM (Associate Editors), Buron A (Assistant Editor) (2014) A dictionary of epidemiology. A handbook sponsored by the IEA, 6th edn. Oxford University Press, Oxford
2. Miettinen OS (2011) Epidemiological research: terms and concepts. Springer, Dordrecht

Part IV
Diagnostic Research

Chapter 9
The Types of Diagnostic Challenge and Needs for Knowledge

Contents

Abstract In the practice of clinical medicine there are *two generic types of knowledge-dependent diagnostic pursuit.* One of these is directed to possible latent presence of a client-specified illness, the other to explanation of a particular sickness (or incidental finding) in terms of diagnoses about its possible underlying illnesses. Relevant to these two types of diagnostic pursuit are, in essence, only *two generic types of knowledge* addressing gnostic probabilities. One of these is knowledge about *diagnostic probability* for a particular illness in a particular domain of case presentations, conditional on the realizations of a particular set of diagnostic indicators (defining a subdomain of the presentation domain). The other is knowledge about the *marginal informativeness* of a particular (set of) added test(s) in a situation of less-than- practically-conclusive probability of the presence/absence of the illness targeted for diagnosis.

Keywords Pre-targeted diagnosis · Complaint-prompted diagnosis · Finding-prompted diagnosis · Diagnosis · Pre-clinical diagnosis · Clinical diagnosis · Differential diagnosis · Diagnostic probability function · Test's performance function · Diagnostic knowledge

O. S. Miettinen et al., *Clinical Research Transformed*,
https://doi.org/10.1007/978-3-030-06176-0_9

9.1 The Generic Types of Diagnostic Challenge

9.1.1 Ruling Out the Presence of a Particular Illness

As diagnostic research has its raison d'être in its service to clinicians' diagnostic challenges, preparation for this species of gnostic clinical research naturally begins with the development of a concrete sense of the generic types of these challenges; and the development of this sense, in turn, most naturally begins with focus on the conceptually simplest type of these pursuits.

Diagnosis poses a minimal challenge to the doctor in instances in which the client presents *no complaint of sickness* and specifies the doctor's tasks, completely. In cases like this, the client is in need of certification of being free of some particular illness(es), typically for employment or insurance. The doctor is told what illnesses are to be (practically) ruled out and, also, by what criteria. In this type of situation the doctor actually does not function as a diagnostician but simply carries out the (pre-specified) fact-finding for diagnosis according to the diagnostic algorithm in the agency mandating this fact-finding.

Alternatively, the client again specifies the illness whose presence is to be ruled out, but the doctor's challenge is to know how to achieve the rule-out diagnosis about it (insofar as it truly is absent).

9.1.2 Detecting a Particular Illness Pre-clinically

More challenging is the doctor's diagnostic pursuit in the case of the other type of client who presents *no complaint of sickness* as the prompting for the doctor's diagnostic work-up. In this type of case the client can be one of the 'worried well,' concerned about possibly having a latent case of a particular illness, one that would be less serious if detected early, before its manifestations in symptoms and/or overt signs. Alternatively, consideration of the pursuit of early, *pre-clinical diagnosis* about a particular illness may be prompted by the doctor's proactive doctoring (teaching; Sect. 1.2.1).

In this situation the doctor's *challenge* is to know how to pursue the rule-in diagnosis, the detection of a latent case of the illness at issue, and to know, also, what to teach the client about the implications of that pursuit (so as to enable the client to take an informed decision about the pursuit).

9.1.3 Explaining a Case of Sickness or Incidental Finding

The typical prompting of a doctor's diagnostic pursuit is the client's – patient's – *complaint about some sickness* (s)he is experiencing – a pain or other symptom (subjective) and/or an overt sign (objective). In a case like this, the doctor may need to first decide whether the patient would be better served by being referred to some other setting or discipline for diagnosis (etc.). If the doctor actually takes on the case, the *challenge* is to achieve the explanation of what illness, if any, is causing the sickness. (The alternative to this is an extrinsic direct cause, iatrogenic perhaps; Sect. 1.2.2).

Analogous to a complaint about some sickness as the prompting of a doctor's diagnostic pursuit is *an incidental finding – abnormal – from some laboratory test* (chemical, radiological, or other). It, like sickness, presents the challenge to identify the illness at the root of the presenting anomaly – as a matter of rule-in diagnosis about an illness explanatory (causally) of the presenting finding.

9.2 The Diagnostic Needs for Knowledge

9.2.1 The Knowledge Needs for Pre-targeted Diagnosis

Let us here focus on the most common generic type of prompting for the pursuit of pre-targeted diagnosis, namely a case of a *positive result of a screening test* for a particular illness. It can be a case of referral from 'mass screening' in community medicine or one arising intrinsically in clinical medicine. This situation is, inherently, one taken to represent an indication for the pursuit of rule-in diagnosis about the illness.

In such a case, the doctor needs to know the answers to these questions:

1. What facts – specifics of that (positive) test result, and clinical (non-laboratory) particulars of the person – are to be routinely ascertained in cases with this presentation?
2. What is the *diagnostic probability* for the illness at issue, conditional on the available diagnostic profile of the case?
3. What *supplementary testing* could now provide for rule-in diagnosis about the illness, and with what probability?
4. What are the *diagnostic probabilities* conditional on the diagnostic profiles enlarged by the supplementary testing?

9.2.2 The Knowledge Needs for Differential Diagnoses

When the diagnostic pursuit is prompted by the need to achieve – by diagnoses about the presence/absence of particular illnesses – explanation (causal) of the patient's sickness, the doctor needs general medical knowledge to answer a series of sequentially-arising questions contextualized by the patient's *presentation* in terms of his/her chief complaint and demographic category:

1. What clinical (non-laboratory) facts are to be routinely ascertained in cases with this presentation? That is, What are the *routine elements in the clinical profile* in such cases? (Cf. Sect. 9.2.1, above.)
2. What illnesses could be explanatory of the chief complaint in this presentation? That is, What is the *complete differential-diagnostic set* in such cases?
3. Concerning any one of those illnesses, What is the *probability* of its presence conditional on the diagnostic profile of the case (purely clinical profile or this supplemented with results from laboratory-level tests)?
4. Concerning cases in which the existing diagnostic profile is not sufficiently pathognomonic (for practical rule-in or rule-out diagnosis about the illness at issue), What *supplementary testing* could make it sufficiently conclusive, and with what probability?
5. What are the *diagnostic probabilities* conditional on the diagnostic profiles enlarged by the supplementary testing?

When the diagnostic pursuit is prompted by an incidental laboratory finding (abnormal), the needs for knowledge are the same as when the prompting is a complaint about sickness.

9.2.3 The Duality in Types of Diagnostic Knowledge about Probability

From the two Sections above it is evident that knowledge about two generic types of *probability* is needed for diagnoses in clinical medicine:

1. In reference to a defined domain, the probability that the illness targeted for diagnosis actually is present, conditionally on the realizations of a particular set of diagnostic indicators (clinical indicators alone or these supplemented by laboratory-based indicators). This is knowledge about *diagnostic probabilities.*
2. Conditionally on the clinical profile in #1 above not implying a diagnostic probability conclusive enough for the sought-for (practical) rule-in or rule-out diagnosis, the probability that a particular (set of) laboratory test(s) would provide for this. This is knowledge about *test performance.*

While these are the two generic types of knowledge about profile-conditional probabilities needed for diagnoses in cases from a particular domain of their presentation in the practice of clinical medicine, the requisite knowledge across the multitudinous possible profiles from the domain in question necessarily addresses the way the probability at issue is a *function* – logistic (Sect. 7.4.3) – of the diagnostic indicators involved (Sect. 4.1).

The duality is, thus, constituted by knowledge of the form of *diagnostic probability functions* versus knowledge about diagnostic *tests' performance functions.* Understanding the former is a prerequisite for understanding the latter, and the two are therefore addressed in this sequence in the Chapters below.

Chapter 10
Harvesting Experts' Diagnostic Probability Estimates

Contents

Abstract Even though meaningful research on diagnostic probabilities hasn't yet really begun (Sect. 3.1.2), diagnostic probability-setting nevertheless is an ubiquitous aspect of actual practice of clinical medicine. The probability estimates are based on *doctors' personal experiences*, first- and secondhand, with cases from the presentation domains they deal with. In respect to whichever one of these domains, some doctors naturally are more experienced and thereby more expert than others. This should make clinical researchers consider harvesting senior diagnosticians' expertise for the benefit of less-experienced diagnosticians and their patients – and also for use in objects design for the research to produce evidence to supplement and ultimately to supersede such expertise. In this Chapter we outline *how empirical values for the parameters in a designed diagnostic probability function can be derived from the reservoir of the 'tacit knowledge' of experts for diagnoses in the function's domain.*

Keywords Diagnostic probability function as the object · Experts' tacit knowledge as the resource · Experts' implicit parameter estimates · Experts' explicit parameter estimates · Treacherousness of experts' experience · The mirage of tacit diagnostic knowledge

O. S. Miettinen et al., *Clinical Research Transformed*,
https://doi.org/10.1007/978-3-030-06176-0_10

10.1 The Elements in the Estimates-Harvesting Mission

10.1.1 Designing the Domain and Form of the Function

In the production of a diagnostic probability function representing experts' 'tacit knowledge' for diagnosis about a particular illness in a particular domain of case presentations, the first phase necessarily is the same as in actual research on a diagnostic probability function; that is, the project begins with designing the form of the function for a designed domain of this. In this first – objects-design – phase of the work, following the development of a suitable definition of the domain of case presentations being addressed, the logit of the probability of the presence of the illness in question is formulated as a linear compound of a particular set of parameters – the coefficients in this compound being a designed set of statistical variates (Xs) based on the diagnostic indicators relevant and accessible in the type of situation for which the function is being developed (Sect. 7.4.3).

Expertise naturally is required in the design of a meaningful and realistic-to-address domain of the function representing experts' tacit knowledge for diagnosis about a particular illness and of the set of diagnostic indicators in it. The *domain* for a function for differential diagnoses needs to be *suitably specific* in respect to the sickness – chief complaint – in its definition, and the *set of diagnostic indicators* addressed in the function needs to be *suitably focused* on the principal indicators, free of undue inclusiveness. While both of these are desiderata of the objects-design for actual research on the designed type of function, they are even more so in the function's construction from experts' profile-specific tacit knowledge.

10.1.2 Estimating the Parameters of the Function

Diagnostic experts in contemporary medicine have not been taught to think about case-specific diagnostic probabilities in terms of realizations of diagnostic probability functions, much less about such functions as the product of their experience with diagnostic encounters in the practice of medicine (clinical). But they do have tacit knowledge for setting these probabilities on a case-by-case basis (without any function from which to read these).

Gnostic clinical researchers have, we hold, the professional *responsibility to seriously consider harvesting diagnostic experts' tacit knowledge* – and, specifically, harvesting it *in the form of diagnostic probability functions*, as this is what ultimately is relevant and required as the inputs to *diagnostic 'expert systems'* [1]. This means their consideration of harvesting experts' knowledge about the magnitudes of the parameters in expertly-designed diagnostic probability functions, even though they haven't been thinking about these.

This might appear to require deducing experts' *implicit estimates* of those parameters from their estimates of the probabilities in particular cases (Sect. 10.2, below). But there actually is an alternative approach to harvesting experts' knowledge about the magnitudes of those parameters, one in which the experts provide *explicit estimates* of parameters that in principle are in their ken, estimates that can be translated into estimates of the parameters in the function at issue (Sect. 10.3).

10.2 Harvesting Experts' Implicit Estimates

In the harvesting of experts' knowledge for the development of estimates of the parameters in a diagnostic probability function of a particular designed form for a defined domain of case presentations, one approach is, as insinuated above, documentation of the values of those parameters that are implicit in the probabilities particular experts actually set in particular cases from the case-presentation domain at issue (Sect. 10.1.2, above).

The *data* assembled in this approach are sets of probability estimates concerning the possible presence of the illness at issue in a series of cases from the presentation domain at issue. The estimates are provided by the members of a *panel of experts* on the diagnosis in cases from the domain, independently from one another. The *cases* can well be hypothetical ones, specified in respect to the domain of presentation and the realizations of the diagnostic indicators that are deemed relevant by the panel of experts collectively.

In the *synthesis of the data*, the case-specific sets of estimates of the individual experts are reduced to their medians. Then, the logits of these medians are addressed in the framework of the General Linear Model (Sect. 7.3). The model's fitting to the data produces empirical values for the parameters in a logistic model for the diagnostic probability function with that same linear compound (of parameters).

A salient feature of our experience with this approach is the recurrent occurrence of *great discrepancies* among the experts' diagnoses. Even for myocardial infarction, experts' estimates of the probability in question range, in some cases, from 0% to 100% [2].

These discrepancies actually are *unsurprising* to us, as the cognitive challenges in informal derivation of these probability estimates (profile-specific) from cases encountered in practice are very daunting, even in the face of explicit layouts of the relevant data from experiences with a very simple type of diagnostic profile [1].

10.3 Harvesting Experts' Explicit Estimates

In Sect. 10.2 above we made two important, closely-related and mutually-reinforcing points, one empirical, the other theoretical. The empirical point was that, in our experience with diagnostic expert panels, experts' estimates of some profile-specific probabilities of the presence of the illness at issue have been strikingly discordant

[2]; and the related theoretical point was that learning about diagnostic probabilities from one's own clinical experience, informally, indeed is an enormous epistemological challenge [1].

Equally-important to note is this: From those points it does not follow that meaningful harvesting of experts' tacit knowledge for quantification of the parameters in diagnostic probability functions (logistic) is impossible. For, *estimates of the magnitudes of the parameters in a DPF (diagnostic probability function) can be derived from experts' experience-based answers to suitably focused, relevant-and-answerable questions about their experiences with the diagnostic challenges at issue.*

In the harvesting of diagnostic expertise, the challenges naturally have to do with estimation of the parameters in the linear compound in the logistic DPF, in the

$$\mathrm{L} = B_0 + B_1\mathrm{X}_1 + B_2\mathrm{X}_2 + \ldots.$$

In the framework of this formulation, the first thing to contemplate naturally is the value of that B_0, which represents the logit of the probability conditional on $\mathrm{X}_1 = \mathrm{X}_2 = \ldots = 0$. Telling examples of the challenges in direct estimation of the magnitude of this parameter are logistic DPFs for adult domains. In these models, one of the Xs would generally represent the patient's age (the numerical value of this), and thus the B_0 in the models would be the value of the probability's logit conditionally on, inter alia, the realization of the variate representing the patient's – an adult's – age being 0! The existence of experience-based expertise in direct estimation of the magnitude of the B_0 in such a model for such a domain obviously is unrealistic to presume.

That problem is resolved by *reformulation of that linear compound* (of the parameters involved) this way:

$$\mathrm{L} = B_0' + B_1(\mathrm{X}_1 - M_1) + B_2(\mathrm{X}_2 - M_2) + \ldots,$$

where M_1 is the mean of X_1 among the cases from the domain of the DFP, and the definitions of M_2 etc. are analogous to this. The magnitude of the B'_0 in this, very different from its counterpart B_0 in the compound's first formulation above, is the value of the logit of the probability addressed by the DFP conditionally on the mean values of all the Xs (implying $\mathrm{L} = B'_0$). The probability underlying this parameter is subject to direct estimation by experts.

The parameters associated with the Xs are the same in these two formulations of the linear compound. They together with B'_0 determine the value of the first parameter in the compound's ordinary formulation:

$$B_0 = B' - (B_1M_1 + B_2M_2 + \ldots).$$

Thus, B_0 is the difference between B'_0 – the logit's value conditional on the mean values of all the Xs – and the linear compound of the parameters associated with the Xs that involves the means of the Xs as the coefficients.

This reformulation of the ordinary L in the DPF implies the set of *relevant-and-answerable questions* to be directed to the members of the panel of experts recruited to a project to develop an expertise-based DPF for the illness at issue in cases presenting from the DPF's defined domain. All of the questions pertain to the experts' experiences (direct and indirect) with *instructive cases* from the domain at issue; that is, with cases from the presentation domain at issue such that the truth about the possible presence of the illness at issue became known to the expert, independently of what the truth was [1].

The question pertaining to that B'_0 is simply this (suitably reformulated): In your experience with instructive cases (as defined above) from the domain at issue, in what proportion of them has that illness actually been present? The answer to this question constitutes the expert's input to estimation of that B'_0 in reference to his/her own experience, the estimate of it being the logit of the (unconditional) proportion P_u given as the answer.

The other relevant-and-answerable questions also refer to those instructive case-presentations from the domain at issue. Some of these questions, like that pertaining to the B'_0, are quite obvious in their meanings. These are the questions about the mean values of the Xs in the the DFP, involved in the production of the expert-specific estimates of the general parameter B_0 (per the relation shown above).

The remaining questions naturally have to do with estimation of the parameters associated with the independent variates in the DPF, the values of B_1 etc., involved first in the derivation of each expert-specific estimate of the B_0 in that function from the value of P_u (as outlined above), and then in association with the Xs in the rest of the DPF.

The estimates of B_1 etc. are best developed in *two stages*: in the first stage, any given one of the indicators is addressed on the premise of it being the only one in the DPF; and then, in the second stage, these first-stage estimates are adjusted for the correlations (relative redundancies) among the indicators involved. In all of this, the focus is on a *DPF that is suitably simple*, in two meanings of this: by involving only the principal ones among all possible indicators, and by representing each of these in suitably simple terms. Thus, involved in the model might be no more than, say, half-a-dozen indicators – the presumedly most-discriminating practicable ones, with each of these represented without any product terms and with no provision for curvature in the probability logit's relation the any quantitative variate.

In that *first stage* of these remaining estimations, a distinction needs to be made between the two fundamental types of independent variate in a regression function (Sect. 7.4).

Concerning the parameter associated with an *indicator-type* X, the relevant-and-answerable question, beyond that about the mean of the variate's distribution (above), is about the ratio of the rates (of prevalence) of the illness being present, contrasting instances of $X_i = 1$ with those of $X_i = 0$ (on the premise of this indicator being used alone). The answer is some prevalence ratio R_i. This answer needs to be translated, first, into estimates of the corresponding rates conditional on $X_i = 1$ and $X_i = 0$, respectively, consistent with the mean of this X_i being M_i and with the unconditional prevalence being the P_u ascertained as the input into the development of the expert-specific estimate of B'_0 (above). Then, the respective estimates of the prevalence-odds are deduced from these two rates. And finally, the estimate of the B_i is produced as the logarithm of the ratio of these two prevalence-odds estimates (contrasting $X_i = 1$ with $X_i = 0$).

The critical element in this is the translation of the expert's three answers – those about the unconditional proportion/prevalence P_u (whose logit is the estimate of B'_0), the variate's mean M_i, and the prevalence ratio R_i – into the two rates of prevalence, R_{1i} and R_{0i}. These rates are the solutions of this pair of equations:

$$R_{1i} / R_{0i} = R_i,$$

$$M_i R_{1i} + (1 - M_i) R_{0i} = P_u.$$

When the variate in question is *quantitative*, and entertained as the only X in the DPF (logistic), the point of departure in the development of an expert-specific estimate of this variate's associated B_i is the already-established estimate P_u of the unconditional probability, which also is the probability's estimate conditional on $X_i = M_i$. This needs to be supplemented with an additional point in the prevalence function. To this end, the expert needs to be asked to estimate the probability/prevalence corresponding to a given deviation d from the mean value of the indicator, say d = 10 y from the mean of age, or d = 10 kg/m^2 from the mean of body mass index (weight in kilograms divided by height in meters squared). In *these examples*, with P_d the answer, the estimate of B_i can be taken to be

$$B_i \text{ est} = (1/10)\{\log[P_d / (1 - P_d)] - \log[P_u / (1 - P_u)]\}.$$

It remains to make *adjustments* of these estimates on account of the correlations (relative redundancies) among the indicators. In this, a distinction needs to be made between the indicators that have to do with risk for the illness (age, say) and those representing manifestations of the illness underlying the presenting sickness. Those risk indicators (generally demographic), different from the manifestational ones, need no adjustment.

Preparatory to the adjustments, the manifestational indicators (having to do with symptoms and signs, possibly including results of laboratory tests) need to be *ranked* according to their (presumed) degrees of discriminating informativeness for the diagnoses (differential) at issue. The estimate of the parameter for the indicator ranked most informative needs no adjustment for redundancy. The estimates of the other parameters need fractional adjustments toward zero, so as to represent their respective degrees of *'marginal' informativeness* in the face of the higher-ranked indicators that have already been accounted for.

A simple yet perhaps commonly-suitable way to do these indicator-specific adjustments of the parameters' initial estimates (expert-specific) is basing all of them on a *single fraction*, say F = 0.8, in an *exponential* manner: F to power 0 (= 1) for the highest-ranked indicator (manifestational); F to power 1 (= F) for the highest-ranked supplementary indicator; F to power 2 (F squared) for the indicator second in the ranking; etc.

The ranking of the indicators (manifestational) and the choice of the scheme of the adjustments for redundancies, while involved in the development of the expert-specific estimates of the indicator-specific parameters (leading to their consequent adjustment of the estimate of B_0 as well) are matters of the expert panel's collective judgement, just as is the adoption of DPF for which the parameters need to be estimated.

Given the expert-specific adjusted estimates of the parameters, the *result on the level of the panel* at large can be derived, simply, as medians of the expert-specific estimates.

10.4 The Select Nature of Diagnostic Experts' Experiences

Insofar as a doctor's expertise in diagnostic probability-setting grows out of his/her own experience with cases from the presentation domain at issue, contributory to learning can only be the cases in which the truth about the nature of the underlying illness became – and in some sense remains – known to the doctor. And, valid learning about the probabilities of the presence (or absence) of each of the illnesses in the differential-diagnostic set, conditionally on the diagnostic profiles of the cases, requires that the truths about the nature of the underlying illness, insofar as they became known to the doctor in question, became known to to him/her independently of what the truth actually was. (Sect. 10.3, above).

The truth about which one of the possible illnesses actually is present in a given case from the presentation domain, becomes known to the diagnostician, firsthand, insofar as attained gets to be rule-in diagnosis about one of the possibilities, implying rule-out diagnoses about the others in the set. By no means is such a conclusive diagnosis generally achieved, or even sought. And relevant to appreciate here is, for one, that the illnesses in the differential-diagnostic set generally are not of equal concern for the attainment of (practical) rule-in diagnosis about it, insofar as the illness actually is present; and for another, that the illnesses in the set are prone to be quite different in the feasibility of the attainment of rule-in diagnoses about them. For instance, in cases of acute dyspnea (in adults), rapid attainment of rule-in diagnosis about myocardial infarction in actual cases of MI is, for both of these reasons, distinctly more likely than is its counterpart about pulmonary embolism in actual cases of PE. And besides, rule-in diagnosis about MI in a case of recent onset of dyspnea is more feasible than that of its counterpart about PE.

While there are such problems – quite notable – with the validity of a doctor's firsthand experience with diagnoses as a source of learning diagnostic probability-setting, they are compounded when secondhand experience is the basis of the learning. For, more likely to come to a doctor's attention secondhand are instances in which the attained rule-in diagnosis was relatively unexpected (given a low probability for it in the clinical diagnosis).

These notes have the burden that, in projects to harvest experts' estimates of the parameters in whatever (carefully-designed) diagnostic probability function, *there is a need to call the experts' attention to these sources of bias* in their experiences with the diagnoses at issue, and to try to cause them to minimize these biases in the estimates they provide.

10.5 Experts' Tacit Knowledge as a Mirage

This Chapter was predicated on the premise – the common belief – that there are expert diagnosticians. This premise we took to have the implication that these experts' tacit knowledge about diagnostic probabilities ought to be harvested for the benefit of less-expert diagnosticians (and their patients).

From what is presented in this Chapter, it is not unreasonable to conclude that our premise – though commonly held – actually is untenable; that the existence experts' diagnostic knowledge worthy of harvesting actually is but a mirage.

To wit, it would not be unreasonable to conclude that the expertise-harvesting effort would not be a worthy alternative for – or even a worthy precursor of – of actual diagnostic research.

References

1. Miettinen OS (2015) Medicine as a scholarly field: an introduction. Springer, Cham
2. Steurer J, Held U, Miettinen OS (2013) Diagnostic probability function for acute coronary heart disease garnered from experts' tacit knowledge. J Clin Epidemiol 66:1289–1295

Chapter 11
Objects Design for a Diagnostic Probability Study

Contents

Abstract The objects design for a diagnostic probability study begins with the design of the *domain* of it: the type of case presentation that gives rise to the diagnostic pursuit. Next is the design of the *illness* whose presence/absence in those cases the study will address. Then comes the design of *the set of diagnostic indicators* that will be addressed in the study, based on their priority ranking for this. The final task is specification of the *statistical variates* for representation of each of the included indicators in the diagnostic probability function (logistic) for the targeted illness, possibly supplemented by variates representing transforms and/or products of these primary variates. We elaborate, on all of this.

Keywords The domain of case presentations · The targeted illness(es) · The diagnostic indicators · The statistical model · Examples

11.1 The Domain of the Case Presentations

A diagnostic probability function, DPF, is meaningless without an *explicitly-defined domain* understood to be its referent. After all, the diagnostic indicators, of which the diagnostic probability is taken to be a function, define subdomains of the function's referent domain (Sect. 9.2.3). Thus, instances in which the Xs involved in a DPF have a particular set of realizations are not defined by this set alone: implicitly

O. S. Miettinen et al., *Clinical Research Transformed*,
https://doi.org/10.1007/978-3-030-06176-0_11

but very importantly, they are defined also by the DFP's domain, by the *chief complaint* and *population category* that are definitional to that domain.

That the definition of a diagnostic study's domain is explicit is, however, not good enough. The definition of the domain of a diagnostic study needs to be *objective* in its meaning. To this end, the definition of a diagnostic study's domain needs to be sufficiently *specific*, and meaningfully so.

Remarkably, neither one of these cardinal requirements for the definition of the study objects' domain was satisfied in a very eminent pair of studies for diagnosis about pulmonary embolism [1, 2]. The domain's definition was merely implicit and altogether non-specific, as it was left to be inferred from in the criterion for the enrolment of cases into the study series, which was the diagnostician's "suspicion" of the presence of this illness.

The domain for this pair of studies, just as for any other study for differential diagnosis about whatever illness, should have been defined not only explicitly and objectively but with a view to specificity of its first-order implications. The definition should in general be such that, for one, the differential-diagnostic set (Sect. 9.2.2) is the same – singular – throughout (the subdomains of) the domain; and for another, such that each set of profile-conditional probabilities (differential-diagnostic) is singular throughout the domain. This generally means that *only a single type of chief complaint* can be used in the definition of the domain.

This is to say, for example, that for a study designed for the advancement of diagnoses about pulmonary embolism (as was the case in the examples above), the domain-definitional sickness must not be, for example, 'chest pain and/or dyspnea' (both acute). For even though PE is a member of the differential-diagnostic set in the context of each of those two symptoms as the chief complaints, the respective differential-diagnostic sets are different, and so also are the profile-conditional probabilities of the presence of PE. These two symptoms, for these reasons, call for their respective separate studies, in their respective separate domains, of the probability of PE (and its alternatives).

Diametrically *antithetical to this singularity principle* is the definition of the domain of a diagnostic study with a view to it being maximally inclusive of the cases of the illness in question. This was, alas, the lead idea in the design of case admissibility into – and hence the domain of – a major study of diagnostic probabilities for myocardial infarction [3]; and in consequence of this, no major advancement of the knowledge-base of the diagnosis about MI was brought about by this major study, not even for cases with chest pain as the chief complaint. This error in the objects design of that major study is a reason why expert diagnoses about MI remain quite discordant in their profile-conditional estimates of the probability, notably in cases presenting with chest pain as the chief complaint [4]; and accordingly, misdiagnosis about this disease has a salient presence among malpractice claims and compensations in the U.S. [5].

11.2 The Illness(es) to Be Directly Addressed

Upon the design of a meaningful domain for a sickness-explanatory diagnostic study, the development of the study's objects design turns to the form of the diagnostic probability function(s), DPF(s), that will be addressed in the study.

In a central role in any DPF, beyond the domain that is its pre-defined referent, will be the illness whose possible presence (in that domain) the function addresses.

In this stage of the study's objects design it is critically important to bear in mind that rule-in diagnosis about one of the possibilities in the differential-diagnostic set is generally tantamount to rule-out diagnosis about each of the other possibilities (cf. Sect. 9.1.3). And also important to appreciate is that, in diagnostic practice, for the needed rule-in diagnosis about one of the possible illnesses it is desirable to target one that is *relatively common* among the possible ones and also subject relatively easy to the rule in, insofar as it actually is present. The design of the illness(es) to be targeted for diagnostic study in reference to the designed domain needs to be guided by these realities in diagnostic practice.

Returning to the example of acute chest pain as the sickness to be explained (diagnostically, in an adult), each of those two considerations in the choice of the illness targeted for diagnostic study points to the desirability of focusing on diagnosis about myocardial infarction, on rule-in diagnosis about it, given that MI actually is the illness that is present (and ipso facto causing the pain).

And as for the other example in the Section above, in cases of acute dyspnea (also in an adult), MI may again be taken to be the target illness of choice for a diagnostic study, instead of the other relatively common illness in these cases, pulmonary embolism, because rule-in diagnosis about PE is distinctly more problematic than that about MI.

The reason why a *single illness* might reasonably be selected as the focus of a diagnostic study in a given domain of case presentations, instead of addressing more of the possibilities, separately in the same project, has to do with practicalities: Whichever one of the possible illnesses is addressed, the truth about its presence/absence needs to be determined in each of the cases enrolled into the study. This is prone to be an imposition on the study subjects, calling for solicitation of the person's informed consent to this service to research; and this imposition would be compounded by the addition of the corresponding work-up in respect to another one of the possible illnesses.

11.3 The Indicators to Be Accounted for

After the design of the domain of the study and the illness that the diagnostic probability function, DPF, will focus on (Sects. 11.1 and 11.2, above), the need is to design the diagnostic indicators that will be accounted for in that function (in terms of the Xs in the DPF; Sect. 7.4.3).

As background for this phase of the study's objects design it is important to bear in mind what, exactly, a DPF in principle is. Designed to address the probability of the presence of a particular one of the possible illnesses (in a case from the study domain; Sect. 11.2, above), the DPF involves involves a discriminant between the presence and absence of this illness (Sects. 7.4.1 and 7.4.3). But in differential diagnosis, given the premise that only one of the possibilities is the reality, that compound is a *discriminant between the presence of the targeted illness and that of an unspecified one of its differential-diagnostic alternatives.*

In consequence of this, the diagnostic indicators to be accounted for in a DPF for the presence of a particular one of the illnesses in the set of the possibilities are not to be thought of, simply, as indicators of risk for this illness or as having to do with possible manifestations of its presence: relevant among these are only those that are *indicators of differential probability* for the presence of the illness at issue and that of one of its alternatives in the differential-diagnostic set.

An instructive example of this principle in application is the judgement that even though age is a major indicator of the (near-term) risk for myocardial infarction, it may be practically meaningless as a discriminant between MI and its differential-diagnostic alternatives (in a reasonably-defined domain for the diagnosis). The same naturally applies to the differential-diagnostic alternatives to MI, such as pulmonary embolism.

On the other hand, those two illnesses have quite different precipitating factors (notably exertion/stress vs. immobilization), and both of these factors therefore have a role in diagnostic discrimination between them and may need to be accounted for in diagnoses about either one of these two illnesses. Hence, while age, for example, may be irrelevant in a DPF function focusing on MI, the function may need to involve accounting for possible precipitation of PE in addition to that of MI; and similarly, a function focusing on PE may need to account for possible precipitation of MI in addition to that of PI itself.

This way of thinking about candidate indicators for the risk segment of the DPF being designed naturally applies to candidates for the manifestational segment of the function as well. But when it comes to actual inclusion of (variates for) these *manifestational indicators* in the DPF, the issue of the degrees *redundancy* among them deserves serious consideration (cf. Sect. 10.3), while among the risk indicators this generally is a nonissue. And a nonissue generally also is redundancy between these two segments of the diagnostic profiles, for the elements tend to be uncorrelated between them.

The relevance of the redundancies among the candidate indicators has to do with priority-setting in their inclusions into, and possible omissions from, the DPF. This is notable in particular if the indicators' inclusions into the set of these are made, as is reasonable, successively and hierarchically, in the spirit of harvesting experts' explicit estimates of the parameters in the (logistic) DPF (Sect. 10.3).

On the other hand, correlations among the independent variates in a regression function does not invalidate the model, because *each of the coefficients of the Xs inherently addresses the marginal contribution* from this variate, contribution conditional on all of the other Xs in the model. (An exception to this is redundancy of the extreme type, in which the realization of one of the variates is determined fully by those of some of the others. In this case the model's fitting to a set of data is impossible).

All of this leads to what amounts to the *core principle* in the design of the set of indicators to be addressed (in terms of the Xs in the DPF) in a diagnostic study focusing on differential diagnosis about a particular illness in a particular domain of case presentations: *Experts* on diagnosis in cases from the domain of the presentations at issue should have a decisive role in the specification of the domain already (under the principles outlined in Sect. 11.1), and then in defining the hierarchy of the diagnostic indicators' inclusion. They need to be interrogated as outlined in Sect. 10.3, and the results of this need to be taken as specifications of the sets of indicators for inclusion in successive DPFs (with none in the first, one in the second, etc.).

In the face of the thus-specified hierarchy for the indicators' inclusion the question becomes, How inclusive should the set addressed in the study be? The broadest answer is that there is *no good reason to include all of the candidates for inclusion*, given that indicators low down in the hierarchy contribute little while accentuating the problem of undue complexity and 'overparametrization' bias (Sect. 8.3). But there can be no general rule-of-thumb about how far down the hierarchy to go with the inclusions.

11.4 The Variates to Represent the Indicators

An introduction to the representation of material entities in terms of statistical variates was given in Chap. 7; and the design of the variates for the indicators in a diagnostic probability function (DPF) was addressed in Sect. 10.3. Some further remarks are in order, however.

For a *quantitative indicator* with a zero-level (in vivo) – such as the daily dose of a medication – the statistical representation could perhaps be, simply, a number proportional to the indicator's deviation from its zero-level. But especially if the datum on the level is subject to appreciable errors, such simple *'dose-response'* modelling could be unrealistic and would need to be replaced *a pair of variates*: indicator of non-zero level and a variate for the product of this indicator and a variate representing the level.

Regarding a quantitative indicator without a natural zero-level it generally is desirable to think of its deviation from a particular *reference level* of it, perhaps the level typical for cases from the domain (cf. Sect. 10.3) or for people in the in the demographic category of the domain – a round-number level in the vicinity of one of those.

The representation of a quantitative indicator in terms of a *variate proportional to the level* of it, whether as such or as its deviation from a reference value, raises the question about the justifiability of modelling the level's role in the diagnostic discriminant in such a simple way. Simplicity is, quite generally and intentionally, an inherent feature of regression models, and even considerable simplifications are, therefore, not only tolerable but also desirable. But if there is good reason to presume that reality would be seriously misrepresented by such simple representation of a diagnostic indicator's level in the logistic discriminant, then a suitable *provision for 'curvature'* in the indicator's contribution to this scoring function is in order. A minimalist yet generally sufficient way to accomplish this is provision for quadratic – parabolic – curvature, by supplementing the variate for the level as such by the inclusion also of a variate that is the square of that 'linear' one.

Once the variates for each of the included indicators have been specified, it remains to consider and decide whether they alone would constitute the set independent variates in the logistic function for the probability of the presence of the illness at issue in the domain defined for the study. The alternative to contentment with this formulation of the model is the view that provision needs to be made for the way in which the diagnostic meaning of the realization of a particular one of the indicators depends on that of a particular other one – on the level of the logistic discriminant. The question is whether the additive representation is adequate, or whether a variate representing the product of the two is needed, as a *'product term'* in the model.

This issue is analogous to that of the consideration of possible provision for curvature in a quantitative indicator's contribution to that discriminant: the simple – simplest possible – formulation presumably is at variance with reality; but good reason for presuming substantial deviation from that simplicity is needed as a justification for not maintaining maximal simplicity of the (designed) form of the function.

Design of the indicators for the DPF all the way to definition of the variates (Xs) to represent them is tantamount to *definition of the particular objects of study*, which are the parameters in the DPF. The *overall object* is the DPF designed as to its form and referent.

11.5 Two Examples of a Study's Objects Design

11.5.1 Diagnosis in Cases of Cough

Patient presentation with the complaint of cough is very common in general practice; and especially if accompanied by fever, it very commonly results in a prescription for an antibiotic treatment [6]. But actually, such treatment in these cases is indicated only on the premise that the underlying illness is pneumonia [7]. In particular, if the illness is acute bronchitis, this commonly is viral rather than bacterial in nature and has, regardless, a self-limiting course [8]; it therefore is not an indication for antibiotic treatment. Thus, in the absence of pneumonia, prescription for antibiotic treatment in cases presenting with cough, even if accompanied by fever, merely contributes to two community-level problems: bacteria's resistance to antibiotics and the cost of healthcare.

In cases of this presentation, the doctor would ideally have access to the requisite knowledge-base for discrimination, on purely clinical grounds, between the presence and absence of pneumonia; that is, ideally a sufficiently conclusive diagnosis about the presence/absence of pneumonia could be based on the diagnostic profile gleaned from history and physical examination alone, without radiography or other non-clinical testing. If pneumonia could be ruled out clinically, obviated would be those tests as well as antibiotic treatment in the case. And the feasibility of reaching rule-in diagnosis about pneumonia clinically would obviate non-clinical testing in cases of pneumonia presenting with cough and fever.

A study on the probability of the presence of pneumonia in cases presenting with cough, well-designed for its objects and methods, could make a contribution to bringing about that ideal, in cases of *a subtype of those presentations* in the practices of diligent doctors. The subtype would be defined by the design of the domain of the diagnostic probability function that would be studied. More than the presence of cough goes into thoughtful definition of the domain for this study, a definition that is explicit and implies the nature of the probability function that is to be studied, a DPF that isn't unduly complicated (Sect. 11.1). Pulmonologists consulted on this matter presumably would advise that *focus on community-acquired pneumonia* would best serve this purpose, especially insofar as diagnoses in settings of general practice are the concern. To this end, the domain would be restricted to cases in persons with no hospitalization for some specified period of time. And in the same vein, the consultants might suggest the domain to be restricted to cases in persons who in fact have been not only out of hospitals but actually healthy (as best is known) for a specified period of time – naturally with the exception of the presenting cough and fever and the upper respiratory infection that may have preceded it. And they presumably would recommend narrowing the domain so as to have the chief complaint to include *fever* in association with the cough, and this in a *previously healthy person*.

The consultants presumably would advise that, in this domain, the *differential-diagnostic set* would include, apart from pneumonia, acute bronchitis as the only alternative to it. And in respect to this differential diagnosis, they presumably would advise that the issues are rather different according to different ranges of *age*, so that undue complexity would be obviated by restricting the domain to cases in persons of, say, 20–65 years of age.

For the domain of the pneumonia versus acute bronchitis differential diagnosis in cases of cough and *fever*, the fever needs to be explicitly defined; and it needs to be high enough to raise the possibility of the case being one of pneumonia. To this end, the consultants presumably would deem it essential that the temperature be measured at the presentation of the case, and that it be at least 38.0° C (100.4 F).

It remains to define the domain in respect to the presenting *cough*. At issue in this is the history of the cough that has continued to the time of the presentation (and presumably will continue beyond). Definitional to the domain the consultants presumably would specify a cough the onset of which was acute. This means that its duration up to the time of the presentation for diagnosis can be specified in terms of a particular number of days, and the domain-defining cough naturally needs to be specified in respect to this period. The consultants need to be asked to consider the range of this time in which the clinically-based differential diagnosis would be realistic to entertain (conditionally on fever being present at the time); and in particular, they need to be asked to suggest the highest-priority range for adoption of the final definer of the study's domain.

With the domain of the study thus specified, the consultants need to be asked to share their expertise about the clinical-level *diagnostic indicators*, definitional to relevant distinctions among subdomains of the specified domain. These indicators address attributes (clinical) in terms of which cases of pneumonia – with or without associated bronchitis – differ from ones of bronchitis without pneumonia (Sect. 11.3). The consultants need to be asked to specify these indicators *hierarchically*, starting with the most important one and thinking about the marginal informativeness (for the discrimination) in introducing the supplementary indicators (Sect. 11.3). Among the candidate indicators naturally are particulars of the cough and the fever.

For each of the indicators the experts are to specify the respective *scales* in terms of which they think about them. The scale of the history about chills, for example, is implicit in the questions the experts would ask about this symptom.

Upon having secured these expert inputs into the study's objects design, the investigators need to decide how far down the rank order of the indicators' inclusion they care to go in the inclusion of these in the diagnostic probability function for pneumonia. And then the investigators, on their own, complete the study's objects design by defining the *statistical variates* representing the clinical entities in the probability function for the diagnoses about pneumonia in cases from the study's domain (Sect. 11.4).

11.5.2 Diagnosis in Cases of Chest Pain

Chest pain is a common complaint in primary-care medicine, most notably in emergency departments of hospitals; and it is a complaint that demands urgent attention, first and foremost calling for expeditious pursuit of clinical (pre-laboratory) diagnosis about *myocardial infarction* in particular.

Diagnosis about MI – practical rule-in diagnosis in particular, insofar as MI actually is at the root of the chest pain – is exceptionally important in the *hours immediately following the onset of the chest pain*, as the opportunity for myocardium-sparing and survival-enhancing thrombolytic therapy is confined to this period. In consequence of this, the study's domain should include this recency feature of the presenting chief complaint. To suitably focus on this timing of the diagnosis, the experts consulted for the design of the study might recommend restriction of the study's domain to cases presenting for diagnosis within, say, 6 h from the onset of the chest pain.

As a further restriction of the study's domain on the basis of the chest pain – with a view to keeping the diagnostic probability function manageably simple to think about and to study – the expert consultants might well suggest confinement of the study to the *type of chest pain* that is rather characteristic of MI without being pathognomonic about this disease. In this vein, the consultants might recommend confining the study to a pain that is substernal in location and dull in kind, characterized by the patient as an 'ache' or a 'pressure.'

In demographic terms, the study's domain would naturally be restricted to some particular range of adult *age*, perhaps to ages in the range from 35 to 65 years.

And, as with the diagnosis about pneumonia prompted by cough with fever (Sect. 11.5.1, above), simplicity and clarity would be enhanced further by domain restriction in terms, also, of the patient's *health prior to the episode* prompting the diagnostic pursuit. To this end, and also to focus on diagnostic indicators that can swiftly yet with reasonable accuracy be addressed under the stress and distraction brought about by the episode, the experts might recommend restricting the domain of the study to persons with no previous cardiovascular disease nor known risk factors for MI. Thus, insofar as the case would be one of MI, it would be entirely unheralded, a case 'out of the blue.'

In the design of the set of *diagnostic indicators* to be accounted for in the diagnostic probability function (specifying the parameters that would be the objects of the study), the lead principle is, again, the need to think not simply about indicators of (near-term) risk for MI and about manifestations of this disease; meaningful diagnostic indicators in this study would serve *discrimination* between MI and its differential-diagnostic alternatives in cases from the domain designed for the study. And the principle closely related to this is, again, that those indicators provide *marginal information* (the burden of which depends on what else is already accounted for). This, in turn, means that the experts are, again, called upon to specify first the indicator which, when available alone, would be the most discriminating between MI and its differential-diagnostic alternatives; then, the one that would be the most informative supplement to this; etc. – up to a manageable number of indicators, say no more than a dozen. It would be reasonable to presume that, apart from history and physical examination, the sources of diagnosis-relevant clinical facts would include the ECG.

The experts might specify the principal *alternatives* to MI to be, in the domain as it was designed, pulmonary embolism and pericarditis. Focusing here on diagnosis about MI with those two alternatives to it, among the *indicators* for the (differential) diagnosis in the domain (such as was sketched above), expert consultants might not include any indicators of (near-term) risk for any of these illnesses (as the role would not be presumed to be sufficiently differential among the possibilities). Among the possible precipitating factors they presumably would consider the inclusion (and ranking) of recent episodes of exceptional stress (physical or emotional), immobilization, and infectious disease. Among symptoms, consideration would presumably be given, for example, to radiation of the pain, dyspnea, tachypnea, and fever. And among signs, a dominant role would presumably be assigned to hyperacute T and ST segment elevations in leads I, aVL, V4, and V6, or alternatively in leads II, III, and aVF (and, with either one of these sets, ST depressions in the reciprocal leads), while in the absence these ECG signs there presumably would be a role for other signs, such as asymmetry of the thickness of the thighs and precordial friction rub.

It deserves note here that while the differentiation of MI from its alternatives in the context of the typical chief complaint – that substernal ache or pressure – has the character sketched above, *the issues are rather different if the chief complaint is, say, dyspnea*. For, even though the alternatives to MI in these cases still include pulmonary embolism, the other possibilities are quite different, as they include pneumothorax and anaphylaxis, for instance.

References

1. PIOPED Investigators (1990) Value of the ventilation/perfusion scan in acute pulmonary embolism. Results of the prospective investigation of pulmonary embolism diagnosis (PIOPED). JAMA 263:2753–2759
2. Stein PD, Fowler SE, Goodman LR *et alii* (2006) Multi-detector computed tomography for acute pulmonary embolism. NEJM 354:2317–2327
3. Pozen MW, D'Agostino RB, Mitchell JB *et alii* (1980) The usefulness of a predictive instrument to reduce inappropriate admissions to the coronary care unit. Ann Intern Med 92:238–242
4. Steurer J, Held U, Miettinen OS (2013) Diagnostic probability function for acute coronary heart disease garnered from experts' tacit knowledge. J Clin Epidemiol 66:1289–1295
5. Brown TW, McCarthy ML, Kelen GD, Levy F (2010) An epidemiologic study of closed emergency department malpractice claims in a national database of physician malpractice insurers. Acad Emerg Med 17:553–560
6. Grijalva CG, Nuorti JP, Griffin MR (2009) Antibiotic prescription rates for acute respiratory tract infections in US ambulatory settings. JAMA 302:758–766
7. Gonzales R, Bartlett JG, Besser RE, Cooper RJ *et alii* (2001) Principles of appropriate antibiotic use for treatment of uncomplicated acute bronchitis: background. Ann Intern Med 134:521–529
8. Boldy DA, Skidmore SJ, Ayres JG (1990) Acute bronchitis in the community: clinical features, infective factors, changes in pulmonary function and bronchial reactivity to histamine. Respir Med 84:377–385

Chapter 12
Methods Design for a Diagnostic Probability Study

Contents

Abstract The designing of the methodology for a differential-diagnostic study involves planning for the formation of the *study base* and for the *documentation* of the relevant facts on this, including the elementary facts' synthesis into the empirical values for the parameters in the designed object function for the study in reference to the designed domain of this function. The design is aimed at the attainment of certain *qualities for the study*, some of them mere desiderata, others more than that: one is a sine-qua-non requirement for meaningfulness of the study's result, and another a requirement for the very admissibility of the study. The process of the designing involves a sequence of topics conforming to that in the actual formation of the study base and then in the documentation of the relevant facts about it, the design decisions on each of them governed by logical principles.

Keywords Essence of the study · Validity of the study · Precision of the study · Efficiency of the study · Ethics of the study · Setting of the study · Case admissibility · Case enrolment · Case documentation · Synthesis of the data

O. S. Miettinen et al., *Clinical Research Transformed*,
https://doi.org/10.1007/978-3-030-06176-0_12

12.1 The Essence of the Study Being Designed

12.1.1 Formation of the Study Base

Any study for the advancement of the knowledge-base of diagnoses in clinical medicine – like any gnostic clinical study – is a project to produce *evidence* about the magnitudes of the parameters in a probability function, pre-designed in respect to its domain and its form in reference to this domain. As evidence about those magnitudes, any such study produces, from experience within the domain in question, an empirical function of the designed form (but with empirical values for the parameters), this together with documentation of the genesis of this result, with inferential statistics associated with the parameters' empirical values (Sect. 8.2.2).

Documented in the study will be experience with *a particular series of case presentations from the referent domain of the objects of study.* This series of cases will constitute the *study base*.

The study base will be *formed* by identification of case presentations from the domain in question, followed by selective enrolment of the identified cases into the study series of these (constituting the study base).

12.1.2 Documentation of the Study Base

The study base is designed to be such that it, upon its documentation, will embody facts that, in the aggregate, will be informative about the magnitudes of the object parameters of the study. To this end, the relevant facts about the study base will be (ascertained and) documented, first on the level of the individual cases in the study base and ultimately among all of them collectively, by synthesizing the case-specific documented facts – the aggregate of the study's *elementary data* – into the *study result*, the diagnostic probability function with empirical content (as to the parameters' values).

The synthesis of the elementary data into the result of the study together with inferential statistics on it does not bring the study process to its terminus; it does not constitute the completion of the study. The statistics and their genesis need to be documented in the study *report*. And scientific research being, inherently, a public enterprise, the actual terminus of the study in question, insofar as it ever will be achieved, will be the *publication* of the study report.

12.2 Quality Aspects of the Study's Design

12.2.1 The Scientific Qualities: Validity and Precision

Thinking about the objects of the study in question, inherently in reference to the domain (abstract) of these, engenders a dream – unrealistic but instructive – about a study that would reveal the actual, correct values of those parameters, perfectly. The methodology of that *truth-revealing study* would assure total freedom from bias – *perfect validity* – of the result; and that study's size would be sufficient – infinite – to provide for *perfect precision* – perfect reproducibility – of its result.

This ideal-but-impracticable study implies that, realistically, a *high-quality design* for an actual diagnostic (or other gnostic) study for clinical medicine represents, as best is understood, a fair fragment of that dreamed-about study. The design, if perfectly executed, provides for study results (the object parameters' empirical values) that are *fully valid* but (unavoidably) *imprecise*.

Validity of the designed study (its methodology) is *more than a desideratum* in the design for the study; a reasonable degree of validity of the study being designed is a *requirement*, a quality to be assured for the study, without compromise with a view to other qualities that are mere desiderata. For, a substantially invalid study is worse than no study, because it is misleading to those – the many – who, just like the investigators themselves, fail to recognize its inadequate level of validity.

The degree of *imprecision* – incomplete reproducibility – of the individual parameters' values in the study result can be highly variable among them. For the precision of the result on any given parameter, a major determinant is the degree to which the indicator at issue varies in the study base: the greater is the variation, the higher is the precision. For parameters associated with binary characteristics among the diagnostic indicators, precision of the result for the parameter's value is maximal if the two realizations are equally common.

The variation of the imprecision among the results on the individual parameters is not relevant for judgements about the imprecision of the values the overall result of the study – the diagnostic probability function from it – gives for the profile-conditional diagnostic probabilities. But it does have bearing on thinking about possible deletion of a particular indicator from the probability function, in particular if it is the result of some onerous test.

The imprecision of the profile-conditional values for the diagnostic probability is highly variable among the various profiles; but it isn't really worth thinking about. For, the value from the result of a valid study, despite its imprecision, presumably is more meaningful than any non-research alternative to it – except that the result from a very small study, however valid, can be less reliable than that from a diagnostic function derived by harvesting experts' estimates of the parameters' magnitudes (Sect. 10.3).

12.2.2 The Economic Quality: Efficiency

Whatever may be the quality of the objects design for a gnostic clinical study, and whatever may be the qualities of the study on the designed objects for it, *it is desirable to achieve the study result economically* – with the smallest possible expenditure of resources, that is. This is to say that a desideratum – non-scientific – to be optimized in the design of a gnostic clinical study is an economic one, that of the *efficiency* with which the study produces its result (of a given degree of validity and precision).

The epitome of an efficient gnostic study is one based on a pre-existing body of data, on the premise that the validity of the study is not thereby compromised. A study designed to be economical is not thereby cheap (i.e., compromised in its scientific quality).

Efficiency for a diagnostic (or other gnostic) study would generally be pursued by a *practical choice of the setting* of the study and *suitably selective enrolment* of admissible cases into the study (Sect. 12.3.4).

12.2.3 The Humane Quality: Ethics

The third and last, but not the least, of the qualities of the design of a gnostic clinical study is its ethics. While precision and efficiency are desiderata, and while a reasonable degree validity is an actual requirement for the meaning of any gnostic clinical study, *impeccable ethics is an actual imperative* in any study involving human subjects. The plan for a study on human subjects is reviewed for ethical acceptability by the Principal Investigator's IRB (Institutional Review Board), and editors of scientific journals generally require such IRB approval for even considering the report's publication.

The issues of ethics in gnostic clinical research generally revolve around two topics: the researchers' obligation to assure that the information garnered for the study on the subjects in it will be kept *confidential*, and their obligation to secure the subjects' *informed consent* for the execution of some aspects the study plan.

The confidentiality obligation in clinical research is akin to that in clinical practice: clinical researchers are bound by it as universally and strictly as clinical practitioners are. On the other hand, while a clinical practitioner can do various things to a patient without the patient's express consent to it, as long as it is done in the interest of the patient alone, doing something in the interest of research is not done in the patient's interest; it requires the patient's informed consent, generally in writing.

Diagnostic (and other gnostic) clinical researchers can obtain (and do obtain even involuntarily) *ethical guidance* from members of their IRBs. But the ultimate guide is the investigators' 'moral compass,' their collective conscience.

12.2.4 The Statistical Pseudo-Quality

Ever since the publication of the landmark randomized trial demonstrating the efficacy of streptomycin in the treatment of tuberculosis [1], paradigmatic for patient-level clinical research on the comparative efficacy of two or more treatments (placebo treatment commonly one of these) has been the randomized trial. That landmark trial was, in its design, heavily influenced by the statistician A. Bradford Hill, who subsequently assumed the role of teaching clinicians about clinical research, treatment trials in the main.

Following Hill's example, other *statisticians,* too, have taken a keen interest in randomized trials on the efficacy of treatments, gradually extending this interest to other areas of patient-level clinical research of the statistical sort.

Preeminent among statisticians' ideas about the design of patient-level clinical studies is statistical 'determination' of the size for the study – the study's *'sample size determination.'* This process is predicated on *two premises.* The first is that the study is being planned as a test of a 'null hypothesis,' eminently exemplified by no difference in efficacy between two treatments. And the second is about the role of the study as the test of that the 'null hypothesis': this premise is that the 'null hypothesis' will be 'accepted' or 'rejected' according as the P-value (Sect. 8.2.2) from the planned testing of the object parameter's null value will be greater or smaller than a certain pre-set value α of 'statistical significance.' This α is the (designed) probability with which the study's result will call for rejection of the 'null hypothesis' insofar as it actually is true. The size determination focuses on the probability with which the 'null hypothesis' will be rejected if the object parameter deviates from its null value by a certain pre-set amount δ.

The 'sample-size' calculation identifies the size of the study with which, conditionally on that degree of deviation from the null state, the probability of the rejection of the null hypothesis (on account of $P < \alpha$) equals a given pre-set value $(1 - \beta)$. This probability is taken to the study's (designed) *'power'* to 'detect' that degree of deviation from the null state.

This 'determination' is subject to serious critique on the level of its premises. Its second premise reflects serious misunderstanding of the way in which clinical research advances knowledge about the correctness/incorrectness of the null value of a parameter: the *P-value* from a study to test a given 'null hypothesis' does not automatically translate into a conclusion – shared conclusion in the relevant scientific community – about the correctness or incorrectness of the parameter's null value; instead, multiple studies on the same topic are commonly introduced and carried out, regardless of the P-values from the previous ones – and even the 'meta-analysis' (synthesis) of the results of all of them does not automatically (on the basis of the resulting P-value) translate into a conclusion about the correctness or incorrectness of the parameter's null value.

Not only is this doctrine about studies' 'sample size determination' conceptually unsound; it is, also, *commonly misunderstood.* While the calculation identifies the size for the study in question needed to achieve a pre-defined degree of 'power' – better would be focus on the level of precision of its result on the object parameter – this calculation is commonly thought of as identifying the optimal size of the study being designed. Even worse is the misunderstanding that it has relevance for interpretation of the study result – despite its imprecision being explicit in the inferential statistics routinely associated with the result (Sect. 8.2.2). Remarkably, the *editorial policies* of many medical journals mandate the reporting of the 'sample size determination' for clinical trials at least [2].

Even if this type of 'sample size determination' is taken to be relevant in the design of hypothesis-testing studies, it should be (but isn't) understood to have *no bearing* on the design of the sizes of gnostic clinical studies, diagnostic or other. For at issue in this research is not hypothesis testing (but, instead, inquiry into the magnitudes of the parameters in pre-designed probability functions).

There can be no statistical theory for optimization of the size of a gnostic clinical study, diagnostic or other. The fact is that, for one, no actual study in this genre is too small to make a contribution to the aggregate of evidence about the magnitudes of the parameters in the probability function at issue; and for another, that no study is handicapped by being too large to make such a contribution.

12.3 Quality Assurance by the Study's Design

12.3.1 Design for the Setting of the Study

The end result of the objects design for a differential-diagnostic clinical study, even in its definition of the domain of the objects of study, does not refer to anything particularistic (i.e., specific in place and/or time). Nevertheless, any study of the (designed) objects of study (characterizing their referent domain, abstract) inherently draws from experience in some particularistic setting of case presentations for it (Sect. 12.1.1).

Any setting of case presentations with a complaint about sickness naturally is one of *clinical practice*, and the first question in the choice of the setting for the study naturally is about the relative merits of in-hospital (tertiary-care) and extramural (mainly primary-care) settings for the purpose.

'Clinical epidemiologists' have repeatedly expressed the notion that research for diagnoses in general-practice settings needs to be conducted in those settings, given that the cases of whatever sickness presenting to general practitioners are, generally, less severe than those presenting in tertiary-care settings. This is a belief about the study's validity-assurance, but it is mistaken.

There is no inherently and uniquely general-practice level of severity of the patients' cough or chest pain, for example, nor a tertiary-care counterpart of these. On both levels of care there generally is a distribution of the severity of the sickness in question, perhaps with relatively mild cases more common in primary-care settings and more severe cases tending to concentrate in settings of tertiary care.

Insofar as this is so, and if the complaint's degree of severity has appreciable relevance diagnostically, it needs to be accounted for in the diagnoses – identically for the different settings of care.

Without accounting for the presentation's severity, if diagnostically relevant, the object function's design would be inadequate for any particular level of care, while upon its inclusion in the function, it is, in this respect, adequate for any level of care.

For the *validity-assurance,* the relevant questions about any candidate setting for the study are these:

1. Can the entries into the study series (study base; Sect. 12.1.1) be made (and omitted) independently of which one of the possible illnesses actually is at the root of the sickness?
2. Can the entries into the study series be made independently of diagnostic indicators other than the ones accounted for in the function in question? For example, in a study for diagnoses based solely on clinical indicators, case enrolment into the study series needs to be independent of the results of any laboratory-level diagnostic tests.
3. Can the documentation of the study series (Sect. 12.1.2) be accomplished in conformity with the study's objects design? For example, can the requisite competence in the clinical fact-finding be assured, being that this generally is, justifiably, a premise in the study's objects design.

These requirements in the study's validity-assurance generally cannot be satisfied by post-hoc abstraction of the routine records of diagnostic practice in any type of setting for patient care. Instead, generally needed is an arrangement for *prospective, protocol-driven case enrolment and documentation, in a setting in which this can be effected* so as to assure that those requirements will be met.

By and large, the assurance of the study's validity calls for its conduct in the outpatient clinics ('policlinics') and/or emergency departments of a group of *academic hospitals*. This, however, does not mean that the study could not be inspired by the diagnostic needs in whatever type of setting for primary care and also designed and directed by *primary-care academics* (given their requisite education in the theory of diagnostic research).

Naturally, the efficiency of the study would generally be enhanced by the involvement of a cluster of settings in relative proximity to the offices of the investigators involved.

12.3.2 Design for the Identification of Cases

For the identification of case presentations from the (designed) domain of these, the design needs to call – and hence to provide – for their identification early enough for prospective processing of them in respect to the (protocol-specified) assessment of admissibility and (admissibility-conditional) consideration of admission into the study series.

There may also be a felt need – notably for valid assessment of the overall prevalence of the illness at issue in cases from the presentation domain – to provide for inclusive identification of the presentations of the cases at issue from the domain at issue; that is, there may be a need to identify *successive cases* for potential enrolment into the study series (Sect. 12.3.4).

12.3.3 Design for the Admissibility of Cases

The cases constituting the study base are enrolled, selectively, from among the cases identified for potential enrolment into it.

A prerequisite for a case's admission into the study base is that it satisfies the criteria of admissibility specified in the study protocol. Some of these are scientific, others extra-scientific.

Scientifically, admissible only are cases that satisfy these validity-relevant criteria:

1. The case actually represents the study's *domain* as to the chief complaint and otherwise. For example, in a study in which the presentation is, to a first approximation, recent-onset cough in an adult, the full specification of the domain may include, for example, elements specific to 'community-acquired' pneumonia (cf. Sect. 11.5.1).
2. In the case's presenting to (one of) the setting(s) of the study there was no role for extraneous diagnostic indicators, that is, indicators not accounted for in the design of the (form of) the DPF (diagnostic probability function) at issue.
3. The case lends itself for valid acquisition of the *relevant information*. For example, the patient needs to be compos mentis and to be fluent in the language of the interviews for the study.

The study protocol is to call for documentation whether these criteria are met.

The additional, *extra-scientific criteria* of admissibility, if any, have to do with the economic desideratum – efficiency – in the acquisition of the result (of a given degree of precision) that the study will produce. For example, if the ascertainment of the truth about the presence/absence of the illness at issue requires follow-up of the patient, inclusion of only local residents serves to enhance the study's efficiency.

12.3.4 Design for the Enrolment of Cases

Regarding the identified admissible cases, the question is whether they should be *targeted for enrolment* into the study base indiscriminately or, instead, somehow selectively. The answer to this question needs to be understood from the vantage of the study's validity requirement, its efficiency desideratum, and also its ethics imperative.

In studying diagnostic probabilities conditional on the profiles of the cases, fully consistent with *validity*-assurance is the admissible cases' enrolment with selectivity based on the diagnostic indicators involved. Thus, for diagnoses conditional on the clinical (pre-laboratory) profile of the case, enrolment can be selective on the basis of the clinical indicators (but must be independent of the results of laboratory-level tests). Likewise, for diagnoses conditional on the results of laboratory-level tests as well (in addition to the clinical items), the enrolment – for determination of the presence/absence of the illness at issue – can be selective on those results (in addition to being selective on the clinical items).

The option of validity-consistent selectivity in the enrolment of admissible cases opens up the possibility to enhance the study's *efficiency* by being suitably selective in the enrolments. One means to this end is selectivity so as to increase the indicators' variability in the resulting study base (cf. Sect. 12.2.2). Another is taking into consideration the case-specific cost of the needed documentation (notably of the determination of the truth about the presence/absence of the illness at issue), insofar as there is appreciable variation in this. Theoretically optimal for efficiency in case enrolments from different subdomains of the study domain is enrolment ratio equal to the square root of the inverse of the ratio of the respective unit costs.

Given that a case is targeted for enrolment, actual enrolment involves the *ethical* predicate of informed consent, especially for solely research-motivated data collection.

12.3.5 Design for the Documentation of the Cases

The purpose of the study's design for *prospective* data-collection (Sect. 2.3.1) is the need for the data to be sufficiently accurate in reference to the time of case presentations.

In the process of the case identification for possible enrolment into the study, the cases are documented in respect to all of the information relevant to their *admissibility* to the study base (Sect. 12.3.3) and regarding the degree of their *desirability* for actual enrolment into the study base (Sect. 12.3.4, above). This is done as stipulated by the study protocol, with a level of discipline that may exceed that of the corresponding practices in the setting in question, in respect to the documentation in particular.

This is the juncture in the study process at which the *targeting* (select) of cases for inclusion in the study base needs to be made and the *informed consent* to study participation needs to be sought. For even if the determination of the truth about the presence/absence of the illness at issue, as conclusively as is required by the study, is part of normative practice in the setting in question, the *solicitation of study participation must not be delayed to the completion of the diagnostic work-up*. With this delay in securing it, the consent to participation could well be dependent on what the truth about the presence/absence of the illness is – resulting in a cardinal case of invalidity of the study base. On the other hand, getting the consent selectively on the basis of the clinical profile, as documented, is fully consistent with validity of the resulting study base (cf. Sect. 12.3.4, above).

12.3.6 Design for the Synthesis of the Data

The primary data, with whatever coding may be involved in this, are translated into the corresponding realizations of the *statistical variates* (Y, Xs) in the *functions* being addressed: there generally would be a set of data for purely clinical diagnoses (with the Xs representing the indicators from history and physical examination), and also for post-clinical diagnoses (with the Xs for the results of laboratory tests included).

Added to this data matrix are the realizations of the variates representing *transforms*, if any, of quantitative Xs and ones defining the *product terms*, if any, that were designed for inclusion in the probability function (Sect. 11.4).

Completion of the data matrix may require *representation of the data missing on some of the cases* (while not missing in others), this modelling approach to the problem generally being much more efficient than the exclusion of all the cases in which at least one datum is missing. Two variates are needed for representation of an indicator for which some of the data are missing: a variate indicating the availability of the datum and the product of this with the variate in question.

With the data matrix complete, any given model is fitted to the data by the use of one of an available software system for this. The result of the study for the designed function involves the fitted values of the parameters in it – upon setting the indicators of the availability of particular data, if any of these were introduced, to indicate presence of the information (with the coefficient of this contributing to the value of B_0).

If the number of parameters in a model is not sufficiently small for avoidance of the bias peculiar to these results (Sect. 8.3) and if, in addition, the intent is that the result be applied as such (in addition to making a contribution to the syntheses of the result from the study at issue with those of some other studies on the function in question), then a supplementary result also needs to be derived, involving appropriate *'shrinkage'* of the profile-specific probabilities toward the value typical of the study series (Sect. 8.3).

References

1. Marshall G, Blacklock JWS, Cameron C *et alii* (1948) Streptomycin treatment of pulmonary tuberculosis. BMJ 2:769–782
2. CONSORT. Transparent reporting of trials. Retrieved 16 Aug 2016 from http://www.consort-statement.org

Chapter 13
The Bayes' Theorem Framework for Diagnostic Research

Contents

Abstract Concerning the knowledge-base of diagnosis, the fundamental tenet of 'clinical epidemiologists' is the one that is traditional in medicine (and manifest in textbooks of medicine): that clinically-relevant knowledge generally is about particular illnesses and their respective manifestations, and that diagnosis-relevant knowledge therefore is about the relative frequencies of various case profiles in the presence (hidden) of the illness in question and that of its alternatives. This also was *the predicate of an article on the theory of diagnosis in Science* (in 1959), which deduced from it the idea that diagnostic probability-setting requires deployment of *Bayes' Theorem.* As this outlook entails quite prohibitive problems of feasibility for diagnostic research, 'clinical epidemiologists' have materially reformulated that theoretical idea, thereby compromising the principles underpinning it. But more fundamentally, *the idea's predicate actually is untenable, and the Theorem is, even in principle, inapplicable for diagnosis and diagnostic research.*

Keywords Bayes' Theorem · The BT doctrine re diagnosis · The doctrine's simplification · The doctrine's extension · The unconditional probability · Research under the doctrine · Untenability of the modifications · Untenability of the doctrine proper · Clinical epidemiology

O. S. Miettinen et al., *Clinical Research Transformed*,
https://doi.org/10.1007/978-3-030-06176-0_13

13.1 Bayes' Theorem about Conditional Probability

Bayes' Theorem is a classic in probability theory. It addresses *the probability of a particular state conditionally on another state.*

With the state in question denoted by the realization Y = 1 for one variate and the condition by the realization X = x for another variate, the Theorem is about Pr (Y = 1 | X = x). It expresses this *conditional probability* in terms of *two probabilities of the reverse kind* – Pr (X = x | Y = 1) and Pr (X = x | Y = 0) – *together with the unconditional Pr (Y = 1).*

One way of formulating the Theorem – the logical truism it represents – is in terms of *odds ratios*:

$$\Pr\left(Y=1 \middle| X=x\right)/\Pr\left(Y=0 \middle| X=x\right)$$
$$=\left[\Pr\left(Y=1\right)/\Pr\left(Y=0\right)\right]\Pr\left(X=x \middle| Y=1\right)/\Pr\left(X=x \middle| Y=0\right).$$

In words: The odds ratio (for Y = 1) conditional on X = x equals the unconditional odds ratio multiplied by the likelihood ratio for X = x contrasting Y = 1 with Y = 0.

In this formulation of the theorem, the *conditioning variate* (X) *need not be a scalar* (uni-dimensional); it can just as well be vector-valued ($X = X_1, X_2, \ldots$).

13.2 The Doctrine about the Theorem for Diagnosis

Bayes' Theorem was brought to the realm of the theory of medical diagnosis in 1959, by Robert Ledley (information technologist) and Lee Lusted (radiologist) in an article in the journal *Science* [1].

In this landmark article, Ledley and Lusted focused, in the main, on diagnostic probability – for a given "disease" – conditionally on the patient's "symptom complex," meaning the manifestational, symptoms-and-signs segment of the diagnostic profile of the case rather than the diagnostic profile at large. Curiously, there was no attention to the risk-related segment of the diagnostic profile.

Their *premise* was that the knowledge-base of diagnosis cannot be of this direct form but is, of necessity, of the *reverse form*: probability of the "symptom complex" conditionally on the disease in question and also on the set of illnesses constituting its differential-diagnostic alternative to the illness at issue. Their *justification* of this premise was the following:

> The reason why medical knowledge takes this form is because [these reverse probabilities are] relatively independent of local environmental factors such as geography, season, and others, and [depend] primarily on the physiological-pathological aspects of the disease complex itself.

This premise led Ledley and Lusted to posit the thesis that translation of diagnostic knowledge, such as it is and will be, into case-specific diagnoses requires the deployment of Bayes' Theorem (Sect. 13.1, above).

The adoption of this outlook required those authors to address, also, the diagnostic probability that is *unconditional* in respect to the symptoms and signs of the case (cf. Sect. 13.1, above). In the terms of their thinking, the probability that is unconditional in this sense (of being prior to considering the "symptom complex") is determined by (and hence conditional on) those "environmental factors" in the quote above, which they also termed the "circumstances" of the case presentation. They said this:

> By 'circumstances' we mean geographic area, local community, season of the year, and so forth. ... [I]n general, nearly all of the patients of an individual physician or clinic will be subject to the same circumstances. Thus each such physician will have his own [unconditional probability for a given disease] which, in general, will be different at different times.

Ledley and Lusted rounded out their presentation – highly formalistic – by describing how an individual doctor or a particular clinical facility can assess the relevant probabilities from the experience with their own patients. (*Sic!*).

13.3 Extension and Simplifications of the Doctrine

'Clinical epidemiologists' have enthusiastically embraced the doctrine of Ledley and Lusted about diagnostic probability-setting (Sect. 13.2, above). Never questioning it, they have only extended the range of the purported applicability of Bayes' Theorem for diagnosis, and they have also simplified all of this.

The *extension* is founded on the doctrine that each item in the diagnostic profile can be thought of as the result of a diagnostic test (cf. Sect. 3.1.2). Thus, they've taken Bayes' Theorem to be relevant and applicable to the translation of the entire diagnostic profile into the corresponding diagnostic probability – given knowledge about the reverse probabilities.

Faced with the challenges (unsurmountable, really) of dealing with the likelihood ratio (Sect. 13.1) for the entire diagnostic profile (à la Ledley and Lusted re the "symptom complex"), with one of the likelihoods conditional on the aggregate of the other illnesses in the differential-diagnostic set, 'clinical epidemiologists' have introduced two simplifications into this.

One of these simplifications has been the decomposition of the likelihood ratio (LR) for the entire profile to the product of the separate likelihood ratios for each of the attributes in the profile. For it is much easier to address those attributes one at a time than collectively.

The *other simplification* has been to not think of the differential-diagnostic alternatives to the illness in question but to take the alternative to the presence of this illness to be no illness at all. This removes the major challenge of thinking about the likelihood (probability) of the case profile conditionally on the presence of one, an unspecified one, of the other possible illnesses at the root of the sickness at hand.

Upon the extension of the application of Bayes' Theorem to the diagnostic profile in its entirety, 'clinical epidemiologists' needed to rethink the *unconditional, 'pre-test' probability* for the presence of the illness in question, the probability prior to accounting for the 'test results' (patient's age, etc.) in case's diagnostic profile. Thus wrote Sackett *et alii* [2]:

> This is a key topic ... How can we estimate a patient's pre-test probability? We've used five different sources for this vital information: clinical experience, regional or national prevalence statistics, practice databases, the original report we used for deciding on the accuracy and importance of the test, and studies devoted specifically to determining pre-test probabilities.

Evidently, this "key topic" remains quite unsettled among the advocates of the Bayes' Theorem framework for diagnostic research.

13.4 The Research under the Doctrine

The research under the doctrine about diagnostic probability-setting in the Bayes' Theorem framework, as this was initially put forth (Sect. 13.2) and subsequently modified (Sect. 13.3, above), is extensively described in a book by Knottnerus and Buntinx [3]. For this reason, and due to its lack of merit (Sect. 13.5, below), it *does not deserve delineation* here.

13.5 The Untenability of That Framework

13.5.1 The Unconditional Probability

The passage by Sackett *et alii* on the various ways they've used to estimate the unconditional, "pre-test" probability that the patient has the illness in question (Sect. 13.3) – the probability of the presence of the illness in a person when nothing is known about the person – is telling: only the last one of the five ways – the results of "studies devoted specifically to determining pre-test probabilities" – makes some sense, though this, even, for only a fleeting moment. For it actually is impossible to imagine a study on the prevalence (probability of the presence) of pneumonia, for example, among *case presentations from an entirely unspecified domain – cases from whatever demographic category presenting with whatever chief complaint.* The same obtains for myocardial infarction, for example, from whatever demographic category presenting with whatever chief complaint. Such unconditional probabilities are not subject to study by any imaginable "studies devoted specifically to determining pre-test probabilities."

This is in sharp contrast with the feasibility of studying the unconditional diagnostic probability in the meaning of this in the *logistic-regression framework* of thinking about, and studying, diagnostic probabilities. Even though that probability is not conditional on any of the attributes accounted for in the diagnostic profile, it is conditional in the sense that all of the case presentations come from the *expressly-*

defined domain of the study. The type of diagnostic study that is natural in the logistic-regression framework for it (Sect. 12.1) provides for obtaining an estimate of the profile-independent overall probability in the defined domain (Sects. 10.3 and 11.3) – insofar as there is any interest in this.

13.5.2 The Case Profiles' Likelihoods

The decomposition of the likelihood ratio into the product of the indicator-specific ones is theoretically untenable, as it *does not account for the correlations* – and their consequent relative redundancies – among the indicators involved. In the logistic-regression framework these correlations are inherently accounted for: each of the parameters addresses its associated variate's informativeness about the probability of Y = 1 conditionally on all of the other Xs in the model.

Untenable also is taking the *alternative* to the presence of the illness in question to be the presence of no illness at all. In the logistic-regression framework the form of the probability function is designed, expressly, for discrimination between the illness at issue and the set of its differential-diagnostic alternatives (Sect. 11.3).

Apart from these theoretically untenable modifications of the original propositions (Sect. 13.1), *those original propositions themselves were in error, and seriously so*. A simple yet compelling example of that doctrine's untenability is this: the *unconditional probability* being specific to each practice (cf. Sect. 13.2), *the actual diagnostic probability* – conditional on the manifestational profile of the case – consequently *is dependent on where the sick person seeks diagnosis*. Thus, in this theoretical framework, a case of ankle sprain inherently leads to very different probabilities of fracture depending on whether the patient presents to, say, a general practitioner, an orthopedic surgeon, or a psychiatrist. In the logistic-regression framework, the diagnostic probability is conditional on the diagnostic profile of the case, this alone, with the nature of the doctor's 'catchment population' entirely irrelevant (as it should be).

And apart from the *very major practical problem* of commonly needing to study the likelihoods (their ratios) for an enormous number of quite complex (vector-valued) profiles, there generally also is a *profound theoretical problem* in this: the very concept of the reverse conditional probability here – the probability of the profile conditional on the presence of the illness in question – is a malformed concept and, as such, generally devoid of meaning. A conditional probability is a meaningful concept only if the condition in it is singular in its meaning. But the likelihoods for the various possible manifestations of pneumonia and myocardial infarction, for example, are very different according to the particulars of the illness in question, and even more obvious is that the probability of hemoptysis, for example, as a manifestation of lung cancer is highly dependent on the size of the tumor, inter alia. In the logistic-regression framework there is no problem about the singularity of the conditions (the realizations of the diagnostic indicators).

13.6 Understanding Doctors' Thinking – Critically

This Chapter has been, in essence, a story – an instructive one – of how a highly formalistic presentation (by Ledley and Lusted) in a highly-esteemed scholarly journal (*Science*) led highly-influential teachers of clinical research ('clinical epidemiologists') to adopt – unjustifiably – a *core tenet* that has seriously misled their teachings.

To recap, the presentation was mainly aimed at "understanding how physicians reason"; but it also gave a justification of sorts for this reasoning. Decades later, once 'clinical epidemiology' in its contemporary version had been launched, its teachers have uncritically shared the essence of the described reasoning and also its purported justification. After all, really new was only the presentation's (reverence-inspiring) formalism (of 'symbolic logic,' i.a.) and, then, the proposition, formally deduced from its premises, that central to the theory framework of diagnostic probability-setting is *Bayes' Theorem.*

That topic of "how physicians reason" – or "how doctors think" ([4], i.a.) – is, to us, one of cognitive psychology rather than of (practice-guiding) *theory of medicine.* In the latter framework, our concern is not to understand, nor merely to know, how doctors reason or otherwise think. In regard to clinical medicine, our most fundamental concern is to gain tenable understanding of a related but very different kind: it is to understand *how doctors should think.* The most elementary features of this normative thinking we present in Part I of this book.

An anathema to those precepts is the reading of a scholarly journal – as evidently has been done by 'clinical epidemiologists' – merely "to believe and take for granted" rather than "to weigh and consider" (Chap. 1). And this critical attitude we present as merely the necessary point of departure in the development of normative thinking in medicine. For, a critically-important prerequisite for genuine critical thinking about clinical medicine, and about directly practice-relevant clinical research, we also take to be suitable educational preparedness for it (Chap. 4), the contents of which this book is about – for the readers to critically weigh and consider.

It bears note that nowhere do 'clinical epidemiologists' argue inappropriateness of the *logistic regression* framework for thinking about diagnostic probabilities and, hence, for designing the objects of diagnostic research.

References

1. Ledley RS, Lusted LB (1959) Reasoning foundations of clinical diagnosis. Symbolic logic, probability, and value theory aid our understanding of how physicians reason. Science 130:9–21
2. Sackett DL, Straus SE, Richardson NS *et alii* (2000) Evidence-based medicine. How to practice and teach EBM, 2nd edn. Churchill Livingstone, Edinburgh, p 82
3. Knottnerus JA, Buntinx F (2008) The evidence base of clinical diagnosis, 2nd edn. Wiley-Blackwell (an imprint of John Wiley & Sons Ltd)
4. Groopman J (2007) How doctors think. Houghton Mifflin Company, Boston

Chapter 14
Research Focused on Diagnostic Tests

Contents

Abstract In the *prevailing theoretical framework* of diagnostic research (Chap. 13, above) the focus is, quite exclusively, on the properties of diagnostic 'tests' (incl. symptoms and clinical signs), properties such as their 'sensitivity' and 'specificity' for the illness at issue. In a study on these properties, the frequency behavior of the 'test' result is compared between a series of cases of the illness and one without the illness. In the here-advocated *alternative theoretical framework* for diagnostic research, the main focus is on the meaning of the diagnostic profile as a whole (Chap. 11), and the only property of note of a diagnostic test (or a set of these jointly) is the probability with which the testing would provide for a sufficiently conclusive post-test probability of the presence/absence of the illness at issue if invoked to supplement the inconclusive pre-test information on the case. Research on this *'power'* of a (set of) diagnostic tests(s) – genuine, laboratory-based – is a simple-but-important extension of studies on diagnostic probability as a joint function of a set of diagnostic indicators. Diagnostic research relevant to *screening* addresses the probability of the test's positive result and the probability of the illness conditional on this.

Keywords Doctrines re properties · Untenability of the doctrines · Research under the doctrines · The relevant property · The relevant research · Screening test as a special case · Clinical epidemiology

O. S. Miettinen et al., *Clinical Research Transformed*,
https://doi.org/10.1007/978-3-030-06176-0_14

14.1 The Prevailing Doctrines on the Research

'Clinical epidemiologists' of the Sackett school think of each of the items in a diagnostic profile as the result of a diagnostic 'test,' including the patient's status in respect to whichever symptom or clinical sign and, even, attributes such as age and gender (while to Feinstein they were realizations of diagnostic 'markers'). And in diagnostic probability-setting, specifically, they think of the properties in terms of the 'test'-specific likelihood ratios contrasting the presence of the illness in question with the absence of this illness (without any alternative illness being taken to be present in lieu of the illness targeted for diagnosis; Sect. 13.3).

If the indicator is a binary one (or its quantitative realizations are dichotomized), the realization that points to (i.e., increases the probability of) the illness in question is thought of as the *'positive'* result, the other result as the *'negative'* one. Thus, if the probability of the presence of the illness in question depends on the patient's gender, then the positive result of the 'gender test' is the one pointing to the presence (rather than absence) of that illness.

The performance properties of a binary 'test' in this framework of thought about diagnosis are the *two likelihood ratios*, the 'likelihood ratio positive' based on the probabilities P_1 and P_0 for the positive result in the presence and absence of the illness, respectively, and the 'likelihood ratio negative,' which is the counterpart of this for a negative result (Sect. 13.3). These likelihood ratios are, naturally,

$$\text{LR+} = P_1 / P_0 \text{ and}$$
$$\text{LR}- = (1 - P_1)/(1 - P_0)$$

for a positive and negative result, respectively, of the 'test.'

These measures are *malformed concepts*, because they are based on conditional probabilities (P_1 and P_0) in which the respective conditions are devoid of singularity and, thereby, of meaning (Sect. 13.5.2).

Even though there logically are no other (performance) properties of a binary 'test' in this framework of diagnostic thought (which is logically untenable; Sect. 13.5), some other measures of the 'accuracy' of diagnostic 'tests' are commonly being addressed in diagnostic research [1]. Preeminent among these is the 'sensitivity'-and-'specificity' pair, based on the same 'conditional' probabilities as are the LRs above:

$$\text{Sensitivity} = P_1 \left(\text{i.e.,probability of the positive result,given presence of the illness}\right),$$
$$\text{Specificity} = 1 - P_0 \left(\text{i.e.,probability of the negative result,given absence of the illness}\right).$$

These two measures – malformed (above) – were adopted by Feinstein already [2], who called them "nosological sensitivity" and "nosological specificity," respectively (as distinct from their "diagnostic" counterparts); and subsequently, Sackett and many, many others uncritically embraced these measures of test 'accuracy.'

These measures are malformed not merely because they share the malformations in the LRs (above). An added, major, malformation in these measures is that, different from the LRs, neither one of them is comparative between P_1 and P_0. A telling consequence of this is the pseudo-meaning of the meaningless: a randomly chosen laboratory test – wholly uninformative about the presence/absence of the illness at issue (as $P_1 = P_0$) – would generally give a negative result in the absence of that illness (i.e., P_0 would be quite small); thus, *any arbitrarily chosen test has, in these malformed terms, a high 'specificity' for the illness at issue, whatever that illness may be!*

***

In the *dictionary of epidemiology* sponsored by the IEA [3], those two properties "of a screening test, a diagnostic test" are defined thus:

> *Sensitivity* is the probability that a diseased person (case) in the population tested will be identified as diseased by the test (syn: true positive probability). Sensitivity is thus the probability that any given case will be identified by the test (syn: true-positive rate).
>
> *Specificity* is the probability that a person without the disease (noncase) will be correctly identified as nondiseased by the test. It is thus the probability of correctly identifying a nondiseased person with the test (syn: true-negative probability).

This dictionary goes on to present the usual fourfold table, with "True status" (Diseased, Not diseased) and "Test results" (Positive, Negative) the marginal headings and numbers a, b, c, and d in the four cells of the table. Sensitivity and specificity are then defined in terms of these numbers, as thought these measures actually weren't probabilities but only statistics (derived from data).

Derived from that table also are, first, "Predictive value of a positive test result" and "Predictive value of a negative test result." The former is specified as the 'true positive' number (a) divided by the number of test positives (a + b); and the latter, correspondingly, as the 'true-negative' number (d) divided by the number of test negatives (c + d).

The final measure derived from that table is *"accuracy."* This is given as the sum of the "true positive" and "true-negative" numbers (a + d) divided by the total (a + b + c + d). Under the "Accuracy" entry in that dictionary, however, said is that "The diagnostic accuracy of a test is usually expressed by its sensitivity and specificity."

***

That dictionary's presentation of the concepts concerning a diagnostic test's properties is fully – and uncritically – in tune with the generally-prevailing doctrines about these. But some *critical notes on these doctrines, additional to the principal ones above*, are in order:

1. *A diagnostic test does not "identify" anything*, including whether the illness targeted for diagnosis actually is present or absent. Even if the test's positive and negative results are pathognomonic about the presence and absence, respectively, of the illness in question, the test does not know this and on this basis translate its own result into the corresponding diagnosis; the doctor may have this knowledge (esoteric) and may, on the basis of this knowledge together with the test result, achieve the (conclusive) diagnosis about the case (Sect. 14.2).

2. *A person with the illness in question is not, thereby, a "case,"* nor is a person without that illness a "noncase." As a matter of the English language, a person can have, for example, a case of hemorrhoids; but this does not mean that a person *is* a case of hemorrhoids, much less that (s)he is a hemorrhoid.
3. A diagnostic test's positive or negative result is not, rationally, a *"true positive"* or *"true negative"* according as the illness in question is or is not present, and otherwise *"false positive"* or *"false negative."* The result is whatever it is, possibly false on account of some error in the testing or in the result's reporting; but *the presence/absence of the illness in question has nothing to do with whether the test result truly is positive or negative* (cf. #1 above).
4. *Proportions derived from the empirical numbers in a fourfold table are not probabilities.* They are, at best, empirical values ('estimates') of probabilities ('sensitivity' etc.).
5. *Diagnostic tests' results, positive or negative, do not have "predictive value."* For, diagnosis is about the present (or the past), not the future; and the result of a diagnostic test is not, in itself in isolation, the basis for setting diagnostic probability for the illness in question – not even in the theoretical framework of 'clinical epidemiologists' (Sect. 13.3).
6. *A diagnostic test is not, generally, an assessment or a determination of whether a particular illness is present; it therefore does not generally have a particular degree of accuracy in such a pursuit.* A diagnostic test typically addresses not the presence/absence of the illness in question but, instead, some determinant of the probability of the presence (or absence) of that illness; it produces a piece of information to the diagnostic profile of the case, not the actual diagnosis (cf. #1 above). It has its particular degree of accuracy in determining that which it actually is intended to determine, namely the realization of a diagnostic indicator.

14.2 The Alternative Outlook on the Research

An alternative to the prevailing dominant, mainly Sackett-adduced doctrines on the properties of diagnostic tests (Sect. 14.1, above) has been implicit in what we've said in this book up to now.

With diagnostic tests taken to be, specially, *laboratory*-level tests (chemical, radiological, ...), they produce information into diagnostic profiles, inputs supplementary to what is gleaned clinically, from history-taking and physical examination (possibly including some non-laboratory clinical tests).

The results of such tests as elements in a diagnostic profile have no special properties, distinct from those of the clinical items in the profile. Each of the diagnostic indicators addressed in a diagnostic profile, if relevant at all, contributes some added, *marginal information* bearing on diagnosis about the presence (or absence) of the illness targeted for diagnosis, the contribution being conditional on the other indicators involved in the specification of the profile, 'marginal' in this sense.

The diagnostician need not know about any 'properties' of any of the indicators involved in the diagnostic profile – about their respective contributions (marginal) to the discriminant in a suitable diagnostic probability function, DPF, should such a diagnostic aide be available. The need is to know about the diagnostic probability conditional on *the profile as a whole*.

***

While, in this alternative theoretical framework, the issue of a test's properties does not arise in the translation of an already-ascertained diagnostic profile into its corresponding diagnosis, it can arise as an input into a *decision about the invocation of a laboratory test*, possibly constituted by a 'battery' of component tests: The diagnostic profile assembled, clinically and from routine laboratory-level tests (if any), may not provide for a sufficiently conclusive ('actionable') rule-in or rule-out diagnosis, and in this situation there may well arise the question about *the probability with which a particular (batch of) added testing would provide for sufficiently conclusive diagnosis* (on the basis of the thus-extended diagnostic profile).

This probability is, in this situation, an important property of the test (or battery of tests) at issue, especially if at issue is testing that is onerous, medically and/or economically.

14.3 The Essence of the Studies

14.3.1 The Studies in the Prevailing Framework

Suffice it here to note the typical essence of a study on the 'sensitivity' and 'specificity' of a particular 'test' ('marker' à la Feinstein) – concerning a particular symptom or clinical sign, say – for diagnosis about the presence/absence of a particular illness.

In a typical study on these properties, the 'test' in question is, in a way, compared with a chosen other, *'reference standard'* test, the positive and negative results of which are taken to serve as proxies for the presence and absence of the illness at issue, repectively. Thus, *in effect, 'sensitivity' is redefined* as the probability with which the result of the 'test' under study accords with the positive result of the other test; and correspondingly, *'specificity' is effectively redefined* as the counterpart of this for the respective negative results.

Critical for the *validity* of such a study is taken to be the *'spectrum'* of the cases of the illness in the group representing its presence. This term was introduced by *Feinstein*, who also specified its denotation: "The individual units admitted as input to a study," he said, "will form the spectrum of the group for which the results are reported." He went on to assert the *principle* that "this spectrum should be broad enough to cover the scope of the phenomena under investigation ..." [2, pp. 61–62]. Sackett *et alii* [4, p. 83] echoed the same principle:

> you will want the diagnostic test to have been evaluated in an appropriate spectrum of patients, similar to the practice population in which the test might be used. ... The article [on a test's sensitivity and specificity] will be informative if the diagnostic test was applied to mild as well as severe and early as well as late cases of the target disorder and among both treated and untreated individuals.

This principle, widely heeded in this line of diagnostic research, is emblematic of the problems with the theoretical underpinnings of the prevailing concepts of the properties of diagnostic tests (Sect. 14.1). At issue here is the *root problem* with them all: those properties' conditionality on the nonsingular concept of the presence the illness in question (Sect. 13.2).

This emphatic concern to have a wide variety of cases of the illness in a study of the 'sensitivity' of a diagnostic test for it, is very noteworthy. For, it reflects recognition that the value of this probability depends, importantly, on the particulars of the illness, as they vary with the manifestational profiles of the cases. But as a diagnostic test's 'sensitivity' for a particular illness is, in this way, a theoretically *untenable concept* (Sect. 13.5.2), it does not become meaningful when *redefined* in reference to the typical probability in whatever "spectrum" of subtypes of the illness.

The probability of positive result of a diagnostic test is a *sound concept* when conditional (not on the presence of the illness in question but) on the pre-test profile of the case; and this is of diagnostic *relevance* insofar as the positive result, as a supplement to an inconclusive pre-test profile, would complete a practically diagnostic post-test profile or at issue is a screening test – as explained in Sects. 14.3.2 and 14.4 below.

14.3.2 The Studies in the Alternative Framework

In the *logistic-regression framework* of thinking about the knowledge-base of diagnostic probability-setting and, hence, about diagnostic research, there are no performance properties of a diagnostic test to consider in diagnostic probability-setting per se, but only in some *decisions about invoking a particular test – an actual test, on the laboratory level* (Sect. 14.2). Specifically, when, upon the routine fact-finding on the case, the probability of the presence of the illness targeted for diagnosis remains less conclusive than that of a practical rule-in or rule-out diagnosis, the doctor may be concerned to know *the probability with which a particular added test (or a battery of these) would provide for a practically conclusive ('actionable') diagnosis.*

Corresponding to the well-established – though questionable – terms denoting the properties of a diagnostic 'test' in the prevailing framework of thinking about these (Sect. 14.1), it would be good to have a *term* – an apposite one – for this still-nameless property of an actual diagnostic test (multidimensional, perhaps). Perhaps *'power'* would do (cf. the statistical concept of a study's 'power' to achieve $P < \alpha$; Sect. 12.2.4). The term would denote the test's ability – in consequence of its result getting to be added to the diagnostic profile – to provide for (practically) conclusive diagnosis. A special, extreme case of this is the pathognomonic property of the results of some tests, providing for categorical ruling in, or out, the illness in question regardless of the pre-test profile (and, hence, regardless of the pre-test probability). The 'power' at issue here is the test's *ability to complete a practically pathognomonic profile* in cases of inconclusive pre-test probability.

For a study of this power of a diagnostic test, the objects' design is bi-phasic. In the first phase it defines the objects of diagnostic knowledge in quite the usual sense of this (Chap. 11): defined by the design would be the *domain* of the study and *the form of the diagnostic probability functions*, DPFs, for the domain. Special would be only the particular *duality in these DPFs*: defined is the pre-test model to be fitted to the data exclusive of the result(s) the test(s) in question, and the post-test model, to be fitted with the inclusion, also, of the latter. The second phase of the study's objects design focuses on the *distribution of the result(s) of the test(s) at issue, conditionally on the pre-test profile of the case* (rather than in the presence and absence of the illness at issue; Sect. 14.3.1, above).

The second phase of the objects design is rather straightforward *if the test is unidimensional and its result binary*, positive or negative. For at issue in this situation is, simply, the way in which *the probability of the positive result* of the test is a *function* of the variates (Xs) definitional to the pre-test profiles of the cases (from the domain of the diagnosis at issue). This function, when evaluated at the pre-test profile of the case, would give the probability with which the testing would produce a positive result in the case at issue, while the post-test DPF would give the post-test probability that the test would provide with that ad-hoc probability of its positive result.

If the test result is not a unidimensional but is represented by the realizations of a *set of variates*, some of these quantitative perhaps, the post-test DPF involves a scoring function based solely the relevant test variates. Instead of a single probability function, as in the situation addressed above, needed now is a set of functions, each of them addressing, as it were, a particular definition of the positive result jointly from the set of test variates in question, based on a particular cut-off point in the score summarizing those variates' realizations.

Thus, whereas the principel practice-relevant property that can characterize a diagnostic test (or a set of these jointly; Sect. 14.2) is the test's power, as a supplement to the available diagnostic profile, to provide for a practically conclusive probability of the presence or absence of the illness at issue, a study of this *does not require any data different from those in a diagnostic study in general, so long as the data on the test(s) at issue are included.* Needed is, instead, mere supplementation of the pre-test and post-test syntheses of the data to the corresponding DPFs, supplementation which in the case of a binary test addresses the probability of its positive (or negative) result, and which in the context of a set of test-result variates is somewhat more involved than this.

14.4 Research on a Screening Test

A particularly remarkable feature of the now-prevailing theoretical framework of research on screening tests is the fundamentally schizoid view of the essence of these. These tests are, for some purposes, actually viewed as such. One thus speaks of, for instance, the PSA test (*sic*) for prostate cancer and the Papanicolau test (*sic*) for cervical cancer. And in this vein, it is commonplace to say, for instance, that an important property of a screening test for a cancer is its suitably high 'sensitivity' to latent cases of the cancer at issue. Yet, there is no serious call for research to quantify the 'sensitivity' of a screening test for a cancer (i.e., the probability of the test's positive result conditionally on latent presence of the cancer). Nor should there be (see below).

For the purposes of research on a screening test's 'properties' in the prevailing theoretical framework of this, the test is not viewed as a source of diagnostic information (with its result a diagnostic indicator, acausal), but as an *intervention* intended to cause (*sic*) a change in the course of a still-latent case of the illness, if present, for the better. In this vein, screening for a cancer is viewed as an intervention to reduce the cancer's case-fatality rate and, thus, mortality from the cancer in cohorts subjected to the 'intervention' by the test. This outlook provides for the prevailing routine of studying the intended 'effect' of a test for cancer screening by means of randomized trials on the 'intervention.' This theoretical framework for screening research is *irrational,* as a diagnostic test cannot rationally be construed as an intervention. Only confusion is the result of it.

Thinking about a screening test's properties in terms of its *'sensitivity'* and *'specificity'* for the illness at issue (Sect. 14.1), which also is commonplace, is not as irrational as is thinking of the testing as an intervention (above); and in this context of concern for possible presence a *latent case* of the illness in question, the issue of the heterogeneous "spectrum" of cases of the illness (Sect. 14.3.1) is much lesser a concern. However, these measures – of the distribution of the result (binary) of a screening test in the latent presence and absence of the illness in question – is not what research centered on such a test realistically and meaningfully is about.

In the theoretical framework of diagnostic research advocated in this book, a screening test – the first element in the pursuit of rule-in diagnosis about an illness that may be latently present – is *not simply a special case* of the generally appropriate way of thinking of, and studying, the relevant performance property of a diagnostic test (Sect. 14.3.2). For, here the pre-test diagnostic profile is inconclusive by definition, and the test is contemplated not as a possible means of completing a diagnostic profile practically pathognomonic about the presence or absence of the illness at issue but as a basis for potentially achieving a post-test probability high enough to warrant further pursuit of the rule-in diagnosis by means of some second-stage diagnostics.

The *relevant research* (diagnostic) on a screening test addresses, for one, the pre-test probability of the positive test result (variously defined perhaps) for a defined domain of case presentations and as a function of the indicators that would be involved in the pre-test DPF (cf. Sect. 14.3.2). Besides, the relevant research addresses the probability with which a particular algorithm of supplementary diagnostics leads to rule-in diagnosis about the illness at issue, conditionally on the pre-test profile of the case together with the positive result of the screening test.

References

1. Knottnerus JA, Buntinx F (2008) The evidence base of clinical diagnosis. 2nd edn. Wiley-Blackwell (an imprint of Wiley), London
2. Feinstein AR (1985) Clinical epidemiology. The architecture of clinical research. W. B. Saunders Company, Philadelphia
3. Porta M (Editor), Greenland S, Hernan M, dos Santos Silva I, last JM (Associate Editors), Buron A (Assistant Editor) (2014) A dictionary of epidemiology. A handbook sponsored by the IEA. 6th edn. Oxford University Press, Oxford
4. Sackett DL, Richardson WS, Rosenberg W, Haynes RB (1997) Evidence-based medicine. How to practice & teach EBM. Churchill Livingstone, London

Part V
Etiognostic Research

Chapter 15
Introduction to Etiognostic Research

Contents

Abstract In the development of a sound orientation to the exceptionally challenging, etiognostic species of quintessentially-applied clinical research, the very first need is to reach a critical understanding of the *meaning* of a case of an illness (or sickness not due to illness) having been caused by a particular factor present prior to this outcome. Closely related to this is the need to achieve a tenable understanding of *what those factors are in principle.* Then comes the pivotal, greatest challenge: the need to reach a true understanding of *how research on this species of causation is possible,* despite the retrospective and unobservable essence of it. Finally, there is the considerable challenge to understand the deduction, from this pivotal understanding, the requisite *essence of etiognostic studies.* This essence remains commonly misunderstood in contemporary epidemiological research, and in etiognostic clinical research in consequence of this.

Keywords Etiognosis vs. diagnosis · Etiogenesis · Etiogenetic factors · Etiogenetic knowledge · Etiogenetic studies · Cohort study · Case-control study · Case-referent study

O. S. Miettinen et al., *Clinical Research Transformed*,
https://doi.org/10.1007/978-3-030-06176-0_15

15.1 Etiognosis vis-à-vis Diagnosis

In the lexicon of medicine we've come to espouse [1], the denotations of some familiar terms are redefined. Salient among these is '*diagnosis*.' According to Stedman's [2], for example, diagnosis is a 'determination' (of the nature of the patient's illness), while to us it is a species of a doctor's esoteric knowing – gnosis – about the health of his/her client (patient or other; Sect. 1.2.2); it is gnosis about the hidden presence/absence of a particular illness, the one targeted for the pursuit of such knowing about it.

In that prevailing conception of diagnosis, the illness underlying the patient's sickness is said to represent the 'etiology' – causal origin – of the case of the sickness. But the 'determination' merely identifies the presence of a particular illness, without addressing whether the illness actually is causal to the case of sickness at issue. That illness could be asymptomatic in the case at issue, with the sickness being caused, for instance, by the patient's use of a medication.

In our conception of it, diagnosis is, expressly, an acausal species of gnosis. Diagnosis as the explanation of presenting sickness is knowing about the presence of an illness potentially causal to that case of sickness (Sect. 1.2.2), and this illness would be simply presumed to be causal to the sickness if it indeed were present. And there is, of course, diagnosis without any sickness being the prompting for its pursuit (Sects. 9.1 and 14.4).

In the prevailing lexicon of medicine, 'etiology' has also another, expressly causal, denotation: the *causal origin of a particular case of an illness or of a particular illness at large*. To us, this is the sole denotation of 'etiology.' This term for causal origin is, however, prone to be misleading, even to those who really should know the concept it denotes [3]. We therefore prefer an alternative, more telling term for this concept: *'etiogenesis'* [1].

As 'diagnosis' in our lexicon of medicine refers, by the '-gnosis' element in it, to a species of doctors' esoteric knowing (gnosis), we need a term for doctors' *gnosis about the etiology/etiogenesis on an illness*. A natural, apposite term for this species of medical gnosis we take to be *'etiognosis'* [1].

Given that the importance of etiognosis – in that meaning of this neologism – is undeniable, it is quite a mystery why this topic – as a species of gnosis along with diagnosis and prognosis – has remained so thoroughly ignored in medicine. A case in point is an eminent textbook on 'evidence-based medicine' [4]. In its index, the numbers of entries devoted to topics beginning with the 'etio-'/'aetio-' prefix and those having to do with diagnosis – all of these having to do with "diagnostic tests" (*sic*!) – is telling: the respective numbers are 0 and 33 (with 15 devoted to prognosis and another 14 to treatment, as though this weren't a concern under prognosis). One notable implication of this seems to be that while there is much evidence taken to be relevant to diagnosis [4, 5], all of the extensive body of work on *'pharmacoepidemiology'* has produced no noteworthy evidence for etiognosis about pharmacoetiogenesis of illness (nor of sickness not due to illness).

15.2 Etiogenesis as a Species of Causation

Causal origin – etiogenesis – of an entity of health is *one the two species of causation that are of concern in medicine*. This species of causation is the sole concern in etiognosis, while the other generally is an orientational and central – but only partial – concern in prognosis: in modern medicine, prognosis is eminently about the prospective effects of treatments (and, secondary to this, about treatment-conditional acausal prospects).

Etiogenesis, to the extent that it is known (as a matter of etiognosis), constitutes *causal explanation* of what has happened, namely: a case of an illness, or of sickness not due illness, has occurred. Etiogenesis is, thus, a *retrospective concept,* from the vantage of the gnosis, in the context of that occurrence. The causation in prognosis, in contrast to this, is a prospective concept from the vantage of the time of the prognostication: it is about the anticipated causal consequences of a treatment that is either contemplated for adoption or actually chosen for adoption (prospective).

15.3 The Essence of Etiogenetic Causation

To say that a certain occurrence, O, which has taken place, was caused by its antecedent A, which was there, is to imply (knowing) that O would not have come about – in the person in question at that time – had A not been there. But the meaning of this requires explication.

For a start, the concept of that counterfactual – *the meaning of the absence* of A – needs to be made explicit. For example, if A is a particular treatment, it needs to be clear whether absence of A means a particular alternative treatment that the patient could have used in lieu of A, or whether it means no treatment. Causal explanation involves an explicit *causal contrast.*

This need to have an explicit – and realistic – alternative to the causal antecedent adduces some limitations on what can be entertained as possible etiogenetic causes. For any given person at any given time, *age* (the accrued time lag since birth) is a given; it has *no alternative* that could be entertained for that same person at that time. The same is true of some characteristics that were present at birth already and have been immutable ever since. *Race* is a clear example of this, and gender also used to be one. *Characteristics like these – demographic – cannot be thought of as potentially having an etiogenetic role.* ('Social epidemiologists' disagree with this, just as they disagree with one another about the essence of this field).

What about a *mutant gene* in this respect? The answer is quite straightforward in respect to any mutation that is 'acquired' post conception: it is an accidental whose having occurred in a given person has the alternative of it not having occurred in that person: acquired mutations therefore are obvious candidates for having etiogenetic roles. This reasoning actually applies to inherited mutations as well: the gametes with the mutation, from which the person in question developed, did have the alternative of being free of the mutation – while they had no alternative to their demographic properties.

Not only does an etiogenetic cause have to have an alternative (counterfactual but realistic); the concept of an antecedent's etiogenetic role involves the *ceteris paribus premise*: an antecedent was causal to a subsequent if the subsequent would not have occurred in the presence of the antecedent's alternative, on the condition that all else that is relevant to the genesis of the outcome had been the same. For example, the concept of a particular treatment having been etiogenetic to a particular case of sickness, with a particular other treatment the alternative to this, is predicated on the premise that all etiogenetically-relevant extraneous treatments – and all other extraneous causes of the outcome too – would have been the same with the alternative treatment as they were with the factual treatment.

Fundamental to all etiognostic explanation is the *overarching premise* that whatever has happened, it was preceded by a sufficient cause of it. The *sufficient cause* generally is, in medicine, a composite of causes which, in isolation, are insufficient to bring about the outcome at issue. But when such a factor actually completes an otherwise insufficient cause, it is a sufficient cause in that situation. Thus, when a fall precipitates a fracture, but only because of the person's heightened susceptibility to fracture (on account of osteoporosis), *the susceptibility factor is a cause – contingently sufficient – just as much as the precipitating factor is.* It thus is not that the latter is the 'primary' cause and the former a 'secondary' or 'contributing' cause.

Etiogenetic causation is, thus, *an all-or-none concept*: an antecedent of the outcome either was, or was not, a cause of the outcome; and besides, a health outcome generally is the consequence (obligate) of more than one solely insufficient but contingently sufficient causes. Thus, a case of illness (or of sickness not due to illness) generally has been caused 100% by each of a number of factors, by a joint action in which each of the components had a critical role. *Apportionment of the causation of a health outcome, with the proportions adding up to 100%, is a mistaken endeavor* in clinical medicine. (In community medicine it is meaningful to say that a given proportion of cases of a particular illness is caused by a particular antecedent; but the sum of such proportions over different causes can be well in the excess of 100%).

15.4 The Species of Etiogenetic Factors

A little anecdote reflects the *common conception of the species of etiogenetic factors:* A youngster is being chided by his parents about the poor grades in his report card from school; and when the parents pause, the youngster asks: Is this *genetic* or *environmental*?

That *perceived duality* in etiogenetic factors is not confined to the teachings in schools; it is a common feature in medical thinking as well. Very curiously, *behavior* is commonly missing in the conception of the species of etiogenetic factors, even in medical thought. It may be seen to have the unspeakable quality of 'blaming the victim' (of the adverse event or state of health).

We replace that genetic species of etiogenetic factors by one of which genetic factors are only a subspecies. This larger category is *constitutional* factors, not only innate (genetic and other) but also acquired – acquired immunodeficiencies and allergies, 'hypertension,' hyperglycemia, obesity, etc. Illnesses too are constitutional entities that can be etiogenetic to other illnesses, ones that are complications of them [1]. But: an early stage of a progressive illness (a cancer, say) cannot be construed to have been etiogenetic to a later stage of it [1].

Environmental factors potentially etiogenetic to illness (and to sickness not due to illness) are ones to which a person is exposed. They are features of a person's environment – in utero, at home, at school, at work, etc. Particularly notable among them are hazardous medical actions to which a person is exposed (in his/her medical environment).

Behavioral etiogenetic factors are, most eminently, features of a person's lifestyle – dietary or medicational, for example. Community-medicine education and regulations are commonly aimed at promotion of healthy behaviors.

Very generally, factors in one of these species influence these in the others; but this has no bearing on the need to think of etiogenesis in terms of these species of possible causes – and to focus on factors possibly involved in the sufficient cause of the case that has occurred.

Causes of etiogenetic causes are matters of medicine only in respect to constitutional factors. Causation of health-hazardous environments and behaviors are not matters of medicine because medical expertise on causation illness (and of sickness in the absence of illness) is confined to processes within the human body and direct causation of these.

As a closing note here, it needs to be recognized that *the term 'factor' is, in this context, used in two meanings*. One of these is exemplified by saying that there are three generic types (species) of etiogenetic factor – constitutional, environmental, and behavioral. In this usage, a factor (etiogenetic) is a *dimension* in which causal contrasts are defined. In another denotation of the term, an etiogenetic factor is a *category* in one of these dimensions (of the person's history as of the time of a particular health outcome) relative to a specified other (alternative) category in the same dimension. For example, in this second meaning of 'factor,' blood pressure 160/100 mmHg is a factor in the etiogenesis of hemorrhagic stroke when the alternative level of the pressure is, say, 130/90 mmHg, but not with, say, 190/120 mmHg as the alternative.

15.5 The Basis for Etiognostic Knowledge

Learning about etiognostic probabilities is profoundly different from learning about diagnostic ones. As for diagnosis, a senior doctor can say that a certain proportion P of patients with the diagnostic profile of the case at issue have, in his/her experience, turned out to have the illness at issue, and that on this basis (s)he estimates the diagnostic probability in the case at issue to be P; the reasoning in this is sound (even though the premise is rather problematic; Sect. 10.4). By contrast, *no doctor can say that in a particular proportion P of cases of a given outcome O with antecedent A, that antecedent has turned out, in his/her experience, to have been causal to the outcome.* (If the outcome at issue is an offence in driving an automobile, the proportion of these cases with blood alcohol level exceeding the legal limit is a matter of police experience, but causal attribution of the outcome to the antecedent is well beyond the capabilities of the police).

The difference at issue here is this: As diagnostic probability is about the frequency of a *phenomenon* (the presence of an illness, conditionally on the diagnostic profile of the case), it is in principle learnable about on the basis of observations on a series of cases presenting for diagnosis; but etiogenetic probability is not about (the frequency of) a phenomenon, as causation, whether etiognostic or prognostic (Sect. 15.2), is not a phenomenon. Causation is, as Kant explains, a *conception a priori*, a *noumenon*, innate rather than learned from experience [6]. Owing to the noumenal nature of etiogenesis, it cannot be learned about on the basis of a mere cases of the outcome-and-antecedent in question, different from diagnostic learning from case presentations for diagnosis (Sect. 12.1.1).

The principle providing for study of clinically-relevant etiogenesis flows from the concept of medical etiogenesis, namely that an antecedent that was present was causal to a case of an outcome if the case would not have occurred in the (counterfactual) presence of the antecedent's defined alternative, ceteris paribus (Sect. 15.3). This means that an antecedent's causal role is manifest in *the outcome's rate of occurrence* in a population with positive histories for the antecedent – in the elevation of this this index rate over what it would have been under the (counterfactual) alternative history. Thus the need is to compare that index rate with the reference rate characterizing a population with the alternative history, adjusting for the ceteris-paribus factors (potential con founders).

If the index and reference rates are R_1 and R_0 respectively, with $R_1 > R_0$ and $R_1/R_0 = RR$, then the experience suggests that the *etiognostic probability* (that the antecedent, when present, actually was causal to the outcome) is

$$\begin{aligned} P &= (R_1 - R_0)/R_1 \\ &= (RR - 1)/RR. \end{aligned}$$

15.6 The Essence of Etiognostic Studies

15.6.1 The Essence of the Objects

The essence of the objects of etiognostic studies is implicit in what was said about logistic regression models for etiognostic research in Sect. 7.4.4 and in Sect. 15.5 above. Below, we make it explicit in reference to an *event*-type outcome.

The adopted model for the event's incidence density in the domain of the study might be this:

$$\log(\mathrm{ID}') = B_0 + B_1X_1 + B_2X_2 + B_3X_3 + B_4X_4 + B_5X_5;$$

ID′: number proportional to the incidence density (ID),
X_1: indicator of the history at issue (the index history),
X_2: indicator of extraneous history on the determinant at issue (history other than the index or the alternative/reference history),
X_3: variate for one of the ceteris paribus – confounder – determinants of the ID,
X_4: product of X_1 and X_3,
X_5: variate for another ceteris paribus – confounder – determinant of the ID.

In the *domain* of the study, various conditions may obtain by its design. A condition a priori generally is the state of being alive.

In terms of this model, the difference in log (ID′) between the subdomain with the index history ($X_1 = 1$) and that with the reference history ($X_1 = X_2 = 0$) is $B_1 + B_4\,X_3$. Hence, the *causal rate (incidence density) ratio* is modelled to be

$$RR = \exp(B_1 + B_4X_3).$$

And this, in turn, means that the *etiognostic probability* is modelled to be (Sect. 15.5, above)

$$\begin{aligned} P &= \left[-1 + \exp(B_1 + B_4X_3)\right] / \exp(B_1 + B_4X_3) \\ &= 1 - \exp(-B_1 - B_4X_3). \end{aligned}$$

In terms of that simple model, thus, the *overall object of study* is that RR function, and the *specific objects of study* are the parameters in it, the ones associated with the indicator of the index history (i.e., B_1 and B_4).

15.6.2 The Essence of the Methods

When at issue is, as usual, the etiogenesis of an *event*-type outcome, the *study base* is an aggregate of population-time, and documented for it is the event's incidence-density ratio, IDR, as a function of some of its modifiers conditionally on some ceteris paribus factors (cf. Sect. 15.6.1, above). The study base is constituted by person-moments, infinite in number, satisfying not only the criteria (scientific) for the study objects' domain but certain extra-scientific requirements as well (e.g., the person being fluent in the language of the study interviews as well as compos mentis).

The study base needs to be approached through the adopted *source base*, within which it is defined. The source base is constituted by the population-time of the selected population's course over a defined span of time, this source population being either open (dynamic) or closed (cohort-type). Cases of the outcome event occurring in the source base are identified, comprehensively, and documented in relevant respects. This first-stage case series is supplemented with a suitable first-stage base series, a suitable sample of the source base. These two series, documented in all relevant respects, are reduced to ones satisfying the criteria of the person-moments (infinite in number) constituting the actual study base.

The *logistic* counterpart of the designed model for incidence density – the log (ID′) replaced by log [P/(1 – P)], where P is the probability of a person-moment in the union of the two study series being one in the case series – is fitted to the data on the two series, and the IDR result is deduced from the result of this fitting (à la Sect. 15.6.1, above).

With the study base the referent not only of the study result but also of the case and base series from it, this general structure of an etiologic/etiogenetic study, when it was first introduced [7], was dubbed the *case-referent* study, to distinguish it from the 'case-control' study. The IEA dictionary of epidemiology [3], however, presents "case-referent study" as a synonym of "case-control study." An apt synonym for 'case -referent study' is 'case-base study.'

15.6.3 The Cohort and Trohoc Fallacies

Epidemiological research on the population level (rather than in laboratories) has been, principally, directed to *etiology/etiogenesis of illness*, with a view to forming the knowledge-base for the practice of epidemiology (i.e., for population-level preventive medicine; Sects. 15.4 and 5.1).

Till the early 1950s, the essence of epidemiologists' etiogenetic studies was the enrolment of a 'case group' of persons with the illness at issue and similar (matched) 'control group' of persons without the illness and comparing these two groups in respect to the frequency of the etiogenetic history at issue.

Then Richard Doll and A. Bradford Hill, without any particular rationale, set out to study the same matter in a different way, which was the entire point of the innovation: they enrolled a cohort of smokers and non-smokers and followed it up to document (for comparison) the rates of incidence of (the detection of cases of) lung cancer in the two smoking-based sub-cohorts.

Having done this, they labelled the earlier studies as *retrospective* and the new type of study as *prospective*. Subsequently, the retrospective study has become termed *case-control* study and the term for the prospective study has become *cohort* study. Feinstein took the retrospective study to represent "inversion" of the "customary logic" represented by cohort studies [8, p. 19]; and on this basis he renamed case-control study "*trohoc*" study ('trohoc' being the inverse – the palindrome – of 'cohort').

In line with all this, the most recent edition of the 'official' dictionary of epidemiology [3] says that "A common feature of a cohort study is comparison of incidences in groups that differ in exposure levels." And it gives as synonyms of 'cohort study' this set: "concurrent, follow-up, incidence, longitudinal, panel, prospective study." If the concept were sound, there presumably would be a single, apposite term for it.

Case-control study that dictionary defines as "The observational epidemiological study of persons with the disease (or another outcome variable) of interest and a suitable control group of persons without the disease (comparison group, reference group)." It gives 'case-referent study' as a synonym; but in the original, and still suitably disciplined conception of the case-referent study [7] there is no "control group" or "comparison group" (cf. Sect. 15.6.2, above).

Trohoc study is not defined in that most recent (sixth) edition of the dictionary. The previous edition (fifth) defined it as "A retrospective case-control study," adding that "the term, proposed by A. R. Feinstein [ref], is the inversion of 'cohort'; its use is rare." The edition prior to that (fourth) had the comment that the use of the 'trohoc' term is "deprecated by most epidemiologists."

Terms aside, truly deprecated should be the *concepts* of both 'cohort study' and 'case-control study,' as they represent the *cohort and trohoc fallacies*, respectively. Suffice it here to point out that both of them are substantially at variance with the essence – singular – of etiogenetic studies, deduced from the very concept of etiogenesis, carefully developed (Sect. 15.6.2, above). Elaboration of these fallacies is available elsewhere [9].

References

1. Miettinen OS (2015) Medicine as a scholarly field: an introduction. Springer, Cham
2. Stedman's Medical Dictionary (2013) Illustrated in color, 28th edn. Williams & Wilkins, Philadelphia
3. Porta M (Editor), Greenland S, Hernan M, dos Santos Silva I, Last JM (Associate Editors), Buron A (Assistant Editor) (2014) A dictionary of epidemiology. A handbook sponsored by the IEA, 6th edn. Oxford University Press, Oxford
4. Sackett DL, Richardson WS, Rosenberg W, Haynes RB (1997) Evidence-based medicine. How to practice & teach EBM. Churchill Livingstone, London
5. Knottnerus JA, Buntinx F (2008) The evidence base of clinical diagnosis, 2nd edn. Wiley-Blackwell. (An imprint of John Wiley & Sons Ltd)
6. Kant I (1990) Critique of pure reason (trans: Meiklejohn JMD). Prometheus Books, Amherst
7. Miettinen OS (1976) Estimability and estimation in case referent studies. Am J Epidemiol 103:226–235
8. Feinstein AR (1985) Clinical epidemiology. The architecture of clinical research. W. B. Saunders Company, Philadelphia
9. Miettinen OS, Karp I (2012) Epidemiological research: an introduction. Springer, Dordrecht

Chapter 16
Objects Design for an Etiognostic Study

Contents

Abstract In the design of the objects of an etiognostic clinical study, the first-order principles are the same as in the context of a diagnostic study; but then, important differences arise from the etiognostic need for knowledge about *causality* in contrast to the acausal knowledge-base of diagnosis. The objects design in reference to the index and reference *histories* is rather challenging, and provision for the *ceteris paribus premise* in the causation's manifestation is even more so. In these design challenges the clinical researcher is, again, guided by theoretical principles together with inputs from experts on the substantive issues.

Keywords Outcome · Domain · Etiogenetic factors · Confounders · Etiognostic · Indicators · Statistical variates · Examples

16.1 The Health Outcome and Its Domain

In an etiognostic study, the mission is to help doctors deal with case presentations calling for etiognosis: a particular type of adverse event of health has occurred in association with a particular type of antecedent, and the need is to set *the probability for the antecedent having been causal (etiogenetic) to the health event at hand.* The etiognostic probability-setting calls for the availability of an etiognostic probability

O. S. Miettinen et al., *Clinical Research Transformed*,
https://doi.org/10.1007/978-3-030-06176-0_16

function, providing an estimate of the probability that the antecedent was causal (etiogenetic) to the outcome, given the particulars of the case within a case-presentation domain to which it belongs (Sect. 15.6.1).

The objects design for an etiognostic study draws from this practice situation one input first and foremost: specification of the *health outcome* (illness or sickness) whose occurrence prompts concern to know about its etiogenesis. This defines the entity of health whose rate of occurrence in relation (causal) to an antecedent will be addressed in the etiognosis-serving study being designed (Sect. 15.6.1).

Once an etiognostic study is specified to be directed to the (rate of) occurrence a particular type of illness (or sickness not due to illness), the next concern in the study's objects design is specification of the study's focus as to the *domain* of these occurrences. The challenge in practice thus calls for studying the rate of occurrence (usually incidence density) of a specified entity of health in a specified domain – in a yet-to-be-specified type of relation (causal) to one or more antecedents.

In the design for the study the *specifics* of the entity of health and the domain of its occurrence, the principles of needed specificity and meaningfulness are the same as in the design of the domains for diagnostic studies (Sect. 11.1).

16.2 The Etiogenetic Factors

An etiognostic study on a given outcome can be designed to address *more than just one etiognostic factor*. The selection of the factors to be addressed is to be guided by the etiognostic concerns that practitioners have in cases of the outcome at issue.

In respect to each particular factor, the design needs to define the *scale* of the histories on it. It is not satisfactory (even though commonplace) to classify histories simply as positive/'exposed' or negative/'unexposed.' (It is awkward, though commonplace, to refer to constitutional and behavioral factors as 'exposures.') If the factor has to do with *the use of a particular medication*, needed generally is specification of the meaning of that 'use' (dosage, i.a.) over a defined period of time (retrospective from the vantage of the time of the outcome; that is, from the time of the etiognosis). This may imply the need to specify separate time-specific factors. In this, a distinction needs to be made between the potentially etiogenetic period and its antecedent time (relevant to modification of the causal rate-ratio).

The design/definition of the *alternative* to that (index) history is not straightforward either; it is not, inherently, merely absence of the index history. For a given (index) history about the use of a particular medication, the chosen alternative could be the use of that same medication at that same time with a different (lower) dosage, say. (A special case of this is zero dosage, so that the alternative to the factual history of the medication's use becomes the counterfactual non-use of it.) Or the alternative could be the use of a different medication at a particular dosage.

This suggests that, in respect to a particular etiogenetic factor, the study can address *various index histories* based on this; and also, that for any given index history, *various alternative/reference histories* can be defined and addressed. Besides, more than just one type of factor can be assessed in any given etiognostic study.

16.3 The Ceteris Paribus Factors

All of the entities involved in the ceteris-paribus premise have the quality of being, by their very nature, at least proxies for extraneous factors that can be etiogenetic to the outcome at issue. Prime examples of these entities – potential confounders – are *age* and *gender*, even though these never are etiogenetic factors (Sect. 15.3): they are proxies to a multitude of etiogenetic factors. Control of them as potential confounders involves no problem on account their proxy status, while the use of a proxy for the etiogenetic histories – say issuance of prescription in lieu of actual use of the medication at issue – is prone to be problematic.

When at issue is the *use of a medication as a potentially etiogenetic factor*, phenomena of health potentially influenced by that medication's use and taking place prior to the outcome at issue, are not, inherently, deserving members of the ceteris-paribus set, for two reasons, both singly sufficient: they are not proxies for anything extraneous to the factor at issue; and they don't necessarily have causal bearing on the occurrence of that outcome.

This raises the question, How is one to think about a *constitutional characteristic that is influenced by the factor at issue and has, on its own, a causal role in the genesis of the outcome at issue?* For example, in a study of an anti-inflammatory medication-use in the etiogenesis of gastrointestinal bleeding, is the degree of the propensity for getting bruises a member of the ceteris paribus set? The correct answer is affirmative insofar as at issue indeed is this propensity – this proxy for reduced adhesiveness of platelets – in terms of the level at which it would prevail in the absence of the factor at issue (anti-inflammatory treatment for arthritis, say). On the other hand, any entity that is an intermediary in the causation under study – as is the level of platelet adhesiveness under anti-inflammatory treatment in that example – obviously is not extraneous factor; it thus is not a confounder in the study, and conditioning on it would obliterate full manifestation of the etiogenesis at issue.

Actual specification of the ceteris paribus set for a study on a particular antecedent in the etiogenesis of the health entity at issue *requires expertise on the etiogenesis at large of that entity.* Of added help can be some of the theoretical ideas in "the new science of cause and effect" [1].

16.4 The Etiognostic Indicators

Given that an etiognostic study focuses on a causal rate-ratio of the outcome's occurrence (Sect. 15.6.1), etiognostic indicators are *modifiers of the causal rate-ratio to be studied.* For the planning for the object function of an etiognostic study in this respect, a first-order principle is to think of any indicator of the (near-term) risk for the outcome at issue as a potential modifier of the causal RR. This means that *the factors in the ceteris paribus set are among the candidates for being treated as modifiers of the RR at issue.* The magnitude of the causal RR generally is a function, also, of some quantitative aspects of the etiogenetic history at issue; but this does not merit consideration as a special case of etiognostic indicators or modification of the causal RR.

When, as is commonplace in clinical etiognosis, at issue is an adverse event's possible causation by something very recent – very recent use of a particular medication, say – an important modifier of the object RR (incidence density ratio) of the event's occurrence is prone to be the amount of earlier, *pre-etiogenetic experience with the factor at issue.* For, those who experience the event in association with the antecedent at issue tend to discontinue their engagements with that factor; and as a consequence of this, those with *much experience* with the antecedent at issue tend to be select in the sense of having a relatively *low susceptibility* to the event resulting from this etiogenetic factor. Thus, for example, the etiognostic probability for recent use (actual) of a particular anti-inflammatory medication in a case of gastrointestinal bleeding is relatively low if the patient has a history of this medication's extensive use prior to its recent, potentially etiogenetic use.

16.5 The Variates in the Model

Most challenging in the design of the variates for the objects-defining etiognostic occurrence relation generally is the specification of the variates addressing the etiogenetic histories. The point of departure in this is the need to appreciate the general triad of the generic types of these histories, in both etiognostic practice and the studies that serve to advance the knowledge-base of this practice: Associated with some cases of the outcome at issue are *index histories* (about the particulars of the factor at issue – use of aspirin, say – which had been present); some other cases are associated with *reference histories* (about the corresponding particulars of the alternative to the factor at issue – use of ibuprofen, say): and yet other cases have *neither one of these two* (study-relevant types). The epitome of this 'other' type of history in an etiogenetic study is a history that remains unknown. *The challenge* is to provide for focus on the rate ratio (causal) between the index and reference histories, without the presence of the 'other' – uninformative – histories obfuscating this focus.

That triad calls for the definition of *two indicator variates for distinction-making among the three of them*. One of these naturally would indicate the index history. To have the other one of these two variates indicate an extraneous (uninformative) history (as in Sect. 15.6.1) is instructive of the general existence of such histories; and it also is essential: the result of the model's fitting is the empirical function with the value of the indicator for 'other' history set to zero.

Commonly needed also are variates addressing the *particulars* of the index and reference histories, involving the indicator of the index history and the complement of this as the respective multipliers.

In the design of the *ceteris paribus variates*, there is no need for the cultivation of simplicity that is so important in the objects design for diagnostic studies. The reason is that these variates in etiognostic studies merely serve the attainment of the rate-ratio's necessary conditionality on those factors, without their associated parameters being among the objects of the studies. These parameters, therefore, do not contribute to the 'overparametrization' problem that tends to plague diagnostic studies (Sect. 8.3) and can be a concern in an etiognostic study as well.

On the other hand, control of *pseudo-confounders* is not inherently innocuous: it can bias the result, including exaggeration of the magnitude of the effect under study.

16.6 Two Examples of a Study's Objects Design

16.6.1 Prednisone Use in the Etiogenesis of an Illness

While etiognosis about the cared-for population's levels of morbidity is a central concern in community medicine (i.e., in population-level preventive medicine) and etiogenesis of illness hence is equally central a concern in population-level epidemiological research (Sect. 5.7.2), etiognosis about individual cases of illness is a much lesser concern in clinical medicine and hence in patient-level clinical research (Sects. 2.2.2 and 5.1).

But *clinicians do face important etiognostic challenges*, most notably in respect to possible *'iatrogenesis'* – medical causation – of cases of serious illness. Illustrative of these challenges is a *patient being treated with prednisone for temporal arteritis* (TA) who suddenly *comes down with a case of upper gastrointestinal bleeding or pancreatitis*. The treatment of the TA is a potential cause of these illnesses, but its *discontinuation* on this basis is *quite problematic*: the treatment serves very important purposes (those of not only controlling the severe symptoms of the TA but also preventing the development of blindness as a complication of this disease); it has no effective alternative; and it cannot be abruptly discontinued without this, in itself, causing serious problems [2]. For an informed decision about starting to taper off the use of prednisone in a case like this, needed is knowledge for the etiognosis, concerning the probability that the medication's use was etiogenetic to the illness that has emerged – as the treatment's discontinuation presupposes knowing that the probability of this is quite high.

To serve the etiognostic probability-setting in situations like this, needed is study, in a suitably-defined domain of population-time, of the incidence density of the occurrence of the illness at issue – upper GI bleeding or pancreatitis (cf. above) – in causal relation to history of prednisone use, under a suitable log-linear model for this (Sect. 15.6.1).

The *domain* might be defined as that of adults without any previous case of the illness at issue and free of any known risk factors for it, to avoid undue complexities in the objects of study (cf. Sect. 5.1).

The *etiogenetic history* of prednisone use (index history) would focus on use that could have been causal to the occurrence of the illness, the time-frame of which the study's subject-matter advisers would specify. They would also advise on other specifics to be accounted for in these histories, notably whether, apart from dosage, distinctions are to be made according to the route of the drug's administration and the continuous versus intermittent (alternate-day) usage.

Given the indication (temporal arteritis) for prednisone's use in this example, the *reference history* would not address the use of an alternative type of medication; it would be the history of no prednisone use in the time-frame of the index histories. (For, as we noted above, in temporal arteritis there is no alternative to prednisone use).

The *ceteris-paribus factors* accounted for (by variates specific to them) in the model for the incidence density of the illness in the domain defined for the study would be extraneous (non-prednisone) risk factors for the illness. By the design for the domain of the objects of study (above), however, this set could be rather empty, with TA itself naturally not among the factors.

Given the essential absence of major risk-factors operative in the domain of (the objects of) the study, they would not constitute a notable source of *modifiers* of the (causal) rate-ratio function implied by the designed model for the event's incidence density in the domain of this. In the main at least, the model would imply the RR to be a function of the particulars of the history of prednisone use, including its use prior to the period in which the use had its role, if any, in the causation of the illness at issue (Sect. 16.4).

16.6.2 NSAID Use in the Etiogenesis of an Illness

Akin to prednisone use, the use of the various NSAIDs (non-steroidal anti-inflammatory drugs) – aspirin, ibuprofen, etc. – also can be etiogenetic to upper GI bleeding. For various indications, the use of one or more of these medications is an alternative, or supplement, to prednisone use; and for the use of one type of NSAID, the use of another one of these medications generally is an available alternative.

When a case of upper *GI bleeding*, say, occurs in association with a history of the use of NSAIDs, the patient's doctor needs to know about the probability that the case was caused by its antecedent use of a particular NSAID (which the patient had used), as this is relevant to the decision about discontinuation of that drug's use and about its possible replacement with the use of other NSAID.

For such etiognoses needed is research on the causal incidence-density ratio contrasting the history of the use of the NSAID at issue with that of the *alternative* at issue – the use of a particular other NSAID. Suffice it here to consider the (simple) situation in which the patient has used only one type of these medications, with the alternative (counterfactual) of having used a particular other anti-inflammatory medication (non-steroidal or steroidal).

Relative to the etiognosis about prednisone use for temporal arteritis (Sect. 16.6.1, above), *the principal novelty* here is the need for the model (log-linear, for incidence density of the illness event; Sect. 15.5.1) to address, also, the history of the alternative NSAID's use in the periods of time of the medication's use in the index histories. Such a function for the incidence-density ratio provides for estimation of the etiognostic probability for the index history at hand when contrasted with the alternative (counterfactual) history of other NSAID use.

16.6.3 The Objects of Two Example Studies

Adverse effects of the use of medications can be an epidemiological (community-medicine) concern, given that they may justify public policy aimed at protection of the public's health by restriction (incl. prohibition) of the medications' availability for doctors' prescription (to say nothing about their availability 'over the counter'). Otherwise, these effects are of clinical concern alone, addressed in etiognosis and prognosis.

Accordingly, in research on the occurrence of adverse effects of the use of medications, a distinction should be made between epidemiological and clinical research (based on which one of the two main branches of medicine – Sect. 16.4 – is being served by the research), and in clinical research of this type between etiognostic and prognostic research. But as it is, this clinical research is now termed *'pharmacoepidemiology'* (cf. 'clinical epidemiology'; Sect. 6.1), and in this research there now generally *is no clear sense of the (profound) distinction between etiognostic and prognostic causality* (Sect. 15.2). Previous studies on the etiognostic topics addressed in Sects. 16.6.1 and 16.6.2 above are illustrative of this culture.

"Steroids and risk of upper gastrointestinal complications" was the title of the report on a study in this 'epidemiological' class, published in a journal of "epidemiology" in 2001 [3]. The aim of this study was said to have been "to estimate the risk of upper gastrointestinal complications associated with use of steroids alone and in combination with [NSAIDs]." Actually addressed were, however, not the magnitudes of those risks, which are matters of prognostic concern; rather, addressed were etiognostically relevant topics: the causal – confounder-conditional – incidence-density ratios for those events, contrasting histories of those medications' use with histories of their non-use, these in a domain free of certain risk factors for those events. However, the temporal aspect of the index histories was taken to be the time since the discontinuation of the steroid's use, rather than the distinction between the etiogenetic time and the time before that (cf. Sect. 16.4). Given that uses of NSAIDs were not excluded from the domain of the study, they should have been treated (not only as obvious confounders but, thereby, also) with other modifiers of the rate ratio addressing the steroids' use (cf. Sect. 16.4). The incidence-density ratio (confounder-conditional) for whichever outcome was not addressed as a function of the particulars of the etiogenetic histories together with other modifiers of it. And the Abstract ended with this non-sequitur, clinical rather than epidemiological: "Whenever possible, antiinflammatory drugs should be given in monotherapy and at the lowest effective dose in order to reduce the risk of upper gastrointestinal complications."

The same authors published, a few years later in the same journal, an article entitled "Risk of uncomplicated peptic ulcer among users of aspirin and nonaspirin nonsteroidal antiinflammatory drugs" [4]. Analogously with that previous study [3], they had "performed a nested case-control analysis [of a general-practice database] to study the association between the risk of these ulcers and the use of aspirin and nonaspirin NSAIDs." The main novelty in the objects of study had to do with *the term to denote the illness event's incidence-density ratio:* in that previous study it was termed "odds ratio," while in this newer study the term for it was "relative risk."

References

1. Pearl J, MacKinsey D (2018) The book of why. The new science of cause and effect. Basic Books, New York
2. Delecoeuillerie G, Joly P, Cohen de Lara A, Paolaggi JB (1988) Polymyalgia rheumatica and temporal arteritis: a retrospective analysis of prognostic features and different corticosteroid regimens (11 year survey of 210 patients). Ann Rheum Dis 47:733–739
3. Hernandez-Diaz S, Garcia Rodriguez LA (2001) Steroids and risk of upper gastrointestinal complications. Am J Epidemiol 153:1089–1093
4. Garcia Rodriguez LA, Hernandez-Diaz S (2004) Risk of uncomplicated peptic ulcer among users of aspirin and nonaspirin nonsteroidal antiinflammatory drugs. Am J Epidemiol 159:23–31

Chapter 17
Methods Design for an Etiognostic Study

Contents

Abstract Etiognostic research is an exceptionally challenging species of gnostic clinical research. Even though such research is of centrally-important service to the practice of epidemiology (community medicine, community-level preventive medicine, i.e.) and already very common, the theoretical underpinnings – concepts and principles – of this research remain quite inadequately understood. An effort is made here to *rectify the main misunderstandings* in etiognostic epidemiological research, with a view to future clinical researchers' preparation for research to advance the knowledge-base of etiognosis – and intervention-prognosis too – in clinical medicine. An important role in that research is now played by *a general-practice database* for clinical research, in the framework of which valid etiognostic clinical research is readily accomplished. This database serves as a *paradigm* for major advancement of the infrastructure for gnostic clinical research at large.

O. S. Miettinen et al., *Clinical Research Transformed*,
https://doi.org/10.1007/978-3-030-06176-0_17

Keywords Example study · Source population · Source base · Study base · Case series · Base sample · Documentation of the series · Synthesis of the data · Report on the study

17.1 An Example of the Elements in the Studies

An instructive example to consider here is the one on the use of steroids, the objects of which were addressed in Sect. 16.6.3, above. In that study [1], the investigators "used data from an ongoing population-based study to assess the risk of upper gastrointestinal complications related to steroid treatment, as well as the potential interaction between steroids and NSAIDs."

17.1.1 Context: The Study's Objects Design

As a matter of general concepts, a *method* is a means to a pre-set end, actual or potential. In suitably purposive patient-level clinical research, the end – the *objective* – generally is to make a contribution to the evidence for the knowledge-base of (a certain aspect of) the practice of clinical medicine (Sect. 2.2), and the *means* to this end is (the implementation of) the designed methods – methodology – of a gnostic study, a piece of gnostic clinical research (Sect. 2.3).

The evidence from a piece of gnostic research is the published result of it, together with documentation of the methodology in its production/genesis. The result has a given (ideally pre-set) form in reference to a given domain (abstract); and from the study in question it has empirical content of that form in reference to the study base, which represented the study objects' domain. Ideally – and realistically just the same – the abstract counterpart of the result of a gnostic clinical study stems from the study's *objects design*; the form is that of an etiognostic probability function for a given domain, or a rate-ratio function (causal) implying etiognostic probabilities (Sect. 16.1.2).

In line with the still-prevailing culture in gnostic clinical research, the report of the *example study* at issue here [1] did not even allude to, much less specify, any pre-designed form-cum-referent of a gnostic probability or rate-ratio function. The *objective* of the study was said to have been "to assess the risk of upper gastrointestinal complications related to steroid treatment, as well as the potential interaction between steroids and NSAIDs" (Cf. Sect. 16.6.3). And the forms of the reported results were not those of any functions. Two *examples of the results* on the occurrence of those "complications" were these: "for current use of oral steroids" the "odds ratio" was …"; and "Simultaneous use of steroids with low-medium and high NSAID doses, respectively, produced odds ratios of …"

17.1.2 *The Selection/Formation of the Source Population*

The investigators exploited – to great advantage – a recent development, namely that some 1500 general practices in the United Kingdom had been, since 1990, in a research-serving routine [2]: those practices "systematically store in office computers clinical information on their patients including demographics, diagnoses and comments, referral information, and all prescriptions issued by them." Included are data on "all referrals to specialists, hospital admissions, and results from these visits."

On this basis, it would have been natural to simply *select* as the study's *source population* the collective *catchment population* of those practices – the population whose members, in their use of clinical healthcare in the framework of the National Health Service of the U.K., would receive their primary care (exclusively) from the general practitioners in those "research practices" and secondary and tertiary care on the basis of these GPs' referrals. But the investigators did not select this population – open, dynamic (Sect. 5.2.1) – as the source population for their study population. They gave no explanation for this, nor for what they did instead.

For the role of their study's source population the investigators *elected to form a cohort* from members of that dynamic population. Membership in this cohort was defined as of April 1993, in terms of being, at that time, not only (alive and) a member of the practices' catchment population but satisfying, also, certain other admissibility criteria at that time: having been a member of the catchment population for 2 years at least and being of age 40–79 years as well as "free of cancer, esophageal varices, Mallory-Weiss disease, liver disease, coagulopathies, and alcohol-related disorders." The size of this cohort was 958,397.

17.1.3 *The Selection of the Source Population-Time*

With the source population thus formed, it remained to select and specify the segment of its course over time that constituted the source population-time – *the source base* – within which the study population-time – the actual study base – was going to be defined. This was set as "the period between April 1993 and October 1998."

17.1.4 *The Identification of the Cases in the Source*

From that source base, the investigators identified all instances of patient referral to secondary or tertiary care that resulted in a rule-in diagnosis about the illness event at issue. From the reports on these referrals, they

> identified [instances of] codes for upper gastrointestinal complications and manually reviewed the information in their computerized patient profiles. To validate the cases we sent the general practitioners a questionnaire for a random sample of 100 patients. We received information on 99 [of these cases] with only one [of them] not confirmed as a case of upper gastrointestinal complications.

Cases "with the source of the bleed/perforation in the esophagus or lower gastrointestinal tract … were excluded."

17.1.5 The Selection of a Sample of the Source

Having thus identified all the cases (2105 in number) of the "complication" at issue that occurred in the study's source base, the investigators supplemented this series of instances (person-moments) by selecting a sample (of size 11,500) of the person-moments (infinite in number) constituting the source base of the study.

This sample from the source base was *matched* to the case series from it by age and gender; but conditionally on age and gender, the selection was random (to make the sample representative of the source base of the study within the age-gender strata of the source population-time).

17.1.6 The Formation of the Study Series, Documented

This first-stage case series and its corresponding base series – both of these having the study's source base as their (shared) referent – were reduced to *instances/person-moments from the actual study base*. This reduction was a matter of excluding the instances in which the person, while having satisfied the domain's exclusion criteria at entry into the source cohort, no longer satisfied these requirements at the time of the contribution to one of the two series of person-moments from the actual study base.

Using the pre-existing database, the two thus-formed study series were *documented* in terms of all that was deemed to be relevant (and available in the database used for the study).

17.1.7 The Synthesis of the Data into Study Results

The data on the actual study series (the second-stage case and base/referent series) were translated into the corresponding realizations of adopted statistical variates. For the production of the *main results* – the incidence-density ratios having to do with medication use that was current at the time of the upper GI event – the *main independent variates* were an indicator of steroids use alone and of steroids use in combination with NSAIDs use. Other variates were defined for "age, sex, calendar year, smoking, antecedents of upper gastrointestinal disorders, aspirin, and anticoagulant use"; and *logistic models* were fitted to these two statistical-type datasets, with the (confounder-conditional) *incidence-density ratios* derived as the exponentials of the fitted values of the parameters associated with the indicator of current use of steroids alone, or steroids use in combination with NSAIDs (Cf. Sects. 7.4.4 and 15.6).

17.1.8 The Reporting of the Study

As background for this study, said in the report (in its opening paragraph) was that "the literature on corticosteroids as an independent risk factor for upper gastrointestinal complications in the general population is limited." Implicitly taking this to be a deficiency in the evidence-base for the knowledge-base of community medicine, the investigators published the report on the study in a *journal of epidemiological research* [1] – in this journal's customary style for etiologic/etiogenetic studies (advancing the knowledge-base of prevention-oriented etiognoses about rates of morbidity in populations served in community medicine; Sect. 5.7.2).

The report's Abstract closed with a *guideline for (not epidemiological but) clinical practice*: "Whenever possible, antiinflammatory drugs should be given in monotherapy and at the lowest level of effective dose in order to reduce the risk of upper gastrointestinal complications."

17.2 The Example Critically Examined

17.2.1 The Source Population-Time

The concept of source population-time did not come up in the context of *diagnostic* research (Part IV). The reason for this is that the study base in diagnostic research never is an aggregate of study population-time but is, always, a series (finite) of person-moments (Sect. 12.7.1 and Chap. 14). In diagnostic studies, the study person-moments are enrolled, selectively, from among identified candidate-cases for this (in the formation of the study series of person-moments); and rather than a chosen source population-time (for the study population-time), in diagnostic studies there is merely the chosen setting for the identification of candidate cases for enrolment into the study series, exploited for a given period of time (Sect. 12.3.1).

For an *etiognostic* study, a source population-time – as the *source base* – is needed. As *one option*, the population for this can be formed, ad hoc, by enrolment of members into a *cohort-type source population* for the study, with the study's source base formed by (the documented segment of) this population's course over a specified period of time. The study at issue here is an example of such formation (active) of the source base (Sect. 17.1, above). An *alternative* for this would have been mere selection/adoption of the practices' catchment population's course over a chosen span of time, notably that of the population – open, dynamic – served by the practices. This would have been the preferable option, more natural.

This design for our example study's *source population was of very high quality scientifically*, as it provided for (a) complete identification of the cases of the illness in question in the source population-time, (b) valid sampling of this source base, and (c) valid ascertainment of the relevant facts on the two series from the source base. Besides, the design for the source base in the framework of this source population was of very high *economic quality*, as the relevant data had been pre-recorded, and in cyberspace at that.

Notable – and instructive – about the designed *source* base of that study is, also, its *size*, which resulted from the size of the source cohort together with the duration of its follow-up: the study's size was *not set by any statistical hocus-pocus* (cf. Sect. 12.2.4). Instead, the investigators, by means of that study, made a contribution of information about the objects of study to the extent that they were willing and able to make it – when among the options was, for example, making no contribution at all.

17.2.2 The Series from the Source Base

The identification of the series of cases of the illness at issue that occurred in the source base was inherent in the choice of the nature of the source base (Sect. 17.2.1, above). No design specific for this was needed nor developed. But the sampling of the source base, by contrast, was designed and executed with great finesse:

> a random date within the study period was generated for each of the members of the [source] cohort. All persons with a random date included in their person-time period of observation (from study entry to end of follow-up) were eligible [to contribute a person-moment to the sample of the source base].

Then, from among these eligible person-moments (958,397 in number) a *sample* (of size 11,500) was drawn, matched to the case series of these by "age (interval 1 year) and gender."

This *matching* in the selection of the sample of the source population-time was, however, a case of *hocus-pocus of the epidemiological kind*, almost as vacuous as the statistical 'sample size determination' alluded to in Sect. 17.2.1 above. Relevant to validity of the source-base sampling in an etiogenetic/etiognostic study is merely the selections' independence of the etiogenetic histories and of correlates of these not accounted for in the conditionality built into the study result for the rate ratio. Thus, a *completely indiscriminate sample of the source base (of all the person-moments in it) would have been just as valid* as the one so artfully selected, given that, in the synthesis of the data, the matching factors (age and gender) had to be – and indeed were – controlled, jointly with all the other ceteris-paribus (confounding) factors. Nor was the matching justifiable on the grounds of the *efficiency* of the study.

17.2.3 The Study Series, Documented

The two series from the source population-time were not used as the actual series for the study; instead, certain exclusions were applied, equally, to the two first-stage series: the admissibility criteria applied at the entries into the study's source cohort were reapplied at the times of follow-up involved in those two series – though not exactly at those times but "in the 2 months after the date [of the person-moment]." Thus, excluded from those first-stage series (from the source base) were instances which, at the point in cohort time that was at issue, no longer represented the study objects' domain (Sect. 17.1.2): the person, while alive, no longer was of age 40–79 and also free of cancer, etc. Besides, discharge from a hospital in the previous 2 weeks became an added criterion for exclusion.

This selective inclusion into the actual study series the members of the study series (the first-stage case and base series whose referent is the source base) is very notable – and highly instructive – feature of the study at issue here. The reduction of the source-base series to the actual study series, performed in that study, *should be a feature of all etiogenetic studies* (Sect. 15.6.2); but it is quite routinely missing from these studies (the essence of which is, still, commonly misunderstood by epidemiological researchers; Sects. 15.6.2 and 16.6.3).

At issue here is a *case-base* or *case-referent* study, not a case-control study, of etiogenesis (Sects. 15.6.2 and 15.6.3). The authors misrepresented this by writing about their "case-control analysis" of the data in it. The formation of the source cohort presumably was motivated by the concern – wholly unjustified – to create the appearance of a 'cohort study' (rather than effecting the appropriate, case-referent/case-based study).

17.2.4 The Synthesis of the Data

Even though the report on the study did not specify the variates involved in the logistic regression model in terms of which the results were derived from the data, it is clear from the form of the reported results that *the model was not correctly formulated* to address "the potential interaction between [the use of] steroids and [that of] NSAIDs" (Cf. Sect. 17.1.7).

In its general usage, the term *'interaction'* between A and B denotes their mutual action, action on each other; the meaning is that A acts on B and B acts on

A. Illustrative of this concept is the love-time interaction pointed out by Euripides: "Love makes time pass. Time makes love pass."

In *clinical pharmacology*, however, interaction between drug A and drug B does not mean that they act on each other (in the human soma). Rather, the meaning of 'interaction' between the two is that the (magnitude of the) effect of the use of one of them depends on the concomitant use/non-use of the other. Thus, steroids-NSAIDs 'interaction' in these pharmacological terms means that the magnitude of the steroids' effect at issue depends on the use/non-use of NSAIDs parallel with the steroids' use (and mutatis mutandis).

In *epidemiology*, the counterpart of pharmacologists' 'interaction' is 'effect modification.' The case in point about this is modification of an etiogenetic rate-ratio having to do with history of use versus non-use of steroids: it has do with this rate-ratio's dependence on the use/non-use of NSAIDs concomitantly with the steroids' use. Study of this modification ("interaction") was one of the two overall objectives in the study at issue here, and study of this modification in the theoretical framework of logistic regression would have required, in the simplest possible terms, supplementation of the indicators for the two types of medication use by a variate representing *the product of the two variates* (Sect. 15.6.1). *Statisticians* call those product terms interaction terms, and regardless of whether any actions/effects are at issue.

Had this "interaction" actually been studied, reported would have been the way in which the steroids-addressing rate-ratio (in the study base, the results' referent) depended on the use of NSAIDs concomitantly with the steroids use, current or discontinued. But *addressed instead was joint use of the two types of medication versus use of neither one of them* – joint action rather than interaction.

17.2.5 The Reporting on the Study

The published report on a gnostic clinical study, etiognostic or other, is the means through which the study advances the evidence-base of knowledge for (an aspect of) clinical medicine. The report on an original study brings forth (previously unavailable) evidence about the magnitudes of the parameters of Nature that, as elements in a gnostic probably function, constitute the objects of the study proper. Actually reported was not a case-control study but a case-referent (case-base) study (cf. above).

The *evidence* from a particular piece of gnostic clinical research is constituted not by its reported result as such – the empirical counterpart of the designed gnostic probability function (or the rate-ratio function that, for etiognosis, implies the probability function) – but *the reported result together with documentation of how it was obtained*, notably in respect to what bears on judgements about its validity. (The precisions of the empirical values of the object parameters are quantified statistically, with measures of this automatically associated with their modern, software-based empirical values; Sect. 8.2).

The report on the example study at issue here [1] had *a number of notable deficiencies*. Some examples of these follow.

The very first problem with the report had to do with specification of what the study was about, resulting in *confusion about whether at issue was an etiognostic study or an intervention-prognostic one* (or neither perhaps). The report's title was wholly enigmatic in this orientational regard, and the one-sentence paragraph about the nature of the study in the report's two-paragraph introductory section didn't clarify this either. It was necessary to study the Abstract to learn that at issue was an etiologic/etiogenetic study, specifically a "nested case-control [trohoc] study" rather than a 'cohort' study, *in the framework of the still-commonplace pair of fallacies about the nature of etiogenetic studies* (Sect. 15.6.2), even though the singular essence of these studies can be (logically) deduced from the very concept of etiogenesis [3]. Different from a 'case-control' study, its first-principles counterpart – a case-referent/case-base study (Sect. 15.6.2) – is inherently "nested" (in the study result's referent, the study base).

This confusion about the general essence of etiogenetic studies took other manifestations as well: the study was said to be "population-based," thereby falsely implying that there was an alternative to this feature of the study; and there was manifest confusion about whether at issue actually was a 'case-control' study or a *'cohort' study*: the listed keywords included no version of the "nested case-control analysis" term used in the Abstract and under "Data analysis," but the listed keywords did include "cohort studies" even though no version of this term actually appeared in the report proper.

"Within our source population," the report said, "we performed a nested case-control analysis." But the referent of the results from this "analysis" was not the study's source population per se nor the source population-time of its follow-up but the study population-time, the study base, imbedded in the source population-time. *The authors evidently did not have the respective concepts of source population and study population*, given that the cohort that served as the source population for the study was described under the rubric "Study population," without the study population addressed under it nor elsewhere.

With this "analysis" performed in terms of fitting logistic regression models to the data, it is a major deficiency in the report that *these models were not specified* as to what the independent variates in them were. The only characterization of them was that they were "*multivariate models*," the meaning of which in statistics is not what was meant by the authors, which was multiple-regression models.

The results of the fittings of the (unspecified) multiple-regression models (logistic) were systematically referred to as "*odds ratios*," in line with what is commonplace in reports of 'case-control' studies involving logistic regression (while 'hazard ratios' is the common counterpart of this in reports from 'cohort' studies involving Cox regression). In truth, however, the results of those model-fittings did not represent odds ratios but were, instead, empirical incidence-density ratios (with the study base as their referent; Sect. 15.6.1).

17.3 General Principles of the Studies' Design

The foregoing on this most challenging species of gnostic clinical research – from the essence of etiogenesis as a species of causation (Sect. 15.2) through the generic nature of the objects of etiognostic studies (Chap. 16) to an example of the objects and methods in an example study on iatrogenesis of an illness, both described (Sect. 17.1) and critically reviewed (Sect. 17.2) – is here rounded out by an epilogue of sorts.

17.3.1 The Essence of the Study Base

With the two study series – the case series and the base/referent series – the structural core of any etiogenetic study on an event-type outcome, and with the study base the referent of both of these (as set forth in Sect. 15.6.2 and illustrated by the example study in Sects. 17.1 and 17.2), *pivotal to understanding of the methodology of etiognostic studies* is appreciation of the general essence of the study base in these studies.

As the example study illustrates, the *instances of admission into the case series* of an etiognostic (or other etiogenetic) study – that is, into the series of all the person-moments in the study base at which a case of the event at issue occurred – need to satisfy, at those moments, *the criteria definitional to the domain of the study* (Sect. 17.1.6). This the investigators understood to be a *transient state* in the example study (ibid.), and so it is in general (as survival, i.a., is a transient state).

This is to say that *the study population* in etiognostic research *inherently is dynamic* (open for exit), *even if the source population is of the cohort type* (closed for exit). Thus, insofar as the term 'cohort study' has any justifiable denotation in reference to an etiogenetic study, it must be that the source population – though not the actual study population – was of the cohort type. Whereas one of the keywords in the report of that example study was "cohort studies," the correct meaning of this would have been the inconsequential one that *the source population* was (made to be) a cohort, while it *could – and preferably would – have been dynamic:* the (existing) catchment population of the practices involved (Sect. 17.3.2, below).

17.3.2 The Definition of the Source Population

The source population for an etiognostic study can be defined directly. An example of this is the way the source population was formed, and thereby defined, in the example study [1] so extensively addressed in this Chapter. While that source population was of the *cohort* type, just as direct can be the source population's definition as a *dynamic* population, such as the resident population (dynamic) for a particular metropolitan area or the population participating in a particular program of health insurance.

Alternatively, a direct definition is given to the way in which cases of the entity of health at issue – the one whose rate of occurrence in relation (causal) to the antecedent of etiognostic concern the study will address (in reference to a defined domain) – will be identified for the study (for its first-stage case series, through select practices of clinical healthcare). Given this aprioristic definition of the case identification, *the source population of the study is thereby defined, indirectly, as the catchment population of this scheme of case identification.* Membership in this population – open, dynamic – is defined by the were-would state of: were a case of that health event now to occur, it would be 'caught' by that scheme of case identification. An example of this in our example study could have been, as an alternative to the formation of the source cohort, the definition of the study's source population as the participating practices' catchment population (dynamic) for cases of upper GI "complication."

With direct definition of the source population and then the source population-time, *valid identification of the cases* occurring in the source base – with their complete identification the general means of assuring that the identifications are independent of the etiogenetic histories at issue – *is prone to be a major challenge,* while valid sampling of such a source base generally is quite feasible (on account of availability of the population's membership lists). Complete case-identification for a directly-defined population can require canvassing all the care facilities in which the population's cases of the event at issue are identified (i.e., rule-in diagnosed) as such.

When direct definition is given to the scheme of case identification, this identification for the (thus indirectly defined) source population and source base is complete by definition, but now *the challenge is valid sampling of the source population-time.* This challenge tends to be greatest when the settings of case identification are arbitrarily scattered. By the same token, this problem tends to vanish when the case identification is of the canvassing sort that it may need to be when the source population is defined directly. When this is done, the distinction between direct and indirect definition of the source population-time vanishes.

The *"research-practices"* setting for our example study here serves to illustrate the *ideal type of setting* for the definition of the source population for an etiognostic study. It is characterized by well-founded ambivalence about the duality constituted by the source population's direct and indirect definitions. In the framework of those practices, *one natural option* would have been to define the source population directly, as the population (dynamic) served by those practices. In this case the generally-challenging case identification from a directly-defined source base would have been, exceptionally, effortlessly and securely complete by virtue of the very nature of that set of practices (as both gate-keepers for all of healthcare and record-keepers for all of it too). *Another natural option* would have been to define the source population indirectly, by making primary commitment to case identification by means of those practices' database, in consequence of which the case ascertainment would have been complete for the source population constituted by the catchment population of those practices for the health outcome at issue. Either way, the practices' database would have been the basis not only for complete case-identification for the study's source base, but for valid sampling of this as well. *The formation of a cohort-type source population was unnatural, uncalled-for, though consistent with validity.*

17.4 The Example Study as a Paradigm

The study we've so extensively considered in this Chapter on etiognostic clinical research has served the purpose of illustrating the nature of the prevailing thinking about the methods of studies on the etiology/etiogenesis of an illness (Sect. 17.1) and, thereby, the shortcomings of the prevailing theoretical underpinnings – concepts and principles – of this research (Sect. 17.2). Besides, there also is something profoundly paradigmatic about this study.

Paradigmatic about that example study is not so much that study per se as the very propitious setting that was available for – and actually exploited in – its design and execution (Sect. 17.1.2, above), a setting prepared and maintained (by others) as a resource for a vast variety of (unspecified) clinical studies – the U.K. General Practice Research Database [2]. This multipurpose resource for clinical research in its general-practice setting serves as a paradigm for the development of its counterparts for other discipline-specific settings of clinical medicine – gastrointestinal, rheumatological etc.

Quite central in our vision of suitably *transformed clinical research* (the theory of which we address in this book) also is the development and maintenance of a *system of clinical informatics* for it (Chap. 25 and App. 2). This system, however, will not be based on practices in a single discipline of clinical medicine – or even in a select set of these – in a non-academic setting. It will cover *all disciplines of clinical medicine, in the hospital systems of a number of first-rank faculties of medicine.*

As at issue are academic hospitals, a well-designed system of clinical informatics (digital) for them serves – well – not only the needs of the care provided in those hospitals. The system's structure and contents – fully consistent with the needs of high-quality practice – are designed to also serve, secondarily yet optimally, the needs of *teaching* the practice.

The practices and teachings in these hospitals naturally revolve around the various *types of case presentation* for gnosis (dia-, etio-, or prognosis) and for care predicated on those insights (into the clients' health). This means that identification and specification of the various types of case presentation constitute the key principle in the design of the *structure ('architecture') of* an optimal system of informatics for both the care and the teaching about it in these hospitals.

Given a case presentation of a given type, the gnostic practice of further fact-acquisition prompted by it, in a teaching hospital in particular, is to be in accord with up-to-date teaching about what is relevant to ascertain for the gnostic profiles of cases from this domain of case presentation. The generic contents in cases of particular types of presentation serve this aspect of teaching in these hospitals.

Once the gnostic profile of a case (from a particular domain of case presentations) is first completed in relevant respects – in accord with the state of the art – the practice and teaching in academic hospitals turns to the profile's translation into *gnostic probabilities.* In this, at present, the teachers involved generally present their respective opinions or guesses about these. But in many of the cases, for diagnosis and prognosis, the *truths* at issue in this ultimately becomes matters of fact, and the system is to document the basis for this, for both the practice and the teaching.

For the purposes of gnostic clinical *research,* the point of all of this is straightforward: a system of informatics that is optimal for patient care and teaching in academic hospitals is, secondary to this, is optimal also for the research that serves to produce the knowledge-base for those academic functions – and, secondary to this, for the development of the clinical 'expert systems' that would guide scientific practice of clinical medicine in settings non-academic as well as academic.

The development of the prototype of such a system of clinical informatics, for cloning in the other academic hospitals participating in the envisioned international program of gnostic clinical research is initially a matter of collaboration between the *epidemiologic* and clinical segments of the faculty in the pioneering role (Sects. 6.5 and 25.2, and App. 2). But thereupon, expertise in *information technology* (incl. 'blockchain technology') will have a critically-important role.

References

1. Hernandez-Diaz S, Garcia Rodriguez LA (2001) Steroids and risk of upper gastrointestinal complications. Am J Epidemiol 153:1089–1093
2. Walley T, Mantgani A (1997) The UK general practice research database. Lancet 350:1097–1099
3. Miettinen OS, Karp I (2012) Epidemiological research: an introduction. Springer, Dordrecht

Part VI
Prognostic Research

Chapter 18
Introduction to Prognostic Research

Contents

Abstract While diagnosis is purely descriptive/acausal knowing and etiognosis is purely causal knowing, prognosis generally is both of these: *causal* in respect to the contemplated or actually adopted treatments and *acausal* conditionally on these. Prognosis generally is first about *survival,* and then about *outcome* or *course* or both conditionally on survival. In thinking about prognoses and also in models for prognostic probabilities, further distinctions need to be made among acute, subacute, and chronic prognoses. And while actual studies for each of these three species of prognosis have their correspondingly differentiated general essence, which fundamentally has to do with the essence of the study base, there generally is an important duality in the way the study base of a prognostic study is constituted.

Keywords Prognosis as gnosis · Survival prognosis · Health prognosis · Time horizon of prognosis · Causal determinants · Acausal determinants · Statistical models · Cohort studies · Non-cohort studies

O. S. Miettinen et al., *Clinical Research Transformed*,
https://doi.org/10.1007/978-3-030-06176-0_18

18.1 Prognosis as a Species of Gnosis

In Chap. 1 of this book we diverged from the common idea of what medicine is about, from the characterization of medicine as 'a healing profession.' We posited the alternative idea that the disciplines of clinical medicine are not healing but *teaching professions*: that the essence of clinical doctors' work – 'doctoring' – is not heeling (which is rare even in modern medicine) but – as the etymology of 'doctor' suggests – teaching the clients about their health. And we naturally took the basis of this teaching to be clinical doctors' esoteric case-by-case knowing about their clients' health, *gnosis*: knowing about what it is (diagnosis), why it is what it is (etiognosis), and/or what it will be (prognosis).

The concept of gnosis, with *prognosis* one of those three species of this esoteric knowing that form the basis of clinicians' doctoring, is *not* manifest in eminent *dictionaries* of medicine (1, 2, i.a.): in them, the concept of diagnosis is presented as one of process (determination), etiognosis is not defined at all, and prognosis is presented as a forecast or prediction of what likely will happen in the client's health.

To us, *prognosis subsumes knowing about unlikely developments as well*, about the probabilities of these; and knowing about a possible development's low probability is not forecasting or prediction of this development.

While diagnosis commonly is the pivotal one among the three species of clinicians' gnoses, *prognosis generally is the principal species of gnosis*, that which matters most, if not solely, to patients and others consulting clinical doctors. A client who is one of the 'worried well' (and hence not a patient) is prone to be looking, specifically, for prognostic teaching – about his/her risk of later coming down with an overt case of some serious illness (a particular type of cancer, say) and about ways (prospective) to mitigate this risk. And a patient presenting with a case of sickness is less concerned with the nature of the underlying illness than with the future course of the sickness and how best this course could be ameliorated.

18.2 The Fundamental Duality in Prognosis

In prognosis there is, in general, a *fundamental duality*, a hierarchical one. It is constituted by prognosis about *survival* and, then, prognoses about *health* conditional on survival.

18.2.1 Prognosis about Survival

Prognoses about a person's future health in reference to whatever point or period of prospective time is predicated on the premise that the person actually will have a future through the time in question; that (s)he will survive throughout that time, at least. For, health – in the broader sense that encompasses ill-health (illness) in addition to freedom from illness – is a topic in reference to the living only. Hence, *meaningful prognosis in the practice of clinical medicine inescapably is, before anything else, about survival* – tacitly at least.

Prognosis about 'survival' through a given span of prospective time is a euphemistic expression for prognosis about death, about it not having occurred by the end of that period. Thus, for example, prognosis as an estimate of the probability of a patient surviving at least another 5 years is the complement of (i.e., 1 minus) the corresponding estimate of the probability of the patient's death occurring within the next 5 years. Survival over a span of time is the consequence of the (continuing) non-occurrence of death over that period; and for survival prognosis, therefore, the knowledge-base is about the *probability of the occurrence of death*, cumulative over the period of prognostic time at issue.

While there naturally is interest in prognostication about death per se, knowledge-based prognosis about death is *focused on one potential cause of death* at a time, the probability of dying from this conditionally on not succumbing to any other, 'competing' cause of death. The probability of dying from whichever one of a set of possible causes can be based on such conditional probabilities of the cause-specific death: If for causes 1 and 2 those probabilities are P_1 and P_2, then the probability of dying from one of them is $P_1 + (1 - P_1)P_2$. For three causes the probability is this plus the complement of this multiplied by P_3; etc.

18.2.2 Prognoses about Health

While survival prognosis is about a single entity of health (the event of death), a similar focus can obtain survival-conditionally as well. In particular, a client expressing worry about his/her risk of coming down with an overt case of a serious illness generally specifies the illness at issue, and the doctor needs to prognosticate the level of the risk for this particular development over particular spans of prospective/prognostic time.

Typically, though, prognosis about health (survival-conditional) is non-singular in respect to the entities of health that are at issue. This non-singularity of the objects of prognosis obtains even in the context of illnesses that are acute in the meaning of their course being of quite short a duration. In these contexts the prognoses focus, for practical purposes, on the possible *outcomes* of the illness at the completion of its course; but even with this focus, there is the need to supplement survival prognosis with (survival-conditional) prognosis about complete recovery and about each of the possible sequelae representing incomplete recovery. And besides, some states of ill-health representing possible *adverse effects of the treatment* of the illness may need to be considered in reference to the time of the completion of the course of the episode.

18.3 The Time Horizons in Prognoses

As prognoses are about events and states in prospective/prognostic time, they have *temporal referents* on the scale of this time, the zero point of which is the time of the prognostications.

In respect to *acute, short-duration illnesses* the time horizon of prognoses inherently is coterminous with the case of illness at issue, and the temporal referent of the prognoses is singular: the time when the course of the illness – a disease or an injury – comes to its end (cf. above). At issue in such fixed-time prognoses can be the possible outcomes not only of the illness itself but also of injuries from its treatment(s).

In respect to *subacute and life-long illnesses* (the latter being neither self-limiting nor curable) the time horizon of some prognoses also are coterminous with the duration of the condition; but the time horizon can also be very short, as in the case of prognosticating the (acute) outcome of surgical treatment of a chronic illness. Such short-term prognoses need to be supplemented by prognoses conditional on short-term survival.

18.4 The Determinants of Prognostic Probabilities

18.4.1 Causal Determinants

Whereas prognosis is a doctor's first-hand knowing – esoteric, probabilistic – about a client's prospective survival and (survival-conditional) health (Sects. 18.1 and 18.2), and whereas a doctor's main prospective concern generally is to effect improvements in these, the medically most-relevant determinants of prognostic probabilities generally are ones having to do with *treatments*, prophylactic and therapeutic. A treatment is supposed to be *negatively-causal* to the outcomes it is intended to prevent (or postpone). And a treatment is, also, of concern in *positively-causal* determination of their adverse outcomes (complications).

As causes of prospective outcomes, the treatments addressed in prognostic studies need to be *explicitly defined* to sufficient extent and detail, over the entire prognostic time horizon in the study; each of the treatments needs to be defined as an *algorithm* that encompasses all of its component treatments.

In an *experimental* intervention-prognostic study there generally is a single treatment-based determinant (involving at least two treatments), and several (types of) outcomes potentially influenced by it are addressed. A *non-experimental* intervention-prognostic study typically addresses a single (type of) outcome, its treatment-related etiogenesis; and more than one such determinant is readily accommodated in such a study.

Causal determinants of prognostic probabilities include, also, factors other than treatments. The species of these are, in principle, the same as in etiognostic research:

constitutional, environmental, and behavioral (Sect. 15.4). The causal contrasts based on these are prospective in prognostic research, in contrast to their retrospective counterparts in etiognostic research (Sect. 15.2).

18.4.2 Acausal Determinants

Conditionally on the choice (contemplated or actual) of prospective treatment and on whatever premises, if any, about causally-relevant prospective lifestyle, prognostic probabilities generally have acausal (non-causal) determinants as well. Preeminent among these, in preventive medicine in particular, generally is the person's *age*; for even though it is a proxy for various unspecifiable/cryptic constitutional causes, it is not a causal factor in itself, as it has no alternative for any actually existing person (Sect. 16.3). And a particularly eminent acausal determinant of prognostic probabilities in therapeutic ('curative') medicine generally is the *indication for treatment*, as the particulars of this, akin to age, are an aprioristic given, with no alternative in the case at issue.

Prognostically acausal indicators *include etiognostically causal factors*: In etiognosis, the histories of etiogenetic interest have alternatives (counterfactual) that could have been the factual ones; but for prognostic purposes these histories have no alternatives; for prognoses they are aprioristic givens, and their prognostic roles are, therefore, acausal. For example, the history (positive) of the use of prednisone in the time period in which it could have been causal to the upper GI bleeding that has occurred can be addressed in causal terms, as the history could have been its defined counterfactual alternative; but prognostically the patient's actual history (*sic*) of prednisone use (as of the time of the prognostication) has no alternative; it thus is an acausal attribute of the patient, akin to age and gender, say.

Further in this vein, a *treatment* is an acausal feature of the case conditionally on a particular category of it; for on this condition it, like gender or age, has no alternative but is, merely, a definer of a subdomain of prognostication – and prognostically relevant as such.

18.5 The Essence of Prognostic Models

In prognostic models, distinctions need to be made according to the *time horizon* of these. Models for *acute* prognoses focus on survival and other outcomes of the course of episodes of short-duration illnesses (such as myocardial infarction) or the short-term outcome of a preventive or therapeutic procedure (such as an injection or a surgery). Those for *subacute* prognoses also address survival and other outcomes of cases; but in addition they address relevant phenomena of health prior to the completion of the course of the case. Models for *chronic* prognoses address the outcome of the course of the illness in terms of the duration of survival and (pre-mortem) outcomes of health as well.

With the exception of models for the outcomes at the end of a very-short-term course, prognostic models need to incorporate *timings* for the outcomes they address, those of death from the illness included. Besides, the models for all interim outcomes within the overall time horizon of prognosis need to be, expressly, *survival-conditional* (cf. Sect. 18.2.1).

And while the models for short-term outcomes are, directly, ones of probability, those for *interim events* of health need to be about the *incidence density* of their occurrence as functions of prognostic time (jointly with the prognostic indicators at the time of the prognostication and the course-influencing choices made at that time). These models imply their counterparts for cumulative incidence (Sect. 5.5.4) and, thereby, for probabilities (cumulative). For *states* of health, the models address their prevalence and, thereby, their probability.

18.6 Types of Prognostic Studies

18.6.1 Prognostic Cohort Studies

Given the inherently prospective nature of the referents of prognoses (from the temporal vantage of the prognostications), it is natural to first think of prognostic studies of the type in which the actual *study population* is a cohort enrolled from the domain of the prognostications the study is to serve, studies in which the actual *study base* is formed by this cohort's prospective follow-up. This feature – quite typical – of prognostic studies contrasts with its counterpart in etiognostic studies, in which only the source population can be of the cohort type, and in which the population-time of this cohort's follow-up constitutes only the study's source base (within which the actual study base is inseparably imbedded).

A prognostic cohort study designed to advance the knowledge-base of decisions about the choice of intervention – an *intervention-prognostic* study of the cohort type, that is – can be *experimental.* In such a study – an intervention '*trial*' – the decisions about the choices among the compared interventions/treatments are not taken in the best interest of the study cohort's members; rather, they are taken with a view to enhanced comparability of the treatment-specific sub-cohorts. *Randomized* assignment of the treatments is a common means to this end in experimental intervention-prognostic cohort studies.

As an experiment inherently is an artifactual construct, there are no 'natural experiments,' intervention-prognostic or other.

An intervention-prognostic cohort study need not be experimental; it can alternatively be *quasi-experimental.* Such a study is, in its structure, like its experimental counterpart (and paradigm) without actually being experimental. In such a study, the sub-cohorts are formed by suitable *selection* of cases/instances of treatment initiation in actual practice of clinical medicine, with the choices of the treatments thus based on perceived best interests of the patients (rather than those of the researchers).

An intervention-prognostic cohort study needs to address the *actual treatment-specific incidence densities* – rather than merely the ratios of these – of each of the event-type entities of prognostic concern in the context of the treatments involved in it. For, this provides for addressing rates of cumulative incidence and, thereby, studying actual intervention-prognostic *probabilities.*

The way this can be done in the framework of the data routinely produced in randomized trials we present in Sect. 20.1.2, in the context of an eminent intervention-prognostic trial.

18.6.2 Prognostic Non-cohort Studies

For a study to produce evidence about treatments-comparing incidence-density ratios – which is the present routine in experimental intervention-prognostic cohort studies – the requisite study population is not inherently a closed one, a cohort: it can be an open one, dynamic. Thus, an alternative to an intervention-prognostic cohort study is an intervention-prognostic study of the etiognostic type. This is a matter of etiognostic studies on particular ones of the outcomes that would be, or are, collectively addressed in experimental studies and other cohort studies on the treatments at issue. These are studies on the effects – preventive or positively causal – of the treatment(s) in the *etiogenesis of the outcomes of prognostic concern.*

These studies are addressed in Chap. 2, in terms of four examples.

Chapter 19
Example: Research on 'Hormone Replacement Therapy'

Contents

Abstract Studies that have addressed the effects of 'hormone replacement therapy' (misnomer) are instructive about the status quo of intervention-prognostic clinical research. An eminent example of these studies is the *Women's Health Initiative* trial addressing the preventive and adverse effects of postmenopausal use of estrogen supplementation 'unopposed' by progesterone use. Understanding the study's report is quite challenging to students preparing for careers in gnostic clinical research and, actually, to all concerned. We here make an effort to make that report comprehensible, and we then explain the ways in which this study can, and cannot, be viewed as paradigmatic for intervention-prognostic cohort studies in general. This 'guided tour' through that report amounts, also, to some 'continuing education' on the epidemiological and statistical foundations of gnostic clinical research in general.

Keywords Hormone replacement therapy · Essentials of the studies · Eminent original study as example · Understanding the report's title · Understanding the report's Abstract · Understanding the report proper · Preferable synthesis of the data · Understanding the report's statistics · Understanding the report on a derivative study

O. S. Miettinen et al., *Clinical Research Transformed*,
https://doi.org/10.1007/978-3-030-06176-0_19

19.1 The Essentials of the Research

19.1.1 The Needs of Practice as the Drivers

In gnostic clinical research, *the investigators' choices of topics to study* should not be based on rankings of the investigators' interests in research on various possible topics. Rather than their own interests, the researchers should be committed *to serving the knowledge needs of practicing clinicians* and, thereby, the health interests of these doctors' clients. For directly practice-serving clinical studies (gnostic), the topics should arise from awareness of the knowledge needs of practicing clinicians and, especially, from *awareness of the salient deficiencies in the knowledge-base of practice* in a given domain of it.

A very major segment of clinicians' clientele is constituted by *women who already are past the childbearing age*, and unique to these women are their age-associated substantially-reduced levels of circulating estrogens and progesterone (as well as androgens, though not testosterone). This hormonal state, universal to this (large) segment of clinicians' clientele, raises a very important question, unique to these women. This question is about the implications of possible adoption of '*hormone-replacement therapy*.' At issue actually is not therapy but either palliation or prophylaxis: The use of 'HRT' early in the postmenopausal status is aimed at relief from the symptoms (hot flashes, most notably) and signs (genito-urinary) of the hormone deficit; but for later use the purpose has been prevention of (fractures-causing) osteoporosis and scoronary heart disease, inter alia. The pursuit of these presumed major benefits from 'HRT' has been hampered by doubts about the reality of them and, especially, by concerns about possible side-effects of 'HRT' (thrombogenic and carcinogenic, mainly), of its long-term use in particular.

Thus *the challenges to clinicians' knowledge* that postmenopausal women uniquely present are not diagnostic nor etiognostic but *prognostic*: they are about these clients' future health, notably as to how the probabilities of various phenomena of health depend (causally) on the choices concerning 'HRT' – conditionally on the women's prognostic profiles.

The doctors' need is to know about those probabilities and, thereby, about the treatment-based differences among them.

19.1.2 The Essential Qualities of the Studies

The Subsection above implicitly underscores, again, the *primacy of objects design over methods design* in gnostic clinical research, the methodology being but the means to the pre-set end of producing evidence about the magnitudes of the parameters (of Nature) involved in the predicate of the study, constituted by the gnostic probability function that has been designed (as to its form) in reference to a selected/designed domain of study. And it illustrates in particular the pursuit of the essential quality of a prognostic study's objects design: the *relevance* of knowledge of the form the designed function in reference to its domain in prognostic practice, notably this quality's accentuation by commonality of client presentations from the function's referent domain together with the importance of the decisions in this domain, taken (by doctors's clients) in the light of (doctors's teachings about) the prognoses, notably about their dependence of the choice of treatment.

The implications of a prognostic study's objects design on (its subordinate) methods design can be profound. If the objects design is devoid of any merit, there obviously is no justification for the study proper, so that its *zero size* is optimal. Somewhat less obviously, this nihilism can be extended to gnostic studies predicated on objects design with whatever identifiable deficiencies subject to correction. In other words, *high-quality (practically flawless) objects design* – assuring definite relevance (for practice) of the type of knowledge formulated in the study's objects design – can be taken to be a *sine-qua-non predicate for the study's methods design*.

When a prognostic (or other gnostic) study's objects design actually justifies studying those objects, *the essential, sine-qua-non qualities of the study's methodology* are its ethics and validity, while efficiency is not such an imperative nor is any pre-ordained degree of precision of the parameters' empirical values (cf. Sect. 12.2).

19.1.3 The Essential Qualities of the Study Reports

For a study addressing prognostic probabilities to actually make a contribution to the aggregate of available evidence about the magnitudes of the parameters involved in a prognostic probability function, a report on the study needs to be produced and also published. Saying this truism is tantamount to saying, just as incontrovertibly, that the published report on a prognostic (or any other gnostic) study is an essential, sine-qua-non part of the study. From this arises the obvious question, What are the essential qualities that are to characterize the study report? that is, What in the report are the counterparts of the object-function's relevance and the evidence-acquisition's validity and ethical justifiability (Sect. 19.1.2, above)?

The elements in the report, if read at all, are read sequentially: the *title* is read first; then, depending on the perceived relevance of that topic to the reader, the report's *abstract* may get to be read in addition; and finally, the abstract may be seen to justify reading – nay, studying – the *report proper*. The purpose of that in-depth study is to actually learn, sequentially and explicitly, three things: first, *what functions were studied* for what domains; then, *how they were studied*; and finally, *what the thus-obtained results were*. Upon critical assessment of the evidence – the results against the backdrop of their genesis – the reader may deem it to justify updating of his/her beliefs about the magnitudes of the probabilities that were addressed.

This sequence in the report's reading bears a resemblance to the sequence in *the genesis of the evidence being reported*: first the object functions were designed for a defined/designed domain; then data on experience in the study objects' domain were collected from the designed study base representing that domain; and finally the study results were derived from these data. The results are consequential only insofar as the essential qualities of their genesis (i.e., of the objects and methods of the study) were satisfied.

While important in the reporting is appreciation of what needs to be reported, and in what sequence, critically-important in the reporting are the *objectivity of the meanings* of what is said and the *veracity of the contents* of that which thereby is communicated. *Clarity* – 'eschewing obfuscations,' that is – also is, clearly, a desideratum to pursue. There are other desiderata to appreciate besides, as will become evident from study of the report on the example study, addressed in what follows.

19.2 Understanding the Report on an Original Study

19.2.1 What to Make of the Title?

One of the eminent original studies on the effects of 'HRT' ('hormone-replacement therapy') has been the one whose report was entitled "*Effects of conjugated equine estrogen in postmenopausal women with hysterectomy. The Women's Health Initiative randomized controlled trial*" [1].

In reading this report, just as any other, the very first challenge is to correctly understand the title of it. The term *'conjugated estrogens'* (plural) the reader may understand, correctly, to denote, specifically, the only mixture of estrogens that is commonly used in 'HRT': the mixture that is inherent in the medication's usual source, namely the urine of pregnant mares. It thus would have gone without saying that the mixture of estrogens used in the study was equine. The reader knowing this to be the source of the medication also knows that a common synonym of that 'conjugated estrogens' term is 'Premarin' – the medication's aptly-telling brand name, derived by conjugating (not various estrogens but) the words 'pregnant' and 'mare.'

The element "women with hysterectomy" in the title implies, surprisingly and incredibly, that the effects of Premarin use that were studied – and left totally unspecified in the title – were taken to be peculiar to women who are not only postmenopausal but also of status post hysterectomy (which implies postmenopausal state but not, in the absence of its associated oophorectomy, low levels of endogenous estrogens). And the term "randomized controlled trial" in the title implies, unjustifiably, that there are also uncontrolled randomized trials. Just as the word "equine" (above), that specification of the hysterectomy status should have been left out of the title as something that is empty of meaning in the context; and likewise the specification of the randomized experiment as a "controlled" one.

A preferable title for the report would have been, for example, "*Efficacy and safety of long-term Premarin use by postmenopausal women: a randomized trial.*"

From this title, the interested reader would understand that at issue are the effects of the estrogen mixture inherent in its routine source (equine); and (s)he likely would also understand (or else learn from the report) that the use of 'unopposed' estrogens (i.e., Premarin use without periodic switches to progesterone use) is contra-indicated in women with intact uterus; and from this title (s)he definitely would understand that at issue indeed is the medication's long-term use and, hence, the hoped-for preventive effects (benefits) and the feared side-effects (harms) of this (exclusive of endometrial cancer).

19.2.2 What to Make of the Abstract/Summary?

The suitably-disciplined reader enticed by the report's title, such as it is, turns to the report's abstract/summary to learn whether study – critical – of the evidence about the effects in the report proper would be worth the effort (quite substantial).

In the abstract/summary of the report at issue here [1], the first two section-headings are "Context" and "Objectives." According to that context specification, the prompting for the design and execution of the study was that the "role" of Premarin use in the prevention of "chronic diseases in postmenopausal women" remained "uncertain," despite "decades of use and considerable research." And the objective is said to have been to "assess the effects" of postmenopausal Premarin use on "major disease incidence rates." (It goes, and was left, without saying that at issue were effects of treatment with Premarin relative to no treatment at all.)

More on the *objects of study* can be gleaned from the contents under other section headings in the abstract/summary. The regimen of the Premarin use is specified under "Intervention," simply as "0.625 mg/d." Concerning the *domain* of this medication's use beyond what was communicated in the report's title and under Objectives (above), the reader can find only that at issue were the treatments' effects when used by women 50–75 years of age, this under "Design, setting, and participants." And those "major diseases" are specified under "Main outcome measures." These are said to include "the primary outcome" (incidence of coronary heart disease), "the primary safety outcome" (incidence of breast cancer), and a "global index of risks and benefits" ("including these primary outcomes plus stroke, pulmonary embolism (PE), colorectal cancer, hip fracture, and death from other causes").

The *design of the study proper* is addressed under two successive headings in the abstract/summary, "Design, setting, and participants" and "Intervention." One learns that the experiment was "double-blind" and that the size of the study cohort was 10,739. The respective sizes of the verum ('HRT') and placebo sub-cohorts are left unspecified, and so too is the designed duration of the treatment and follow-up. The average duration of follow-up is stated, parenthetically, under "Results."

Nothing in the abstract/summary is said about *the designed methods' implementation*, most notably the participants' adherence to the assigned treatments (experimental).

An extensive section on "Results" follows. In it, the main content is "estimated hazard ratios" in conjunction with their 95% confidence intervals for "[Premarin] vs placebo for the major clinical outcomes." These are supplemented by two points: "For the outcomes significantly affected [by Premarin use], there was an absolute excess risk reduction of 6 fewer hip fractures per 100000 person-years. The estimated excess risk for all monitored events in the global index was a nonsignificant 2 events per 10000 person-years."

The closing section of the report's abstract/summary, entitled "*Conclusions*," goes beyond the report on the study per se: it relates what the study's Steering Committee made of the evidence accrued in the study, namely that, "The use of [Premarin] increases the risk of stroke, decreases the risk of hip fracture, and does not affect [coronary heart disease] incidence in postmenopausal women with prior hysterectomy over an average of 6.8 years. A possible reduction in breast cancer risk requires further investigation. The burden of incident disease events was equivalent in the [Premarin] and placebo groups, indicating no overall benefit. Thus, [Premarin] should not be recommended for chronic disease prevention in postmenopausal women."

***

This abstract/summary of the report of a very high-profile study serves to bring to focus some of the salient features of the prevailing culture in prognostic research. It is, thus, quite instructive about this culture. But it also *gives rise to a number of suggested improvements in this culture:*

1. For any prognostic study, whether purely descriptive-prognostic or both descriptive- and intervention-prognostic, the *context* naturally is *the prevailing state of the knowledge-base* of the prognoses in question. For an intervention-prognostic study, such as the study at issue here, the context thus is not the "role" of the intervention in the pursuit of its aims, whatever may be meant by this; and in particular, the context cannot meaningfully be described as the role having remained "uncertain" – as though it could be otherwise. More specifically, the context of any practice-relevant prognostic study is the need for improvement in the knowledge-base of prognoses of a particular kind. Hence, nothing needs to be said about this in the abstract or summary of the report. A delineation of the status quo of the knowledge-base belongs in the opening section of the report proper.
2. Any correct statement of the *objective* of a gnostic clinical study also is meaningless. For it goes without saying that the objective of such a study is to advance the state of knowledge about the objects of the study (through the production of new evidence, original or derivative). Instead of the objective of the study, therefore, the abstract/summary in the report on the study should give some specification of the nature of the *objects of study* beyond the mere allusion to these in the title of the report. And the objects of study should be a topic unto itself in the abstract/summary and not left for construction from bits scattered under various subheadings in it.

3. The objects of intervention-prognostic studies naturally have to do with *outcomes* of the treatments addressed in the study. These are events and states of health, such as stroke and osteoporosis. They are these entities as such, on the individual (rather than population) level, just as are the treatments (Premarin and placebo treatments in this study). The "outcomes" addressed in an intervention-prognostic clinical study thus are not properly specified as the "incidence" (and/or prevalence) of the entities that actually were the outcomes (of 'HRT') that were addressed. Rates of occurrence of these individual-level phenomena are addressed. Rates in prognostic clinical research not for their own sake but only as a basis of learning about prognostic probabilities (Sects. 6.2 and 7.4.5).
4. Just as the objects of an intervention-prognostic clinical study would properly be delineated under a single subheading (Objects; cf. # 2 above) in the report's abstract/summary, the *methods* deployed in the study also are best sketched under a single subheading (Methods). Distinctions commonly need to be made between the design of the methods and what they actually got to be; but regardless, the entirety of the methodology is, in principle, at issue in both of these. The "Design, setting, and participants" subheading in the abstract/summary at issue here is, incontrovertibly, a less-than-adequate alternative to 'Methods,' elements of which include the choice of the setting of the study and the enrolment of participants into the study cohort. The design versus reality duality can, and selectively needs to be, addressed under the Methods subheading. In the context of an experimental intervention-prognostic cohort study addressing chronic treatments, exemplified by the study at issue here, this distinction is particularly important in respect to the adherence to the assigned treatments and the completeness of the designed follow-up. Hence, a statement about the adherence to the assigned treatments would have been important to make, but wasn't made, in this report's abstract/summary.
5. The *results* of an intervention-prognostic study do not deserve extensive display in the report's abstract/summary. For, no devotee of 'evidence-based medicine' should, just as no clinical scientist would, take the methods-cum-results contents of the abstract/summary of the report of a study, to constitute the evidence from the study. Learning from a study requires thorough and critical study of the report itself; and it requires thus-attained affirmation of the relevance of knowledge of the form of the results (per objects design) and of the validity of the results' empirical content (per the design and execution of the methods); and if such affirmation actually is achieved by studying the report proper, it remains to integrate the new evidence with that which was available before.
6. To the extent that results nevertheless are displayed in the abstract/summary of a report on an intervention-prognostic study, they should not be couched in statistical jargon alien to clinicians and should not reflect statistical misunderstandings, serious ones in particular. Thus, in the context of a study whose objective purportedly was to assess Premarin treatment's effects on "incidence rates" (rather than prognostic probabilities), those results should not be presented as being about "estimated hazard ratios," which the reader may not understand to denote empirical incidence-density ratios. And even if this is

understood, it remains to understand the meanings of "estimated excess risk" and "absolute excess risk reduction." In any event, seriously mistaken and misleading is equating Premarin versus placebo empirical differences in the incidence rates of particular outcomes, whenever 'statistically significant' at the chosen level (arbitrary, unstated), as implying "outcomes significantly affected by the treatment." (Cf. Sect. 8.2.2.)

7. The product of a gnostic clinical study cannot be discovery of the truths about the magnitudes of the parameters that it was designed to assess (by means of the designed methodology of the study); the product is, merely, evidence about these magnitudes – quite possibly materially invalid/biased and in any case quite imprecise, including in the study at issue here. This evidence, insofar as it is deemed to have the requisite levels of relevance and validity, is useable as input to the report's readers' updatings of their respective opinions about those magnitudes, to these inferences about them. Very important to appreciate is this: the evidence does not provide for conclusions about the magnitudes of treatment effects, not even on the qualitative level of whether some effect, in a particular direction, actually exists (in the abstract). Thus the inclusion of the "*Conclusions*" section in the abstract/summary of the report on the study at issue here, though commonplace in reports on human-level clinical studies, was a violation of an important and incontrovertible principle, quite irrespective of what was "concluded."

19.2.3 What to Make of the Report Proper?

In the report proper, as (inexplicably) is commonplace, the section headings are quite different from those in the abstract/summary.

The *state of knowledge* about the effects of Premarin use by postmenopausal women, such as it was at the time this study was designed and launched, is described in the first paragraph of the report's first section, left untitled. The description, in its entirety, is this: "Proven benefits [of "estrogen therapy" in "postmenopausal women"] include relief of vasomotor symptoms and vaginal atrophy and prevention and treatment of osteoporosis. Observational studies primarily examining unopposed estrogen preparations [i.e., Premarin alone] have suggested a 30–50% reduction in coronary events [refs.] and an 8–30% increase in breast cancer [refs.]." This statement is not focused on the use of Premarin alone, nor on women in status post hysterectomy.

Nothing is said about *the rationale for launching this study in that context*. Said is, simply, that this "randomized, double-blind, placebo-controlled clinical trial" was "undertaken to determine whether [Premarin] alone (for women with prior hysterectomy) … would reduce cardiovascular events in mostly healthy postmenopausal women." And while the background statement (above) is quantitative, this is merely one of hypothesis-testing (qualitative) – and implies irrelevance of the results of the "observational" studies.

Thus, as remains commonplace in intervention-prognostic studies, the report's introduction (untitled and sketchy) gives a very sparse account of the objects of study; and *nowhere in the report is there any indication of the objects of study having been the magnitudes of prognostic probabilities in causal relation to Premarin use*, much less these as they also depend on prognostic time and prognostic indicators at the time of the prognostications (and their associated decisions about the adoption of the treatment).

But, as also is commonplace in the reports on intervention-prognostic studies, *much more on the objects of study is implied by the study's reported methods and results.*

Under *Methods*, the first subsection is entitled "Study population and randomization." From it one can learn the criteria for the *domain* of the prognostications and treatment decisions that are at issue. Specified is the range of age at entry into the study in addition to the status post hysterectomy; and added to this is that, "Major exclusions were related to competing risks (…), safety (…), adherence and retention concerns (…), or …" An added item about the objects study, revealed in this subsection of Methods, is that the compared *treatments* were Premarin with the dosage 0.625 mg/day and "a matching placebo."

The designed *duration of the treatments* is revealed, quite incidentally, in the "Statistical power and analyses" subsection of Methods: the treatments were going to be without any scheduled ending. However, in the subsection "Maintenance/discontinuation of study medications" under Methods there are specifications of provisions for some indications-based temporary *reductions of the dosages* and even for temporary *withholding the treatment* altogether on account of the occurrence of myocardial infarction or stroke or certain other illnesses. But: "The decision to resume study medication after MI or stroke was left to the *discretion of the clinical center, individual participant, and her health care clinician*." Besides, "Study medication was *permanently discontinued* in women who developed breast cancer; deep vein thrombosis or … ; … ; … ; … ; or who were treated by their personal health care practitioners with prescription estrogen, testosterone, or selective estrogen receptor modulators."

From the subsection of "Outcome ascertainment" (under Methods) one learns, for a start, that the "*outcomes*" addressed in the study involved cardiovascular diseases, cancers, and fractures – well more than what is specified in the report's introductory section (cf. above). And one learns, also, that the outcome specifications in the abstract/summary indeed were incorrect, that the "outcomes" of study concern indeed were particular illnesses rather than rates of "incidence" of these. While CHD and breast cancer are designated in the abstract/summary as the "primary" outcomes for efficacy and safety, respectively, this is affirmed in the "Data and safety monitoring" section under Methods for the former but contradicted for the latter. From the subsection "Statistical power and analyses" of Methods one learns that the *generic meaning of "outcome"* in the study was, more specifically, "the first postrandomization diagnosis of the designated event."

The inputs to readers' understanding of the objects of this study is rounded out by some unheralded items in the *Results* section of the additional report proper. One of these additional concerns of the investigators had been "intermediate cardiovascular end points," encompassing blood levels of lipid and cholesterol fractions and triglycerides, as well as blood pressure. Another had been "Time trends," in terms of "cumulative hazards" or "cumulative hazard rates." Yet another had been the question of "whether selected participant characteristics modified [Premarin] effects on major clinical outcome event rates."

Having thus pieced together a conception of the objects of this (very eminent) intervention-prognostic study – from various sections of the report in the (still-routine) absence of a section devoted to this topic pivotal to any gnostic clinical study – the reader who deems them relevant needs to identify the elements in the study's methods design and, especially, in the design's execution that had a critical role in determining the quality of the study proper (Sect. 19.1.2).

***

In studying the report in regard to *validity assurance* in this intervention-prognostic trial, the reader needs to be mindful of what the compared treatments actually were; that is, about the study's objects design's failure *to define the compared treatments as algorithms for the entire time horizon of the prognoses* at issue and, thereby, for the entire duration of the follow-up of the study population (Sect. 18.4.1). For, as described above, much of the decision-making about medication after various health events was not stipulated by the study protocol.

Even though the compared treatments – randomly assigned – were thus designed to (unjustifiably) provide for non-adherence to them, the methods design – in respect to the selection of the study subjects and the communications with them in the course of their follow-up – did include *means to enhance adherence* to the assignments among candidates for admission, "recruited by population-based direct mailing campaigns ... and national media awareness programs." However, *the attained degree of adherence to the assigned (and agreed-upon) treatment turned out to be quite wanting*: the reader learns (under Results rather than Methods) that "At the time of study termination, 53.8% of women had already stopped taking study medication," as assigned. "Some women initiated hormone use through their own health care clinician: 5.7% of women in the [Premarin] group and 9.1% in the placebo group by follow-up year 6." (This difference is noteworthy in this purportedly double-blind study.)

The methods of *randomization* and *blinding* are covered by saying that "The computerized randomization and blinding procedures have been described [ref.]." Given the large size of the study cohort (and equal allocation to the two treatments), the distribution of the baseline characteristics of the two sub-cohorts could be expected to be very similar. Yet, extensive data affirming this are given, gratuitously, in the "Baseline characteristics" subsection under Results (rather than Methods). On the other hand, even though, the attainability of successful blinding of whether the treatment involved Premarin or placebo was not obvious at all (cf. above), nothing is said about this.

Regarding the *documentation of the "outcomes,"* the report describes (under "Outcome ascertainment" in the Methods section) how "Designated outcome events were evaluated by review of medical records by centrally trained physician adjudicators at each clinical center who were blinded to the treatment assignment and symptoms related to study medication. Final adjudication of key cardiovascular and cancer outcomes, as well as hip fractures and deaths, was performed centrally by equally blinded [Women's Health Initiative] physician adjudicators, neurologists, or cancer coders." But no point is made of the fact that such adjudication does not resolve the implications of *differential initiations of the pursuits of the diagnoses*, possible insofar as the blinding indeed was unsuccessful (as is suggested by the evidence alluded to above and the existence of "symptoms related to study medications").

As would be expected, the report elaborates, in the "Statistical power and analyses" section of Methods, on the *design of the study's "sample size,"* this specifically as to how many women "would be needed to be randomized to have 81% power to detect a 21% reduction in CHD [coronary heart disease] rates over a projected 9-year average follow-up". Said is that the thus-derived size of the study cohort – 12,375 women – "would provide 65% power to detect 20% reduction in hip fractures." The elaboration goes on from this, with the implication that all of this, including the resulting "sample size" – specific down to five significant digits – is somehow relevant to the meaning of the results and/or the confidence intervals associated with these – presented in the report's abstract already. Nothing is said – whether under Methods or Results – about the relevance of the statistical calculation of the study population's target size (cf. Sect. 12.2.4), focused on learning about hip fractures (*sic*!).

This statistical section (under Methods) makes also a number of other points: For the "primary outcomes," the "hazard ratios" and their 95% confidence intervals were derived by means of "Cox proportional hazard analyses [ref.], stratified by age, prior disease, and randomization status ... Cumulative hazard rates were estimated by the Kaplan-Meier method for each designated outcome. ... To acknowledge multiple testing issues, adjusted [confidence intervals] were calculated using group sequential methods, and for secondary outcomes a Bonferroni correction based on the data and safety monitoring plan ...The possibility of important subgroup effects was explored by testing for interactions in expanded Cox models." The implication is that practitioners of 'evidence-based medicine' and other readers of *JAMA* understand not only the meaning but also the relevance (for validity) of all of this.

***

As for the necessary *ethics-assurance* (Sect. 19.1.2), the report includes the content that is expected in the framework of the prevailing culture in intervention-prognostic clinical studies. There is, first, the statement that "the protocol and consent forms were approved by the institutional review board for each participating institution (see end of this report), and all women provided written informed consent." At the end of the report are, in small print, sections on "Authors/WHI steering committee," "Financial disclosures," etc., including "Funding/support and role of the sponsor." But *there actually is nothing about that which was taken to qualify the consent as "informed"* – based on well-informed and impartial, effective teaching the potential participants about the status quo of the knowledge-base of postmenopausal use of Premarin. It would have been relevant to report, for instance, what the women were told about the "suggestion," from "observational" studies, of "a 30% to 50% reduction in coronary events" with the countervailing "8% to 30% increase in breast cancer with extended use," and about the meaning of this background for mounting the trial.

Whatever may have been the information on the *status quo* of knowledge about the effects of Premarin use by postmenopausal women, underpinning the "informed" consents to participation in the study, it presumably also included another element: assurance that there is no need to worry about the emergence, unbeknownst to the participants in the course of the study, of *new evidence*, from within the study itself or without, that the harms from Premarin treatment actually overweigh its benefits. The information the investigators provided on this, to the satisfaction of the participants, presumably was that the established way to deal with possibly worrisome new evidence, were it to emerge in the course of the study, is to *keep it secret to the participants* and all others too, except for the study's "Data and safety monitoring board."

In this now-conventional framework of the ethics of intervention-prognostic trials, *the participants had no role in decisions about discontinuation of their participation* in the light of emerging new evidence about efficacy or of safety, considering this in the context of their individual utility/disutility valuations. The decision was made on a 'higher level,' on behalf of the participants; and it wasn't going to be made judgmentally but statistically: "Statistical monitoring boundaries on O'Brien-Fleming group sequential procedures [ref.] with asymmetric boundaries for benefit (1-sided .025 upper boundary for CHD) and adverse effects (1-sided.05 lower boundary). The adverse effect boundary for the 6 monitored outcomes [incl. CHD] incorporated a Bonferroni correction. The Bonferroni correction was not applied to breast cancer because it was the primary safety outcome. Early stopping was to be considered if a disease-specific boundary was crossed and … Additional aspects of the monitoring plan have been published [ref.]." The implication of reporting this is that, knowing these specifics the reader will understand the trial to have been meticulously ethical. In point of fact, though, the typical reader doesn't understand any of this.

The *decisions of that Board* are outlined as the first topic in the Results section of the report, under the subheading "Trial Monitoring and Early stopping." The last one of the board's meetings, "using data through November 30, 2003, did not lead to a consensus recommendation. None of the predefined stopping boundaries had been crossed, … On February 2, 2004, following subsequent reviews with additional advisors, the NIH [National Institutes of Health] decided to stop the intervention phase of the trial. … ," as it found that Premarin use "does not appear to affect the risk of heart disease, the primary outcome of the study," and that the "increased risk of stroke was similar to the risk reported from the [concomitant] estrogen plus progestin trial. … On March 1, 2004, participants were informed of the trial termination and advised to stop taking their study medication."

For an experimental intervention-prognostic study to be *genuinely ethical*, the subjects' decisions to participate in it need to be truly informed, in all relevant respects. There is the decision to enter into the trial, informed by what is knowable at that time; and upon the entry, there is prone to be needs for decisions about continuation of the participation as the information available at entry into the study is updated (including from the study itself); and there may also be changes in the subject's valuations of the treatments' relative benefits and harms, relevant to the continuation of the consent. *In a genuinely ethical intervention-prognostic trial there is no need for ethics-oriented (or other) 'stopping rules.'*

* * *

The *Results* section begins with the (methodological) subsections "Trial monitoring and stopping," "Baseline characteristics," and "Follow-up, adherence, and unblinding," followed by one on sample-based results concerning "Intermediate cardiovascular disease end points." The *actual results* – concerning the health events at issue – are addressed under three subheadings: "Clinical outcomes," "Time trends," and "Further analyses."

The subsection on "Clinical outcomes" opens with the point (about the objects of study) that "The primary outcome for this trial was the rate of CHD," which contradicts the point under Methods that one of the outcomes of study concern was CHD, this event as such, not the rate of its occurrence. Results on the various outcome events (CHD, etc.) are presented in a table entitled "Clinical outcomes by randomization assignment," and the text about these is a set of very brief comments.

Concerning CHD, said is that "These data rule out a reduction in CHD rates with [Premarin] of more than 25% during the trial period." This statement presumably is based on the result for fatal and nonfatal CHD combined, for which the "hazard ratio" is given as 0.91 and the "nominal 95% CI" as 0.75–1.12. The suitably-educated reader is surprised about this interpretation of a 95% confidence interval, specifically the idea that the lower bound of such an interval "rules out" values smaller than that. But much more importantly, though, such a reader presumably is taken aback by the major discrepancy between this ruling out, merely, of quite large effects and the utterly nihilistic counterpart of this in the report's abstract/summary, namely that Premarin has no effect on CHD occurrence in usage such as in this study. Puzzling also is the number of CHD events used in deriving that result with its CI, as it is smaller than the sum of the numbers given for CHD deaths and nonfatal MIs.

For *stroke*, by contrast, the overall number is larger than those for fatal and nonfatal cases combined. For stroke overall, the "hazard ratio" in the table is 1.39 with the associated "nominal 95% CI" of 0.97–1.99. The comment on this also is a single sentence, though more elaborate: "The incidence of stroke was increased by 39% in the [Premarin] group (44 vs 32 per 10000 person-years, $z = -2.72$, $P = .007$), which crossed the adverse effect monitoring boundary for the 14th planned interim analysis (defined as z = –2.69)." So the 39% higher rate in the Premarin group is mistaken to have been "increased" by 39% (as an effect of the treatment); and curiously, a distinction is not made between thrombotic and hemorrhagic strokes.

The corresponding result for invasive *breast cancer* in the table is 0.77 in conjunction with the interval 0.59–1.01. The comment on this is: "Invasive breast cancer, the primary safety outcome for this trial, was diagnosed at 23% lower rate in the [Premarin] group than in the placebo group (26 vs 33 per 10000 person-years) and this comparison narrowly missed statistical significance (P = .06)." Analogous with the statement about stroke would have been to say that the incidence of invasive breast cancer was decreased by 23% in the Premarin group.

Regarding *fractures* – with results separately for hip, vertebral and total – the opening statement is that "Use of [Premarin] reduced the rates of fractures by 30% to 39%," those three "hazard ratios" being shown as 0.61, 0.62, and 0.70. For hip fractures, the interval associated with the 0.61 is 0.41–0.91. Again, *empirical differences are attributed to effects of the treatment*, and *quantitatively at that*, with no regard for wanting validity and precision – and for evidence from other studies.

Under "*Time trends*," a figure shows "Kaplan-Meier estimates of cumulative hazards for selected clinical outcomes," and in the text is made this point (i.a.): "Tests for trends with time since randomization were computed for all of the monitored and composite outcomes using Cox proportional hazards model with a time-dependent treatment interaction term. Coronary heart disease was the only outcome with a statistically significant trend (P = .02) …" *The meaning of this is obscure even to readers well familiar with Cox regression.*

Under "*Further analyses*," the opener is that "Exploratory analyses were conducted to determine whether selected participant characteristics modified [Premarin] effects on major outcome event rates." The first point along these lines is this: "There were no significant interactions between [Premarin] and race/ethnicity or body mass index on risk of [the various outcome events] (data not shown). Of particular interest for all outcomes was age at enrolment (Fig. 5). The only treatment x age interaction reaching statistical significance was for colorectal cancer (P = .048), for which increasing age was associated with increasing risk with [Premarin] use. The effect of prior disease on cardiovascular event rates was also evaluated," with plenty of numbers following. And finally, "Sensitivity analyses were conducted to provide an indication of the potential [*sic*] impact of lack of adherence to assigned study medication," with results of these following. Whatever the intended meaning of all of this, clear is the fact that *prognostic probabilities were not addressed at all*, not even the averages of these.

***

Following the Methods and Results sections comes the third and final one, entitled *Comment*. The beginning is nothing new relative to what has been said already about the nature of the study and about its main results. Then the results are discussed in comparison with those from other studies. The points include these: "The lack of effect of [Premarin] on CHD risk is substantially different from the favorable reports from observational studies that motivated this trial"; "the observed adverse effect of [Premarin] on stroke is consistent with ..."; and "The trend toward a reduction in breast cancer incidence was unanticipated and is opposite that observed in ... [and] also appears contrary to the preponderance of observational study results [refs.]." That purported "lack of effect" etc. represent, again, *failure to appreciate that effects of treatment – including lack thereof – are not observable in intervention trials*.

Under the subheading "*Limitations*," allusion is made to the "high rates of discontinuation of study medications," with the associated remark that "Sensitivity analyses suggest that the lack of adherence to assigned study medication may have diluted the [Premarin] effects, both positive and negative, relative to what might be observed with full adherence, but did not distort the overall balance of effects." *That such dilutions did occur, to considerable extent, should have been obvious without any "sensitivity analyses."*

The other subheading under Comment is "*Clinical implications*." The first of the two paragraphs repeats, for the final time, that "[Premarin] did not affect CHD rates but did increase the risk of stroke ... and reduced the risk of hip fractures, ... "; and that it "appeared" to reduce the risk of breast cancer. This is supplemented with the point that "The totality of monitored effects, ... , suggests an overall balance of risks and benefits and importantly no effect on total mortality." But, no data were shown, and the overall "balance of risks and benefits" left undefined.

The second, final paragraph under "Clinical implications" summarizes the authors' view of the study. It opens with the (very upbeat) observation that "Based on these findings, women now have usable estimates for the benefits and harms of [Premarin] alone." And it closes with this: "Overall, these data support the current US Food and Drug Administration recommendations for postmenopausal women to use [Premarin] only for menopausal symptoms at the smallest effective dose for the shortest possible time [ref.]." *A critical reader is much less sanguine about the clinical implications of this (very high-profile) trial.*

***

Like the abstract/summary of the report on this very eminent intervention-prognostic study, published in an equally eminent medical journal, the report proper also is quite instructive about the prevailing culture in these studies; and it, too, indicates *needs for improvements* in the culture. Some of the impressions in and lessons from studying this example report are these:

1. In comparison with the report's title and abstract/summary, the report proper on this experimental intervention-prognostic cohort study – exemplifying the prevailing culture in this – is rather more challenging to understand, principally because of the way it is organized (in this example just as in general). Understanding of what, exactly, the objects of this study were requires synthesizing what is said in the report's untitled introduction as well as under both Methods and Results; and as for the methods, important information on

them is found not only under Methods but also in the Results section. The example well illustrates that *understanding of the report on a study like this, and indeed on any gnostic clinical study, would be greatly enhanced by adopting the structure consisting of Background, Objects, Methods, Results, and Commentary.* That Background section would focus on, and specify, what gnostic challenges (of clinical practice) are at issue and what the state of their requisite knowledge-base is. The Objects section would focus on, and specify, what probability functions were studied, and for what domain(s). The Methods section would specify how the study base came into being and the way in which the empirical values of the parameters in the object functions (specified under Objects) were derived (in reference to the study base), distinguishing between the methods' design and the de-facto methods. The Results section would simply give the results, that is, the obtained empirical values of the parameters that were studied, these together with measures of their precisions (confidence intervals or standard errors). And the Commentary section would focus on reporting whatever further facts about the study are relevant for readers' full understanding of the evidence from it (regarding the magnitudes of the object parameters).

2. Understanding of the report of this study would have been enhanced further by *more disciplined writings in other terms as well.* In broadest terms, the reporting vacillates between the study being about hypothesis-testing (qualitative, concerning the existence/non-existence of effects in particular directions) and its being about estimation (quantitative, of the magnitudes of particular parameters); and whereas the concerns in practice are quantitative, estimation should have been the sole concern in this study as well. Likewise, the report is unsettled about the very entity that the testing or estimation is about, as the meaning of "outcome" vacillates between events of health per se and the rates of their incidence; and in this, the (epidemiological) term "incidence rate" is abruptly replaced, without any explanation, by "hazard rate" (adopted from the jargon surrounding 'Cox regression').
3. A third obstacle for understanding the report proper also is worthy of note here: the *statistical inputs* to it beyond jargon such as that "hazard rate" and its cognate "cumulative hazard." The statistical "analyses" (syntheses) of the data could have been *more intuitive and thereby more comprehensible* than the ones that were based on 'Cox regression' and 'survival analysis' à la Kaplan and Mayer (Sect. 19.2.4, below); and understanding of the report would have been enhanced by refraining from expounding various *questionable statistical doctrines* and from repeating common *misrepresentations* of elementary statistics.
4. Despite these (and other) unnecessary obstacles for understanding the report proper on the study at issue here, study of it illustrates *the importance of studying the report beyond the abstract/summary of it.* The prime example of this, already noted in the foregoing, has to do with the "conclusion" about the "primary outcome" and is worthy of repetition here: Presented in the abstract/summary is the utterly nihilistic "conclusion" that "The use of [Premarin] … does not affect CHD incidence in postmenopausal women with hysterectomy over an average of 6.8 years," while in the report proper the corresponding statement is that "No

significant effect of [Premarin] was observed on CHD rates compared with placebo [meaning that there was no statistically significant difference, at the P = 0.05 level, between the Premarin and placebo groups in CHD rates] (40 vs 54 per 10,000 person-years) (Table 3). These data rule out a reduction in CHD rates with [Premarin] of more than 25% during the trial period."

19.2.4 More Comprehensible Synthesis of the Data

As we noted in Sect. 19.2.3 above, understanding this eminent study [1] is unduly challenging in respect to the statistical aspects of it; and we insinuated that part of the problem is the less-than-intuitive way in which the data were synthesized into the results of it and into measures of the imprecision of these. So we here present what would have been a more comprehensible treatment of these aspects of the study – and would be so in intervention-prognostic studies in general, as long as they, like this one, are not predicated on pre-designed prognostic probability functions as the overall objects of study.

Understanding of these statistical aspects of the study at issue here would have been greatly enhanced, we suggest, by *not addressing any 'statistical methods' or anything else statistical in the Methods section of the report, and starting the Results presentation in respect to, first, the "primary" one of the outcome events with the actual treatment-specific incidence densities of its occurrence in the experience of the study base* (constituted by the study cohort's follow-up for this event, as specified under Methods). This would have been a matter of presenting these CHD rates, R_1 and R_0, for the Premarin and placebo (index and reference) sub-cohorts:

$$R_1 = 177/(36{,}100\,\text{p}-\text{y}) = 49.0/(10{,}000\,\text{p}-\text{y}),$$
$$R_0 = 199/(36{,}900\,\text{p}-\text{y}) = 53.9/(10{,}000\,\text{p}-\text{y}),$$

where 177 and 199 are the index and reference numbers of CHD events (total, from Table 3), and the amounts of population time are the sizes of the respective sub-cohorts multiplied by the average duration of follow-up (6.8 year). (This overall average is used here, as the treatment-specific averages are not given in the report.)

These rates imply, in an utterly straightforward way, the *incidence-density ratio* for the Premarin versus placebo contrast:

$$\text{IDR} = 49.0/53.9 = 0.909 = 0.91,$$

this result being the very same as the "hazard ratio" (0.91) given in the study report as a product of "Cox proportional hazards analysis."

To obtaining the corresponding *95% confidence interval* – as an expression of the (im)precision of this result – the intuitive approach is that of *'test-based' confidence intervals* [2]. Central to this is the statistic for testing the 'statistical significance' of this result's deviation from the corresponding parameter's null value, *IDR* = 1. The obvious basis for this testing is to focus on, say, the index number of CHD cases (n = 177) as a realization of a binomial distribution of this index number out of the total number of CHD cases, N = 177 + 199 = 376. The null number corresponding to that binomial realization (n = 177) is N multiplied by the null probability that a case arises from the index (rather than reference) segment of the study base, this probability obviously being the index proportion of the study population-time, 36.1/(36.1 + 36.9) = 0.495; that is, the null number corresponding to that 177 is 376(0.495) = 185.9. And the null variance of the index number of cases is 376(0.495)(1 – 0.495) = 94.0, the corresponding standard deviation being the square root of this, 9.69. Thus the realization of the *Gaussian test statistic* is:

$$z = (177 - 185.9)/9.69 = -0.918.$$

Based on this z together with the result at issue (IDR = 0.909), then, the test-based 95% CI around the result is [2]

$$\exp\{[\log(0.909)](1 \pm 1.96/z)]\} = 0.74, 1.01.$$

This result is essentially identical with the "nominal" 0.75–1.12 in the report, derived by means of "Cox proportional hazards analyses".

The *rationale* for this statistic may be evident from its structure: The logarithm of the rate ratio is taken to have a Gaussian replication-distribution, just as in Cox regression; and the point is that the null standard-deviation of this distribution can be taken to be [log (0.909)] / z, which assures that the upper confidence limit is the null value – 0.00 for the ratio's logarithm, 1.00 for the ratio itself – when z = – 1.96, implying one-sided P = 0.025. The corresponding 'Wald statistic' would not involve first-principles null variance but, instead, one in which the unit variance is based on the empirical proportion, 177/376 = 0.471. In these terms, z = – 0.923, and the resulting interval would be 0.74–1.11 (cf. 0.74–1.12 above).

As other examples of this, let us consider stroke and breast cancer. For *stroke*, the compared rates were these: R_1 = 158/(36.100 p-y) = 43.8/(10,000 p-y) and R_0 = 118/(36.900 p-y) = 32.0/(10,000 p-y). These imply IDR = 43.8/32.0 = 1.37, corresponding to "hazard ratio" 1.39 in the report on the study. For the 95% CI, the first-principles test static's realization is z = 2.57, and the test-based 95% CI thus is exp{[log (1.37)] (1 ± 1.96/2.57)} = 1.08, 1.74 – essentially identical with the "nominal" 1.10–1.77 in the report.

For invasive *breast cancer*, the index and reference numbers are 94 and 124, respectively, translating to IDR = 0.77, the very same as in the report. For the test statistic the realization is 1.88, and the 95% CI becomes exp{[log (0.775)] (1 ± 1.96/1.88)]} = 0.59, 1.01, also the very same as "nominal" interval in the report.

***

As for the "Kaplan-Meier estimates of cumulative hazards for selected outcomes" presented in the report's Fig. 3, they represent (empirical values for) rates of *cumulative incidence* of the events being addressed, these for the compared sub-cohorts' course over time post randomization. Before addressing the essence and prognostic relevance of these rates, we'll show how they can be derived from the data that are given in that Figure, and this we'll do strictly in the framework of rates of incidence specific to periods of prognostic time – without any reference the "Kaplan-Meier method" (which wasn't explicated in the report). We'll focus on CHD in this.

For the successive 9 years of the study cohort's follow-up, the numbers of study subjects in the Premarin and placebo sub-cohorts that entered the successive years of still-continuing follow-up, this without yet having experienced any CHD event, were these (per that Table 3):

Year	1.	2.	3.	4.	5.	6.	7.	8.	9.
Premarin	5310	5219	5147	5067	4978	4874	3934	2248	999
Placebo	5429	5336	5254	5171	5072	4959	4015	2331	1106

The corresponding numbers of *person-years of follow-up* in those successive years can be approximated (very closely) by averaging the numbers at the beginnings of the successive years. These numbers are:

Year	1.	2.	3.	4.	5.	6.	7.	8.
Premarin	5265	5183	5107	5023	4926	4404	3091	1624
Placebo	5383	5295	5213	5122	5016	4487	3273	1719

In the first year, 26 first cases of CHD occurred in the Premarin sub-cohort (per Table 3), and the *incidence density* of these events thus was 26/(5265 p-y) = 49/(10,000 p-y). All the rates specific to treatment and year of follow-up, derived this way and expressed as the number of cases in 10,000 p-y, were these:

Year	1.	2.	3.	4.	5.	6.	7.	8.
Premarin	49	53	43	42	61	70	42	37
Placebo	43	44	48	53	48	58	86	99

The *integral* of these rates over the 8 years is the sum of all of these rates multiplied by 1 year. For the Premarin sub-cohort, this integral is: (49 + 53 + … + 37)/10,000 = 0.0397. For the placebo group the corresponding result is 0.0479. These integrals translate into their corresponding values for *cumulative incidence* [2, 3]: 1 – exp. (– 0.0397) = 3.9% and 1 – exp. (– 0.0479) = 4.7%. These results are in good accord with the corresponding readings from the graphs in the report's Fig. 3.

***

A word on the big picture of this Section (on "more comprehensible synthesis of the data") may be in order. The first-order, dominant point of departure in this Section was that which the investigators themselves, in their way, derived from the study data (which was empirical values for certain parameters together with certain measures of the imprecisions of these). For our synthesis of the data to those ends, an added, subordinate point of departure was very different from what the investigators used as the direct basis for the rate-ratio results etc. *Rather than the detailed data, the direct basis for our synthesis of the data were the results of their reduction, such that it did not compromise the information in them to those ends of the investigators.* This two-stage process – data reduction followed by statistics-derivation based on these – was the basis for the attained – and very desirable – greater *comprehensibility* of the way the results, and the measures of their (im)precisions, were derived from the assembled primary, individual-level data. And beyond comprehensibility, these syntheses of the data have the desirable quality of *reproducibility by the reader* (as illustrated here).

A needed supplementation to this may be a word on the concept – quite subtle – of *cumulative incidence* of events of CHD etc. here, explication beyond what may be autonomously inferred from the derivation of its values here (and the introduction of this in Sect. 5.5.4). A rate of an event's cumulative incidence over a span of time has to do with a *cohort-type population*, and it is related to the probability that a member of the cohort – typical of the members at entry into the membership – will experience that event in that period of prognostic time. The subtlety of this rate, and of the probability related to it, is the conditionality of it in prospective terms: as the rate is derived from the integral of the event's incidence density over a period of the cohort's prospective course, it is predicated on the *premise (counterfactual) that all of the cohort's members survive to contribute person-time up to the time of the event's occurrence (within that period of prospective/cohort time) or else throughout that period*; and the value of this rate is derived on the basis of time-specific incidence densities on the *premise* that, despite the terminations of follow-up for reasons other than the event's occurrence, those input rates are valid representations of the rates that would have materialized in the (counterfactual) absence of those terminations of follow-up for extraneous reasons.

19.2.5 Understanding the Statistics on the Results

In the field of statistics, the *concept of statistic* is a dual one: in one meaning of the term, a statistic is a number derived from a set of data, while in another meaning it is the functional form of this derivation (specifying how the number is a function of the data). Our focus here is on the former, the ad-hoc concept of statistic. Examples of statistics in this meaning of the term are the values for various incidence-density ratios reported from the study at issue here, and so also are the 'confidence intervals' associated with these ratios in the report. Other examples are the P-values in the report. (Cf. Sect. 8.2.)

All of these (and other) statistics, in this meaning of the term, are commonly thought of as representing results of statistical-type studies; but we prefer to restrict the *denotation of 'results'* of gnostic clinical studies to the values that are derived from the study data for the parameters that constitute the objects of the study. And while these statistics are, in the field of statistics, termed estimates – point estimates as distinct from interval estimates (as a synonym for 'confidence intervals') – of the parameters' values, *we prefer to term them empirical values of the parameters*; for, the concept of estimate of a parameter's value is, to us, one of belief about the magnitude in question, and by no means is that belief generally based solely on – and hence equated with – the ad-hoc result on it. (Cf. Sect. 8.2.)

With the concept of the results of a gnostic (or other statistical-type) study thus restricted (to the obtained empirical values of the object parameters), the *statistical products of such a study* are constituted by the *results* of the study in conjunction with *statistics on them*, notably 'confidence intervals' (or 'standard errors' for their construction) as measures of the results' imprecision/irreproducibility and P-values as measures of their consistency with the parameters' null values.

As an example of understanding/misunderstanding the statistics on the results of the study being studied here [1], let us consider the statistics on the causal – Premarin versus placebo – incidence-density ratio for the "primary outcome," first event of CHD. The reported statistics were these: result ("hazard ratio") 0.91, and 95% 'confidence interval' ("nominal," as a measure of that result's imprecision/irreproducibility) 0.75–1.12. The investigators' understanding of this pair of statistics was, as we've pointed out, that "These data rule out a reduction in CHD rates with [Premarin] of more than 25% during the trial period" (an utterly nihilistic version of this being presented as a "conclusion" in the abstract/summary). This statement evidently reflects the investigators' belief that values of this parameter outside the 95% 'confidence interval' ("nominal") for it are excluded by this study, for which "significance was set at the.05 level."

Given that the investigators believe – as is implied by the term "95% confidence interval" – that one can be 95% confident that the parameter's value is within that interval, *they must assign not 5% but 2.5% probability to values below the interval's lower bound* (and another 2.5% for values higher than its upper bound). For this type of ruling out, "at the.05 level," the basis should have been the lower bound of a 90% two-sided interval or of 95% one-sided interval, which is 0.77 rather than 0.75.

The larger point about this is that *the concept of X% confidence interval in statistics is not, contrary to the implication of that term, that one can be X% confident that the parameter's value is contained* within that interval. The concept in statistics has to do, not with any confidence about the parameter's values but, instead, with the construction of it: an 'X% confidence interval' (misnomer) is an interval *so constructed that in X% of its valid constructions from valid data it contains the parameter's* (unknown) value (Sect. 8.2.2). Thus, one can be X% confident that the parameter's value is contained within an 'X% confidence interval' only insofar as those validity conditions obtain and, very importantly, *nothing at all is known about the parameter's value apart from this (valid) measure of the imprecision of the only relevant result* on its magnitude (this in the absence, also, of any substantive insight into that magnitude).

Now, what about that duality of *"nominal"* versus *"adjusted"* 'confidence intervals in the report being studied here? Two notions of multiple hypothesis-testing are at the root of this duality, both of them commonly held yet arising from (common) *misunderstandings within statistics proper.*

One of these notions has to do with *sequential testing* (for 'statistical significance') by the study's "Data and safety monitoring board." The notion generally has been – and continues to be – that such repeat testings increase the probability of finding a 'statistically significant' difference (between the compared sub-cohorts, in the frequency of the event at issue); and that, therefore, the P-value derived after these testings in the usual way has become only "nominal" and requires adjustment for the sequential testing – and so does the 'confidence interval.'

In point of fact, however, the information in the study data had not been compromised, at all, by the sequential testings in the course of their accrual. This has been shown formally [4]; but it could be understood intuitively as well. For, the sequential testing did not change the data; they were what they would have been without those testings.

The other basis for that "nominal" versus "adjusted" duality in the study at issue here was the fact that the probability of finding a 'statistically significant' difference in any given study increases with increasing number of the types of entity for which the testing is applied in the study; that *multiple comparisons* in a single study leads to 'statistically significant' differences purely 'by chance' – that in this study, for which "significance was set at the.05 level," 5% of the comparisons would have been expected to show a 'statistically significant' difference in the absence of any Premarin effect. This perceived problem was dealt with in the usual two ways. One of these was advance specification of the "primary outcome" for efficacy, and for safety too, with the idea that, on this basis, the 'multiple-comparison problem' will not arise in respect to the events of principal concern. For the "secondary outcomes" the solution was the application of an adjustment – the 'Bonferroni correction' – to the P-values and confidence intervals.

Here, too, a spurious problem was being 'solved.' As in the context of sequential – and thereby multiple – testing in respect to a single type of event (outcome), the perceived problem in the context of testing multiple types of event in a single study is rooted in the concern to prevent multiplicity of testing from unjustifiably increasing the probability of finding a 'statistically significant' difference in the study. This concern is misplaced. Just as the information ("nominal") regarding the type of event at issue is not 'diluted' by (however multiple) previous testings about it in the study (cf. above), so *the P-value ("nominal") regarding a given event is not diluted by (however multiple) other events are addressed in the study.* And quite obviously, the burden of the evidence from the study in regard to a given event is not enhanced, in the least, by the investigators having designated, in whatever meaning of this but "in advance" of the availability of the data, this event as being of "*primary*" concern to them; and the "adjustments" of the statistics on the "secondary" outcomes for multiple comparisons is unfounded just the same.

In this context of the relevance spuriously attached to advance designation of the "primary" contrast(s), it is of note that a notion closely related to this is the doctrine (just as spurious) that the *study size* should be determined in advance of the study instead of allowing the accrued evidence to determine whether to continue adding to it. In conformity with this, the design of the size of the study at issue here is described in the report on it, with no word on the relevance of this (actually none) on the validity of the results (after results-dependent termination of the follow-up contributing to the reported evidence).

19.3 Understanding the Report on a Derivative Study

In the Sections above we struggled to understand the report on a study in a major medical journal, on a major study concerning a major topic in clinical-level preventive medicine [1]. It was a study in which *"conclusions" were drawn, as is commonplace, solely from the evidence intrinsic to that study, even though evidence from other sources was available as well.* It therefore is instructive to study and try to understand *its related-and-contemporary derivative study on the same object(s)*, one in which the evidence from prior original studies was synthesized. So we take up a study entitled *"Postmenopausal hormone replacement therapy: scientific review"* [5]. "This review was initiated to aid the current USPSTF [U.S. Preventive Services Task Force] in making new recommendations that will be released this fall [2004]."

While that *original study was focused* on effects of 'unopposed' estrogens (in the usual meaning of this, namely Premarin alone) in women who were of status post hysterectomy (in addition to being postmenopausal), *this focus is not a feature of any part of the report on this all-purpose derivative study* on the effects of 'hormone-replacement therapy.' Emblematic of the quality assurance in this derivative study is the falsehood that it drew from "all published studies if they contained a comparison group of HRT nonusers and reported data on HRT use and clinical outcomes of interest." For in the report's "Table 1. Hormone replacement therapy (HRT) and cardiovascular disease and thromboembolism studies," under the column heading "Type of study," some of the entries are "case control" – presumably referring to etiogenetic studies of the type that actually did not "contain a comparison group of HRT nonusers" (but, instead, a group free of CVD or TE). (Cf. Sect. 15.6.3.)

As those orientational notes indicate, the *effort to make sense of this derivative study scarcely would be instructive enough to justify delving into its particulars*, such as "fixed and random effects models" fitted "using the Bayesian data analytic framework," with "inference on the parameters … via posterior probability distributions." For, while *gratuitous hypertrophy of incompletely-understood statistics* obfuscated the design of, and reporting on, the original intervention-prognostic study (Sects. 19.2.4 and 19.2.5), this aberration of research culture evidently is notably *accentuated in this derivative study;* and essential in educational preparation for gnostic clinical research is not learning the myriad of ways in which it can, and does, go wrong but the theory that defines the way of doing it correctly (cf. Sect. 4.2).

More on the derivative studies surrounding the trial at issue here is given in Chap. 22.

References

1. The Women's Health Initiative steering committee (2004) Effects of conjugated equine estrogen in postmenopausal women with hysterectomy. JAMA 291:1701–1712
2. Miettinen OS (1976) Estimability and estimation in case-referent studies. Am J Epidemiol 103:226–231
3. Miettinen OS (2008) Survival analysis: up from Kaplan-Meier-Greenwood. Eur J Epidemiol 23:585–592
4. Cornfield J (1966) A Bayesian test of some classical hypotheses – with application to sequential clinical trials. J Am Stat Assoc 61:577–594
5. Nelson HD, Humphrey LL, Nygren P *et alii* (2002) Postmenopausal hormone replacement therapy: scientific review. JAMA 288:872–881

Chapter 20
Prognostic Probability Functions from Clinical-Trial Data

Contents

Abstract In the eminent intervention-prognostic cohort study (experimental) addressed in Chap. 19 above, the data were synthesized in a manner that represents the prevailing state-of-the-art in clinical trials at large; for, the core results on the various outcomes were derived by means of *Cox regression*, and they were, thus, treatments-comparing "hazard ratios" – incidence-density ratios, that is – for the various entities of the investigators' concern. Very notably, prognostic probabilities were not addressed in that particular study, nor are they being addressed in other clinical trials, as the Cox model (for "proportional hazards") does not provide for this. But, as we show in this Chapter, *prognostic probabilities, including their functional dependence on prognostic time (jointly with treatment and prognostic indicators), actually can be studied in another theoretical framework* for clinical trials (and their quasi-experimental counterparts). In this approach to clinical-trial data, theory of the other species causal gnostic studies – etiognostic studies (singular in their true essence; Sect. 15.6.2) – is brought to bear on intervention-prognostic studies. This brings *logistic-regression models* into preeminence in the data-synthesis of intervention-prognostic cohort studies (Sect. 15.6) and in prognostic non-cohort studies (non-experimental; Chap. 21).

O. S. Miettinen et al., *Clinical Research Transformed*,
https://doi.org/10.1007/978-3-030-06176-0_20

Keywords Cox regression · Alternative sampling · Incidence density proper · Logistic regression · Examples · Basic models · Augmented models · Model fitting

20.1 Introduction to the Synthesis of the Data

20.1.1 The Prevailing Type of Synthesis

For whichever type of outcome event in a clinical trial (or a quasi-experimental intervention-prognostic study; Sect. 18.6.1), the concern is with the occurrence of cases of that event in the *study base* for that type of event, formed by the study cohort's follow-up. The study base for the event at issue is the study cohort's aggregate of population-time of follow-up for that event, constituted by its members' individual 'waiting times' for the occurrence of that event, of the first case of it when recurrence is possible. Each member of the study cohort contributes to the study base for the event at issue up to the time of that event's occurrence under the follow-up or else to some other, intended or unintended, termination of his/her follow-up. Thus, *while a single cohort is followed, the aggregate of population-time constituting the study base is specific to each of the various types of event addressed in the study.* So it was, also, in the study [1] addressed in Chap. 19 above.

In *Cox regression*, which was central to the syntheses of the data in that example study, the occurrence of any given type of event in the study base is addressed with focus on the '*risk sets'* identified from the data assembled in the study cohort's follow-up. These sets are formed around each of the identified cases of the event at issue; and each of these sets is constituted by the person-moment of the event's occurrence (the first for the person involved) together with all the other person-moments in the cross-section of the study base (for that event) at that point in cohort/prognostic time (measured from entry into the cohort).

The *data* associated with the person-moments in those sets naturally specify whether at issue is the event's occurrence (Y = 1) or non-occurrence (Y = 0) and what treatment was assigned to the person at entry into the cohort (at prognostic T = 0); and besides, they can specify (by the realizations of the other Xs involved) select aspects of the person's prognostic profile (at T = 0), but the timing of the set (on the scale of cohort/prognostic time) is not among the data; for, the *Cox model* – of "proportional hazards" – postulates that the "hazard ratio" – *incidence-density ratio* – in reference to the compared treatments, or whichever contrast based on the prognostic variates, is *constant throughout the prognostic time-horizon of the study.*

The results synthesized from the study data by means of Cox regression, well illustrated by the example study addressed in Chap. 19 above, are, inherently, of the form of those incidence-density ratios for the various events being addressed. This is a salient limitation inherent in the Cox-regression approach to the synthesis of the data assembled in clinical trials (and their quasi-experimental counterparts). For, *constancy of incidence-density ratios, treatments-comparing or other, is not realis-*

tic to presume in intervention-prognostic research; and much more importantly, *prognostication in the practice of clinical medicine is not about treatment effects in terms of those ratios*; it is about various possible events – and states too – in terms of the respective probabilities of their occurrence, *these prognostic probabilities as functions of the choice of treatment, causally, jointly with prognostic indicators and prognostic time, acausally* (Sect. 18.4).

There thus is a burning *need for an alternative to Cox regression* as the theoretical framework for the synthesis of the data in clinical trials, and indeed in prognostic cohort studies in general. The need is for an alternative that provides for the advancement of the knowledge-base of prognostic practices in terms of *prognostic probability functions* that accord with the true needs of practice (Sect. 4.1). *We present* the essence of such a theoretical framework in Sect. 20.1.2 below, and explicate it further in the rest of this Chapter.

20.1.2 The Needed, Novel Type of Synthesis

While in Cox regression, for the synthesis of clinical-trial (or other prognostic) data in regard to an event-type outcome, the pivotal element is *the series of the cases of the event* at issue, such a series is pivotal also in the alternative to it that we're here proposing – nay, advocating. But we introduce a critically-important novelty into the documentation of this series: the *timing* of each of the cases on the scale of prognostic time. This datum naturally is available in the database of any clinical trial.

And while in Cox regression the case series is supplemented with the sets of probes into the study base in terms of the cases' associated (synchronic) other members of the 'risk sets' of person-moments, we replace these by a *single sample of the study base at large*, not time-matched to the case series nor otherwise restricted/discriminate but a *completely representative* (stochastically) of the entirety of person-moments (infinite in number) constituting the study population-time, the study base. For this base series, the same data are abstracted from the study's database as for the case series (the timings of these probes included), the requisite data being available for these purposes in the database just as are the data needed for Cox regression.

Given these two series, with Y = 1 and Y = 0 for the case and base series, respectively, but the Xs identically defined – in reference to the type of treatment; time since the treatment's initiation; and the prognostic indicators' realizations – a *logistic model* for Pr (Y = 1) is fitted to the thus-constituted data. The result of the fitting is a linear compound of the empirical values of the parameters in the logistic model (Sects. 7.4.1 and 7.4.5).

Two things about this *logistic-regression result* are critically important to understand (Sect. 7.4.5). First, that it *addresses* the logarithms of ratios in which the numerators are the numbers of cases from the various strata of the study base and the denominators are the respective numbers of base probes from these – these denominator numbers being proportional (stochastically) to the respective amounts of population-time in the study base. Thus, if c and b are the sizes of the case and base series, respectively, the logistic function expresses the counterparts of the logarithm the c/b ratio – of this overall *quasi-rate* – specific to each of the strata defined by the Xs. (The values implied by the logistic function do not generally represent those stratum-specific values exactly as they are in the data; for they reflect the 'smoothening' that is inherent in the results of model-fitting).

The second critically-important thing to understand in this context is that the exponential of the linear compound from the logistic model-fitting, exp (L), represents the various Xs-specified *quasi-rates.* Once this important subtlety is understood, it is easy to understand how the result of the logistic model-fitting provides for the corresponding result for the actual *incidence-density*, ID, of the event's occurrence in the study base, that is, for that ID as a function of those Xs. For the needed transition from the quasi-rates to actual incidence-densities, needed is replacement of the denominators of the quasi-rates by the corresponding amounts of actual population-time in the strata of the study base:

$$\mathrm{ID} = \left(\mathrm{b} / \mathrm{B}\right)\exp\left(\mathrm{L}\right),$$

where b is the size of the (representative) base series and B is the size of the study base proper.

This access to result in the form of actual incidence-density as a function of prognostic time implies access to the event's *cumulative incidence* over prognostic time and, thereby, to empirical values for the *probabilities* of its occurrence in various spans of prognostic time (Sects. 5.5.4, 7.4.5, and 18.5) in addition to their dependence on the choice of treatment and the realizations of various prognostic indicators.

This approach to prognostic probabilities for event-type entities of health has a ready extension the *states* of health. Instead of a case series coupled with a representative base series, needed is merely a *single series of person-moments* somehow covering the range of prognostic time of study interest, selected independently of the presence/absence of the state in question (at whatever chosen times). For these person-moments, the datum on the presence/absence of the state at issue (implying Y = 1 or Y = 0) can be ascertained from the study's database, in addition to the data abstracted from it for studying the probabilities for event-type entities. The linear compound L, obtained by fitting a logistic model for Pr (Y = 1) to the data, represents the result function for the logit transform of the probability of the state in question being present, conditionally on the Xs. The corresponding *function for the prognostic probability* itself is non-linear (in the parameters).

$$\Pr\left(\mathrm{Y} = 1\right) = 1 / \left[1 + \exp\left(-\mathrm{L}\right)\right].$$

20.1.3 Notes on the Needed Type of Synthesis

The Section above (20.1.2) reflects the truism (per Sect. 20.1.1) that in the synthesis of the data from a prognostic cohort study – a randomized trial, say – on the occurrence of an event-type outcome in prognostic (prospective) time, the focus needs to be on the *incidence density* of that event's occurrence in the *study base specific to that event*; and the Section above emphasizes that, in the thus-focused synthesis of the data, *it is essential to account for the timings of the events' occurrence* so as to obtain a first-stage result on this rate of the event's occurrence as a function of prognostic time (i.a.). For, this function is the requisite basis for the corresponding result for cumulative incidence of the event's occurrence as a function of prognostic time (i.a.), this function providing empirical values for the cumulative probabilities of the event's prospective occurrence (Sect. 18.2.2).

Besides, the Section above shows how the *actual incidence-density function* – and not merely the corresponding function for incidence-density ratio – *can be derived from the routine type of database in clinical trials* (and, naturally, in their quasi-experimental counterparts as well). Involved in it necessarily is the case series together with a suitable – representative – base series, with the causal (treatment-focused) histories documented for both, just as in an etiognostic study (Sect. 15.6) and in a non-cohort intervention-prognostic study (non-experimental; Chap. 21).

With all of this understood, the question may arise, *Is the Cox model subject to the requisite modifications* – so as to address incidence-density ratio as a function of prognostic time as well (and not merely as a function of factors, choice of treatment included, whose temporal referents are prognostic T = 0), and this in such a way that it provides for obtaining the corresponding result for incidence-density proper? The short answer is No.

20.2 Example of the Needed Type of Synthesis for Incidence Density

Whereas Sect. 20.1 above was an introduction to the theory of studying intervention-prognostic probability functions on the basis of the data routinely collected in clinical trials on treatments' comparative effects, and whereas internalization of that didactic content may call for examples of the theory in application, we here provide such examples. *These examples we build around the eminent trial* [1] *extensively addressed in* Chap. 19 *above*, in two stages. In the *first stage* of this (in Sects. 20.2.1 and 20.2.2), we show how initial, exploratory results can be derived without any regression, from the *etiognostic vantage* we advocate for these studies. And in the *second stage* (Sect. 2.2.3) we address logistic regression synthesis of the case-base data into incidence-density functions of prognostic time.

20.2.1 'Tabular' Replication of Cox-Type Statistics

In the trial addressed in Chap. 19 [1], it may be recalled, the expressly designated "primary" efficacy and safety outcomes of the use of Premarin by postmenopausal women were (rule-in diagnosed) cases of coronary heart disease (acute) and breast cancer (invasive), respectively. For these, the respective results from Cox regression were these: for CHD, the "estimated hazard ratio" – the empirical incidence-density ratio – was 0.91, with the imprecision of this in terms of 95% 'confidence interval' reported as the range from 0.75 to 1.12; and for breast cancer, correspondingly, Cox regression yielded "0.77 (0.59–1.01)."

We now set out to replicate these CHD statistics on the basis of the relevant data (reduced) reported from that study, doing this in the *case-base (case-referent) framework* we're advocating. And for good measure, in Sect. 20.2.2 we replicate the corresponding statistics for breast cancer as well as for stroke. This extends the introduction to this alternative approach given in Sect. 19.2.4 by that specificity to the case-base structure of the data abstracted for the trial's database.

In the study base for *CHD*, the number of identified *cases* of this event was 376, and the numbers among these associated with index (Premarin) and reference (placebo) histories were (per the report's Table 3) 177 and 199, respectively (177 + 199 = 376). From the case series, thus, the numerator *inputs to the index and reference quasi-rates* in the study base (the study result's referent) for CHD were 177 and 199, respectively (Cf. Sect. 19.2.4).

In a *representative sample of the study base* for CHD, the numbers of the probes (person-moments) associated with index and reference histories, respectively, would have been proportional (stochastically) to the population-time sizes of the index and reference segments of the study base in the various segments of follow-up time. These are not given in the report on the study, but given are (in Figure 3) the respective numbers of subjects entering the successive years of follow-up in the study base for CHD. Pairwise averaging of those successive numbers in the Premarin and placebo cohorts yields reasonable estimates of the year-specific amounts of population-time in the study base for the first 8 years of follow-up (Sect. 19.2.4) and the amounts (small) for the 9th year can reasonably be extrapolated. *Proportional to those amounts of population-time* are the following numbers, showing what would have been the *distribution of the base sample* – unrestrictedly representative – of *size* equal to 1% the number of person-years of follow-up for CHD:

Year	1.	2.	3.	4.	5.	6.	7.	8.	9.	Total
Premarin	53	52	51	50	49	44	31	16	5	351
Placebo	54	53	52	51	50	45	32	17	5	359

With this sample, the *index and reference quasi-rates* (proportional to the index and reference incidence-densities in the study base) for CHD would have been 177/351 and 199/359, respectively, *their ratio* being 0.910 = 0.91 – this *incidence-*

density ratio being, as expected, the very same as the "hazard ratio" reported from Cox regression. (Based on the first 8 years, without those extrapolations to the 9th year, the result is the same: the index and reference quasi-rates are 177/346 and 199/354, respectively, their ratio being 0.910 = 0.91).

From the 'etiognostic' 2×2 table with these IDR-implying numbers in the cells of it and the marginal totals 376 (number of cases), 719 (number of base probes), 528 (number of index cases and probes), and 558 (number of reference cases and probes), for a grand total of 1086, the inferential statistics are derived in the usual way of etiogenetic epidemiological studies: For the 'observed' number of index cases (177), the corresponding null number is E = 376(518)/1,086 = 132.81, and the null variance (hypergeometric) is the product of the marginal totals divided by T^2 (T – 1), where T is the grand total. This number is V = 61.52, whose square root is 7.84. Thus the Gaussian test statistic has the realization of z = (177 – 182.81)/7.8 4 = – 0.71. The corresponding 95% interval (test-based) for the IDR thus is exp [(log O. 91)(1 + / – 1.96/0.741)] = 0.71, 1.17. (Cf. Sect. 19.2.4).

With that base sample (representative) – only twofold relative to the case series – the result (IDR = 0.91) would have been somewhat less precise than it was without the sampling (Sect. 19.2.4). With the base series tenfold relative to the case series (b = 10c = 3510), the 95% interval associated with the result (IDR = 0.91) would have been from 0.74 to 1.12. (In this context, the result's imprecision would have derived almost totally from the size of the case series).

Given that this example was intended to consolidate elementary understanding of the approach we're advocating for the synthesis of the data from clinical trials (Sects. 20.1.2 and 20.1.3), the essentials of its instructive burden may be summarized in the following three propositions:

1. Whereas the Cox-regression approach to clinical-trial data produces *results* in terms of incidence-density ratios – commonly, as in the example study [1], a single value for any given type of event – these results can be derived from the database for Cox regression in a manner that flows directly from *first principles of etiogenetic/etiognostic studies* (Sect. 15.6), *without any regression-type modelling* and its consequent computer-based model-fitting.
2. Whereas as the imprecision of those (single-valued) rate-ratio results from Cox regression is routinely expressed in terms of 'confidence intervals,' which the computer output from the model-fitting commonly gives, these statistics, too, can be derived, in a straightforward way [2], from the (simple) inputs to the (first-principles) derivation of those results in the alternative theoretical framework herein advocated – with a base series tenfold in size relative to the case series sufficient to capture practically all of the information in the study base.
3. These understandings suggest replacement of Cox regression by *logistic regression* in the synthesis of the data from clinical trials into those (simplistic) statistics now commonly derived by means of the Cox-regression approach, given the well-established status of logistic regression in etiogenetic studies. And as this etiogenetic/etiognostic viewpoint – with representative sampling of the study-base – is germane to the data-synthesis we advocate for intervention-prognostic

studies (Sects. 20.1.2 and 20.1.3), the larger implication is our call for the replacement of Cox regression by logistic regression in these studies.

20.2.2 'Tabular' Results on Incidence Density Proper

In seeking to understand the here-advocated transition from Cox regression to logistic regression in the synthesis of the data from a clinical trial, the key thing to come to grips with is *the essential novelty* in this: addressing, in the synthesis, the way the *incidence-density proper* – rather than incidence-density ratio – of the event in question is, according to the data, a function of *prognostic time*. We here illustrate this pivotal aspect of the synthesis of the data in the framework of such case-base (case-referent) abstraction of the data as we're here advocating (Sect. 20.1.2). In this, we extend, still in the 'tabular' framework, our treatment of the example addressed in Sect. 20.2.1 above.

Just as we in Chap. 19 addressed the data from the example trial [1] in a 'tabular' manner to derive the statistics reported from Cox regression for a single-valued incidence-density ratio, we here approach the data in respect to the *time trend in the incidence density* proper of each of the three outcomes in a similar two-stage manner: first by means of suitable reductions of the detailed ('raw') data, and then in the framework of logistic regression.

For the 'tabular' approach at issue here, the *first-stage reduced data are imbedded in the case and (representative) base series* pertaining to the outcome at issue, and the first concern here is to suitably *reduce these data further* so as to get a sense of the event's incidence density as a function of prognostic time – and so as to further cultivate this habit of informative data-reduction in the reader and to help him/her better understand the statistics from the fitting of a logistic model to the detailed data (and to learn to check those statistics' consistency with the data).

So we consider, again, the "primary" effectiveness outcome, *CHD* (coronary heart disease). The report on the study [1] gives the distribution of the cases (N = 376) by time after entry into the study cohort, in terms of 1st year, 2nd year, etc. (Figure 3), separately by the two types of treatment (N = 177 with Premarin as the treatment, 199 with placebo). The corresponding distribution in the (representative) base series would have mirrored the relative amounts of population-time of the study population's follow-up in those successive years. These can be estimated by averaging the numbers (in that Figure 3) of participants entering successive years of follow-up for CHD (Sects. 19.2.4 and 20.2.1, above). Here we again consider these estimates for a base series of size equal to 1% of the number of person-years in the study base for CHD.

We thus have these data (already to some extent reduced) on the *case and base series* in respect to CHD, relevant to getting a sense of the *temporal pattern* in the rates:

Year of follow-up		1.	2.	3.	4.	5.	6.	7.	8.	9.
Case series	(N = 376)									
Premarin	(N = 177)	26	27	22	21	30	31	13	6	1
Placebo	(N = 199)	23	23	25	27	24	26	28	17	6
Base series	(N = 710)									
Premarin	(N = 351)	53	52	51	50	49	44	31	16	5
Placebo	(N = 359)	54	53	52	51	50	45	32	17	5

To make the pattern to emerge more clearly, we reduce these data even more:

Years of follow-up		1. – 3.	4. – 6.	7. – 9.
Case series	(N = 376)			
Premarin	(N = 177)	75	82	20
Placebo	(N = 199)	71	77	51
Base series	(N = 710)			
Premarin	(N = 351)	156	143	52
Placebo	(N = 359)	159	146	54

From these data on the distributions of the case and base series we deduce, for those three periods of prognostic time, the respective index (Premarin-associated) and reference (placebo-associated) *incidence-densities for CHD*. As an example of this (per Sect. 20.1.2), let's focus on the *first 3 years* of follow-up: The *quasi-rate* of CHD occurrence under (assigned) Premarin use was 75/156. Thus the *incidence density* of these cases' occurrence was – given a sample of size 351 + 359 = 710 from the study base of size 71,000 p – y – [710/(71,000 p – y)]75/156 = 0.48/(100 p – y) = 48/(10,000 p – y). Thus derived from the data above, the index and reference incidence-densities for CHD in those three periods of follow-up (prognostic time) were these:

Years of follow-up	1. – 3.	4. – 6.	7. – 9.
Premarin cohort	48/(10,000 p-y)	57/(10,000 p-y)	38/(10,000 p-y)
Placebo cohort	45/(10,000 p-y)	53/(10,000 p-y)	94/(10,000 p-y)

From these data (suitably reduced) on the temporal trends, it is evident that in the *placebo cohort* there was a trend, one of substantial increase, in the CHD rate from the first period to the third. (A doubling of the rate over mere 6 years of increase in the placebo-cohort's age is surprising). In the *Premarin cohort*, by contrast, there appears not to have been any such trend, nor a declining trend, notably when keeping in mind that the experience in the third period was relatively small.

Let's look more closely at that temporal pattern of the rate in the *Premarin cohort*, as the third-period result seems to be so out of line with the first two. For this it is necessary to quantify the *imprecisions of those three rates*; and this we'll do in terms of the routine measure of it in all of the foregoing, and in general too: the 95%

'confidence' (imprecision) interval. Statistical models are needed for the production of these statistics (just as any other 'inferential statistics') from study data. *The focus in this needs to be on the numbers of CHD cases* in the three periods, those 75, 82, and 20 above. These can be viewed as realizations of *Poisson*-type distributions. In deriving confidence intervals for them, use can be made of the fact that the *square root* of a Poisson-distributed variate has *variance 1/4* irrespective of the distribution's mean. Thus, for those numbers' square roots, the 95% intervals have the boundaries of these values minus/plus 1.96(0.50) = 1.0. For the first period, the boundaries on the square-root level are 7.7 and 9.7, the squares of which are the 95% limits 59 and 94 for the number of cases in the first period, the corresponding quasi-rates being these numbers divided by the corresponding number of base probes, 156 (cf. above).

Thus derived, the 95% intervals for the *quasi-rates* in the three successive periods were: 0.38–0.60, 0.46–0.71, and 0.28–0.65. So, all three of the time-specific quasi-rates for the Premarin cohort were well consistent with the overall quasi-rate for this cohort, 177/351 = 0.50; and therefore, the *actual rates*, given above, were *consistent with the overall rate* for this cohort, 50/(10,000 p-y). But whereas the rates in the placebo cohort were, by contrast, very clearly increasing with prognostic time – from 45 to 94 per 10,000 person-years from the first triad of years to the third – it is clear that *the incidence-density ratio (theoretical) was not constant* over the follow-time of the trial, and that, therefore, it is unjustifiable to reduce those time-specific results for this ratio to its overall counterpart, (177/351)/(199/359) = 0.91 – which was the result reported from the study [1], derived under the "proportional hazards" model of Cox regression (cf. Chap. 9 and Sect. 20.1.1).

As for *breast cancer,* the distribution of the study base by year of follow-up turned out to be the very same as for CHD. The sample – representative – of this, considered for the illustration here, was again taken to be 1% of the number of person-years constituting the study base. The first-order reduced data, analogously abstracted from the report [1], are these (cf. CHD above):

Year of follow-up		1.	2.	3.	4.	5.	6.	7.	8.	9.
Case series	(N = 218)									
Premarin	(N = 94)	9	11	13	18	10	16	6	6	5
Placebo	(N = 124)	7	20	15	22	24	18	12	6	0
Base series	(N = 710)									
Premarin	(N = 351)	53	52	51	50	49	44	31	16	5
Placebo	(N = 359)	54	53	52	51	50	45	32	17	5

These we again reduce to the corresponding data for the three successive periods of prognostic time:

Years of follow-up		1. – 3.	4. – 6.	7. – 9.
Case series	(N = 218)			

Years of follow-up		1. – 3.	4. – 6.	7. – 9.
Premarin	(N = 94)	33	44	17
Placebo	(N = 124)	42	64	18
Base series	(N = 710)			
Premarin	(N = 351)	156	143	52
Placebo	(N = 359)	159	146	54

For the Premarin cohort, thus, the incidence density of breast-cancer diagnoses in the first period was 710/(710,000 p-y) 33/156 = 21/(10,000 p-y). And for each of the two cohorts in each of the three periods the rates were these:

Years of follow-up	1. – 3.	4. – 6.	7. – 9.
Premarin cohort	21/(10,000 p-y)	31/(10,000 p-y)	33/(10,000 p-y)
Placebo cohort	26/(10,000 p-y)	44/(10,000 p-y)	33/(10,000 p-y)

Despite their imprecision, these rates (empirical) give *an indication of the corresponding rates generally being lower among Premarin users* than among comparable non-users – which, if true, would mean that Premarin (a mixture of estrogens) actually retards, rather than accelerates, the growth of this estrogen-dependent cancer. This would be *quite odd*, as evinced by the fact that the investigators had designated breast cancer as the "primary" outcome to be addressed with a view to existing concerns about the safety of sustained use of Premarin (as a prophylactic against CHD, i.a., in postmenopausal women).

20.2.3 Incidence Density's Time Function per Logistic Regression

With the foregoing addressing the data-reduction preliminaries, with some inferential statistics added, we fitted a logistic-regression model to the minimally-reduced data on CHD incidence specified above, the realizations of the treatments' duration being, in units of years, 0.5 for the 1st year, 1.5 for the second, etc., but only 8.25 for the 9th year (as the sparse experience presumably was concentrated in the earliest part of that year).

The model – for the logarithm of the quasi-rate (number of cases per number of base probes; Sect. 20.1.2) – involved Y = 1 and Y = 0 for the case and base series, respectively, and this linear compound of parameters (four in number):

$$\mathrm{L} = B_0 + B_1\mathrm{X}_1 + B_2\mathrm{X}_2 + B_3\mathrm{X}_3;$$

X_1: indicator of assignment to treatment by Premarin,
X_2: time since the assignment of the treatment (number of years),
$\mathrm{X}_3 = \mathrm{X}_1\mathrm{X}_2$.

The fitting of this model to those data produced these usually-sought-after (but somewhat redundant) statistics (along with much usually-bypassed esoterica): "*Estimate, Std. Error, z value, and Pr (>|z|),*" with inordinate numbers of significant digits. Our interest here is in those "estimates," which to us are the real results among them, as they are the object parameters' empirical values (biased and imprecise) produced by the study.

The model's fitting yielded this linear compound (representing the logarithm of the quasi-rate; cf. above): L = − 1.029 + 0.327X_1 + 0.116 X_2 − 0.111X_3. Thus the respective results for the quasi-rate's logarithm for the Premarin (X_1 = 1) and placebo (X_1 = X_3 = 0) cohorts were these:

$$\begin{aligned}\text{Premarin}: L_1 &= -1.029 + 0.327 + (0.116 - 0.111)X_2 \\ &= -0.702 + 0.0049X_2, \\ \text{Placebo}: L_0 &= -1.029 + 0.116X_2.\end{aligned}$$

Given these results from the fitting of the regression model, it is interesting to consider *how well their implications jibe with the rates derived above by tabular means* for the three successive 3-year periods of follow-up and shown above. Deriving the regression counterparts of those rates involves the quasi-rates that are the exponentials of those linear compounds evaluated at the midpoints of those ranges of time, at values 1.5, 4.5, and 7.5 of X_2. These regression-based results are:

Prognostic time (X_2)	1.5	4.5	7.5
Premarin cohort	50/(10,000 p-y)	51/(10,000 p-y)	51/(10,000 p-y)
Placebo cohort	43/(10,000 p-y)	60/(10,000 p-y)	85/(10,000 p-y)

The agreement of these rates with their tabular counterparts (above) is good, notably in the light of the imprecisions of those tabular rates (quantified above).

That same model's fitting to the corresponding data on *breast cancer* produced this linear compound (representing the logarithm of the quasi-rate): L = − 1.344 − 0.353X_1 + 0.0763 X_2 + 0.0250X_3. For the Premarin and placebo cohorts, respectively; this result implies

$$\begin{aligned}L_1 &= -1.697 + 0.101X_2, \\ L_0 &= -1.344 + 0.076X_2.\end{aligned}$$

The respective functions for the *incidence-density proper* (of breast cancer) are these:

$$\text{Premarin cohort}: \text{ID} = [1/(100\text{p}-\text{y})]\exp(-1.70 + 0.10X_2).$$
$$\text{Placebo cohort}: \text{ID} = [1/(100\text{p}-\text{y})]\exp(-1.34 + 0.076X_2).$$

Regarding these functions' *consistency with the data*, shown below are, for the three successive 3-year periods of follow-up, *the 95% intervals/ranges for the numbers of cases per 10,000 person-years* (repeating what was given above) together with the *results from those functions* at typical points in those rages of time, namely at 1.5, 4.5, and 7.5 years post randomization:

Years of follow-up	1. – 3.	4. – 6.	7. – 9.
Premarin cohort			
Tabular 95% range	14–29	22–41	19–50
Regression result	21	29	39
Placebo cohort			
Tabular 95% range	19–35	34–55	19–51
Regression result	29	39	46

The results from the regression-model's fitting to the detailed data (as detailed as were available from the report on the study) are seen to be well consistent with the time-specific results from the reduced data.

Against the backdrop of those rather thorough treatments of the data on CHD and breast cancer, a less-detailed treatment of the data concerning *stroke* will suffice for the ultimate purpose common to all the examples here, namely illustration that it is feasible to go beyond the Cox-regression result and to synthesize the data into *incidence density as a function of prognostic time* jointly with the choice of treatment – and, by obvious extension, as functions of prognostic indicators as well – in tabular terms and by means of logistic regression.

For each of the successive 3-year periods of follow-up, shown below are two types of result for the *number of cases of stroke per 10,000 person-years* (derived by calculations analogous to those in the examples above): first, the tabular quasi-rate multiplied (in accordance with the size on the base series in relation to the size of the base proper) by 1/(100 p-y), with the resulting number per this amount of population-time translated to the corresponding number per 10,000 person-years by multiplication by 100; and second, the corresponding result with the quasi-rate derived, as in the two examples above from the exponential of the linear compound from the fitting of the same logistic model as above, evaluated for those periods at times 1.5, 4.5, and 7.5 years, respectively (just as above).

The respective results were these:

Years of follow-up	1. – 3.	4. – 6.	7. – 9.
Premarin cohort			
Tabular result	37	48	60
Regression result	37	48	63
Placebo cohort			
Tabular result	31	34	37
Regression result	29	35	42

To say that the agreement is good would be an understatement.

The result of the model's fitting (for the quasi-rate's logarithm) was this:

$$L = -1.344 + 0.221X_1 + 0.0631X_2 + 0.0242X_3$$

overall; and for the Premarin and placebo cohorts, respectively, they thus were these:

$$L_1 = -1.123 + 0.0873X_2,$$
$$L_0 = -1.344 + 0.0631X_2.$$

20.2.4 Notes on the Examples Above

A few *concluding notes* in the three Sections above may serve to consolidate the learning from them:

1. It is notable that the *tabular-type exploration of the treatment-specific temporal trends* in the outcome events' incidence-densities over the study cohort's follow-up, illustrated by the examples above, was absent from the report on the very high-profile study [1] from which the data for those examples were drawn; and especially, that it has been missing from the syntheses of clinical-trial data in general. This is regrettable because, different from the fitting of a regression model, such exploration would provide the investigators – and their readers likewise – the necessary *'feel' for the data*, notably in regard to the obviously-important matter of the rates' relation to prognostic time.
2. Those *tabular preliminaries* to model-based synthesis of clinical-trial data *would indicate whether the Cox-regression premise of proportional hazards* is tenable for the experience at issue. To wit, for the three successive periods of follow-up time in the example study we here addressed, the respective ratios of the thus-calculated rates were 1.1, 1.1, and 0.4 for CHD; 0.8, 0.7, and 1.0 for breast cancer; and 1.2, 1.4, and 1.6 for stroke; and we showed how to quantify the imprecisions of the empirical rates as well as of their ratios.
3. When these preliminaries are preparatory to data-synthesis into a result expressing, for a given type of event, the incidence-density of its occurrence as a function of various determinants of this rate (incl. prognostic time), it is good to deploy, in these preliminaries already, the *case-base (case-referent) approach* that is integral to that ultimate, regression-based synthesis of the data and to that end requires, specifically, the use of a *fully representative (rather than somehow stratified) sample of the study base* (specific for the outcome in question). In the examples above, the size of the base series was kept small for the convenience of the illustrations, but it actually should be (and readily can be) made much larger

than the size of the case series, consequent to which the results' imprecision derives solely from the case series (its limited size).

4. *It is critically important to understand what the linear-compound result of the fitting of a logistic-regression model to case-referent (case-base) data represents*, namely: the logarithm of the ratio of the numbers of instances (person-moments) in the two series – this quasi-rate proxy for incidence density – specific to the strata of the study base defined by the variates (Xs) involved in the compound. For, *from this fact flow two essential corollaries*: first the obvious one that the exponential (antilog) of that linear compound represents the quasi-rates themselves in the various strata of the study base (the study result's referent); and then the more subtle but ultimately critical one, that this exponential multiplied by the size of the base series divided by the size of the actual study base (in amount of population-time) translates that quasi-rate function into the corresponding function for the incidence-density proper – provided that the distribution of the base series over the strata of the study base accords with the respective stratum-specific proportions of the overall population-time of the study base. These understandings are the foundation of the here-advocated logistic-regression synthesis of clinical-trial data into the outcome events' incidence-densities as functions of prognostic time, inter alia, and thereby into prognostic probability functions.
5. While we calculated some inferential statistics in those preliminaries, from the statistics arising from the fitting of the regression model to the data on each of the three types of outcome, we took actual interest only in the parameters' "estimates," meaning their *fitted values*, empirical in this meaning. There were *three reasons for this focus*. First, in respect to the main issue – the treatments' relative effects – the inferential statistics associated with the parameters' empirical values were redundant with their counterparts from the preliminaries. Second, they were devoid of ready interpretability, as three parameters were involved in the result on those effects in respect to any given outcome. And third, the purpose of the regression syntheses of the data is not to serve some inference about each of the parameters involved but to obtain an empirical function for the outcome's prospective incidence-density – as a basis deriving the corresponding cumulative incidence functions (interpretable as cumulative probability functions, with certain subtleties involved; Sect. 18.2).
6. As a little closing note here, *the counterparts of the reported "odds ratios"* – incidence density ratios – for CHD, breast cancer, and stroke – 0.91, 0.77, and 1.39 – can be derived by fitting the logistic model, involving simply $L = B_0 + B_1X_1$ with X_1 the indicator of (assignment to) Premarin use. The exponentials of the resulting values for B_1 are: 0.91, 0.77, and 1.37. But these should be taken to be very uninteresting, given the prognosis-serving focus here, which calls for addressing incidence density itself, and thereby cumulative incidence and probability, as a function of prognostic time, inter alia.

20.3 Intervention-Prognostic Probability Models

20.3.1 The Basic Model for Incidence Density

In this Chapter we've explicated the connection between the logistic model for the union of the case series (complete) and base series (representative, relatively large) from the study cohort's follow-up, most recently in the fourth one of the concluding statements in the closing of Sect. 20.2.2 above. And we here underscore how well the same – simple, bare-bones – model described the incidence densities of all three of the outcome events addressed in those very different examples (cf. concluding note number 2 above).

So *we propose that the basic model for logistic-regression synthesis of the data assembled in two-treatment experimental intervention-prognostic 'cohort' studies be taken to be the one we used in those examples.* It involves, as has been seen, this four-parameter linear compound:

$$\mathrm{L} = B_0 + B_1\mathrm{X}_1 + B_2\mathrm{X}_2 + B_3\mathrm{X}_3;$$

X_1: indicator of assignment to index treatment (1 if index treatment, 0 otherwise)
X_2: *prognostic time* (numerical value),
X_3: $\mathrm{X}_1\mathrm{X}_2$.

This basic model can readily be expanded by inclusion of *prognostic variates* (analogously to the basic Cox model).

It is instructive to consider this basic model in the further-simplified situation involving the indicator of the assigned treatment (X_1) but no provision for prognostic time (nor for prognostic indicators), juxtaposing this to the corresponding Cox model (involving X_1 alone). Our basic model, when involving X_1 as the only independent variate, implies

$$\mathrm{ID} = (\mathrm{b}/\mathrm{B})\exp(B_0 + B_1\mathrm{X}_1).$$

The Cox counterpart of this is:

$$\mathrm{ID} = h_0 \exp(B_1\mathrm{X}_1),$$

where h_0 is the incidence density conditional on $\mathrm{X}_i = 0$ for all i, here conditional on $\mathrm{X}_1 = 0$.

Two *implications of this equivalence* are of note. First, that our approach provides for studying that h_0 of the Cox model, while Cox regression itself does not. It is, simply, (b/B) times exp (B_0). And second, that insofar as interest is in presumedly time-invariant incidence-density ratio – which is what Cox regression inherently postulates – our approach provides for addressing this. It is, simply, the exponential of B_1 (in the logistic $L = B_0 + B_1X_1$, involved in the basic model reduced by removing the terms for prognostic time).

The results under those two (utterly-reduced) models for the synthesis of data from clinical-trial data, derived in our example study [1] by Cox regression, we replicated without any regression in Sects. 19.2.4 and 20.2.1; and here we present the results of their replication with the approach we advocate, here involving $L = B_0 + B_1X_1$ and data on the two series as described in Sect. 20.2.1. At issue for each outcome is the result on (presumedly time-invariant) incidence-density ratio together with its 95% 'confidence' (imprecision) interval.

For *coronary heart disease*, the fitting gave for B_1 the result – 0.0946 with 'standard error' 0.128. Thus the result for the incidence-density ratio was exp (–0.0946) = 0.91, and the 95% interval was exp [–0.946 ± 1.96(0.128)] = 0.72, 1.17 – while the result from Cox regression was reported [1] to be (that same) 0.91 with the 95% interval (the somewhat narrower) 0.75–1.12. The use of a larger base series would have reduced the width of the interval from the logistic approach (cf. Sect. 20.2.1).

For *breast cancer*, the fitting gave $B_1 = -0.255$ as the rate-ratio's logarithm, with 0.156 as this logarithm's 'SE.' For the rate ratio proper, this implied the value 0.77, with 95% imprecision limits 0.57 and 1.05 – corresponding to the "0.77 (0.59–1.01)" from Cox regression on the detailed data.

And for *stroke*, the fitted value for B_1 was 0.314, with 'SE' 0.143. Thus, the result for the rate ratio was 1.37, with 95% limits 1.03 and 1.81 – corresponding to "1.39 (1.10–1.77)."

As these examples illustrate, the results from Cox regression can be replicated by means of logistic regression, applied to the data on the case and base series as outlined in Sect. 20.1.2, notably with a base series that is sufficiently large.

20.3.2 The Basic Model for Cumulative Incidence

That basic model for the event's incidence density (ID) in the study base implies the corresponding basic model for cumulative incidence and, thereby, for prognostic probability. To this end there is the *need to integrate the incidence density over the span of prognostic time at issue*. For, the cumulative incidence is the complement of (i.e., 1 –) the exponential of the negative of this integral [2]. We'll first consider the informal version of this integration, focusing on the three examples in Sect. 20.2. Like in the report on the trial, we'll consider the entire span of prognostic time in the study, for which the report shows (in its Figure 3) "Kaplan-Meier cumulative hazards for selected clinical outcomes."

For *CHD*, the fitting of the basic model (Sect. 20.3.1, above) gave for the Premarin cohort, these numbers of cases per 10,000 person-years – cases per 10,000 years – for the successive 3-year periods: 50, 50, and 51 (cf. Sect. 20.2.2). The integral of those rates over all three of these periods is their sum multiplied by

3 year. The result of this calculation is 453/10,000 = 0.0453. The corresponding value (empirical) for 9-year cumulative incidence (and cumulative probability) is 1 − exp (−0.0453) = 0.044. For the *placebo* cohort, the corresponding triad of numbers is 43, 60, and 85, the corresponding integral of the rate is 0.0564, and the cumulative incidence rate is 0.055.

For *breast cancer*, the corresponding numbers of cases per 10,000 person-years (10,000 years) were 21, 29, and 39 for the Premarin cohort, and 29, 39, and 46 for the placebo cohort. The cumulatives resulting from these are 0.026 and 0.034, respectively.

And for *stroke*, the corresponding numbers were 37, 48, and 63 for the Premarin cohort, and 29, 35, and 42 for the placebo cohort. These translate into the respective cumulatives of 0.043 and 0.031.

Formally, the integral of the reference rate ID_0 = (b/B) exp (B_0 + B_2X_2] from $X_2 = 0$ to $X_2 = t$ (in years) is (b/B) [exp (B_0)](1/B_2)[−1 + exp (B_2t)]y. For the index rate, B_0 in the reference integral is replaced by $B_0 + B_1$, and B_2 by $B_2 + B_3$.

For CHD, the index and reference ID functions were

$$ID_1 = \left[1/(100y)\right]\exp\left(-0.702 + 0.0049X_2\right),$$
$$ID_0 = \left[1/(100y)\right]\exp\left(-1.029 + 0.116X_2\right),$$

as informally derived above. The corresponding integral of ID_1 from 0 to 9 years is (1/(100 y)[exp (−0.702)](1/0.0049)[−1 + exp (0.044)] y = 0.45, essentially the same as with the informal calculation above, translating into 1.01[1 − exp (−0.45)] = 0.45, also essentially the same as the informal informally-derived result above. Thus verified, the resulting basic cumulative incidence function for CHD conditional on assignment to Premarin use is the following over the period from T = 0 to T = t:

$$CI = 1.0\left[-1 + \exp\left(0.0049t'\right)\right],$$

where t′ is prognostic time (t) in terms of the number of years (i.e., as t/y). The other basic probability functions can be derived analogously from the results of the fitting of the basic logistic model (above).

20.3.3 Augmented Models for Prognostic Probabilities

For actual prognostic probabilities, the basic regression-model for the synthesis of the data from a clinical trial (Sect. 20.3.1) would need to be augmented in two ways, one trivial, the other rather challenging. The needed trivial augmentation is a matter of including B_4X_4 etc. as terms representing prognostic indicators. The needed but rather *challenging augmentation* is a matter of moving, in the modelling for incidence density, from description of the event's actual rate of occurrence in the study base to the intended-but-unattained, practice-relevant counterpart of this: the pattern of incidence that would have obtained in the study base *had there been full adherence* to the treatments to which the study subjects were assigned.

The study we've been using as the source of examples of clinical-trial data [1] exemplifies, also, the importance of correcting for the non-adherence bias in the results. In that trial, as now is commonplace, "The rate comparisons were based on the intention-to-treat principle using failure time methods," without correcting for the biases arising from the study subjects' not following through with their intention to be treated according to the (randomized) assignments. But the corrections really were called for, as "At the time of study termination, 53.8% of women had already stopped taking study medication" and "some women initiated hormone use through their own health care clinician: …"

For synthesis of the data in reference to *full adherence* to the assigned treatments, needed is replacement of the histories of the assigned treatments by their counterparts for the *actual treatments,* suitably defined. For example, if the effect of Premarin use in the etiogenesis of *CHD* (in the meaning of MI) is thought of in terms of 'HRT' enhancing thrombogenesis alone (exclusive of atherogenesis), relevant in the histories is only 'recent' use of 'HRT,' suitably defined. And on this premise, then, the indicator of assignment to the verum treatment would be replaced by an indicator of 'recent' treatment of this type.

As another example, if the 'HRT' effect in the etiogenesis of *breast cancer* (overt) is thought of in terms of the cancer's promotion alone (and not its initiation), the relevant history might be taken to be the proportion of the time since the randomization that 'HRT' was used. The result in reference to this proportion becomes the result for full adherence with this history variate's values 1 and 0 for the index and reference histories, respectively.

Introduction of *confounding at baseline* (T = 0) by this transition from the assigned treatments to the actual ones should not be seen as a problem, given that all potential confounders are members of the complete set of prognostic indicators, practically all of which are accounted for in the prognostic probability functions designed as the objects of the trial. And *prospectively emerging confounding* can be controlled in terms of variates with the case and base series' person-moments their temporal referents.

20.4 Fitting a Prognostic Probability Model to Clinical-Trial Data

The central theme in this Chapter has been the need to address, in each clinical trial for the advancement of the knowledge-base of clinical medicine, an expressly-designed *prognostic probability function* for each of the types of outcome event documented in it – the designed function for any given type of those events expressing the adopted way of thinking about its cumulative probability over prognostic time, conditionally on the type of intervention (assigned or actual) and the realizations of the prognostic indicators documented at prognostic T_0 (the time of entry into the trial cohort).

In a clinical trial addressing such a function, the study base (specific to the outcome in question; Sect. 20.1.1) is documented in respect to the event's *incidence density* in it, the way this rate is a function of prognostic time, the type of intervention, and the set of prognostic indicators (Sects. 7.4.5 and 20.1.2), jointly considered.

The documentation of the study base for the event's incidence density involves, it may be recalled (Sect. 7.4.5), first the identification of two series of person-moments. One of these is the series of the person-moments at which a case of the event in question occurred. This case series is supplemented by the selection of a special type of base series: one constituted by an unselect, (stochastically) *representative sample* of the study base. Then, the person-moments in both of these series are documented in respect to the outcome at that point ($Y = 1$ and $Y = 0$ for the case and base series, respectively), and the variates representing the determinants of Pr ($Y = 1$) for particular points in the union of these two series (i.e., the Xs for prognostic time at the person-moment, its antecedent intervention, and the prognostic indicators at T_0). Finally, given this database, the logistic-regression counterpart of the designed model for the event's incidence density (Sect. 7.4.5) is fitted to the data.

The question may arise, Why is one to use this variant of logistic regression in a study of an event's incidence density, introducing the challenge of representative sampling of the population-time constituting the study base? Why not the familiar and facile *Poisson regression*? The reason is the limitation in the applicability of the latter, having to do with the extent of its requisite stratification of the study base and the numbers of events within the individual strata. To wit, in the trial addressed in this Chapter [1] there were 376 cases of CHD, the outcome event of main concern in respect to efficacy. With the study base stratified by not only treatment (two categories) and prognostic time (five categories, say) but also the prognostic indicators at the baseline (say three for age and two for each of five other indicators of the risk), even the average number of cases per stratum is very small (with those strata, $376/2 \times 5 \times 3 \times 32 = 0.4$). So the Poisson regression quickly breaks down by untenable paucity of cases of the event in at least some of the strata.

The novel challenge in the implementation of the here-advocated 'MSH regression' – as a replacement of Poisson regression and Cox regression – in an intervention trial is only the production of its database (involving the realizations of Y and the Xs) on the c + b data-points (on c cases of the event and b base-probes). For, fitting the logistic model to these data is straightforward by means of any one of the existing statistical software-packages for this.

Identification and documentation of the case series is a simple extension of its counterpart in Cox regression: the difference is only that it here involves the datum specifying the event's timing (the time to its occurrence from prognostic T_0).

The person-moments constituting the *base series* can be chosen by means of a two-stage process. In the first stage of the selection of a base probe, a member of the trial cohort is chosen with probability proportional to the size of his/her contribution to the population-time of the study base; and in the second stage, then, a point in this person-time fragment is chosen as a realization of a uniform distribution over that span of time. The thus-selected points of the study populationtime are documented analogously with the points in the case series. (The base series may involve more than just one point in a given person's contribution to the study base).

The software for the production of this dataset for fitting the logistic model for a given type of outcome event is already available [3], and so also are examples of its application [4].

References

1. The Women's Health Initiative steering committee (2004) Effects of conjugated equine estrogen in postmenopausal women with hysterectomy. The Women's Health Initiative randomized controlled trial. JAMA 292:1701–1712
2. Miettinen OS (1976) Estimability and estimation in case-referent studies. Am J Epidemiol 103:226–235
3. Bhatnagar S, Turgeon M, Saarela O, Hanley J (2017) Casebase: fitting flexible smooth-in-time hazards and risk functions via logistic and multinomial regression. R package version 0.1.0. https://cran.r-project.org/web/packages/casebase/index.html
4. Casebase. http://www.medicine.mcgill.ca/epidemiology/hanley/software/

Chapter 21
Non-experimental Intervention-Prognostic Studies

Contents

Abstract Study of the effects of interventions is of central concern in prognostic clinical research; and experimental intervention-prognostic studies – *clinical trials* – are being held as paradigmatic for their non-experimental counterparts. *We here expand this paradigm beyond the now-common type of focus in its objects, and then delineate the non-experimental alternatives* to these. This we follow with rather extensive treatment, descriptive and also critical, of some *carefully-chosen non-experimental studies* on the effect that was the focus of the principal effectiveness concern in the trial we've extensively addressed in the preceding two Chapters.

Keywords Experimental paradigms · Essentials of the studies · Examples of the studies · Overview of the examples

21.1 The Four Levels of the Experimental Paradigm

Two features of the study addressed in Chaps. 19 and 20 above [1] are illustrative of *the broadest outlook now animating research for clinicians' prognoses*. For one, that study – just as the other one of the two studies constituting the Women's Health Initiative [2] – was not about the health-prospects at large of a particular class of clinicians' clients as such; it was, specifically and solely, about the possibility of *changing those prospects* (whatever they may be) for the better, by means of a particular type of clinical intervention; that prognostic study focused on the effects

O. S. Miettinen et al., *Clinical Research Transformed*,
https://doi.org/10.1007/978-3-030-06176-0_21

(prospective) of a particular type of intervention. And for another, that study reflects the (common) *belief that experimental intervention-prognostic studies have, inherently, validity superior to that of their non-experimental counterparts*, and that, therefore, evidence from them trumps whatever may have been produced non-experimentally. Thus, categorical "conclusions" were drawn from the results of the trial we've been using as the example, without any regard for the ample evidence from its antecedent non-experimental ("observational") studies.

In this orientational framework for intervention prognostic clinical research, and in regard to the usual concern for an event-type outcome, *four levels of experimental paradigm for non-experimental intervention-prognostic studies* can be identified (per Chaps. 19 and 20, above), *based on what actually is addressed* in regard to that event's incidence in the study base:

Level 1. On the most elementary level addressed in respect to any given outcome event is its *incidence-density ratio* (causal), comparative between the sub-cohorts and representing the randomly assigned *intended treatments*. The model can incorporate variates for *prognostic indicators* as modifiers of the IDR but not prognostic time. This is what the now-commonly-deployed Cox model is all about (Sect. 20.1.1).

Level 2. On the next level, produced in the trial are results for any given outcome-event's IDR (comparing the intended treatments) with specificity not only on its dependence on prognostic indicators (à la Level 1, above) but on *prognostic (cohort) time* as well. This is achieved by invoking the *case-base/case-referent viewpoint* in the documentation of the IDR in the study base, the viewpoint of etiognostic studies. Replacement of the Cox model by *logistic modelling* is involved in the synthesis of the data with this important enlargement of the objects of study (Cf. Sect. 20.1.2).

Level 3. On the third level, the trial produces for any outcome event a result addressing its *incidence density itself*, this as a joint function of all three of the generic types of its determinants – prognostic time, choice of intended intervention, and prognostic indicators. The key to this is dual: for one, deployment of the etiognostic viewpoint on the synthesis of the data, as on Level 2, above; and for another, doing this with the special feature that provides for studying actual incidence densities (determinant-conditional) and not merely the ratios of these: selection of the *base series as a representative sample* of the study base for the outcome at issue. On this level, the trial provides for addressing cumulative incidence and, thereby, *prognostic probability functions* (Cf. Sect. 20.3).

Level 4. On the fourth, most advanced level, the intention-to-treat principle, still plaguing any Level 3 trial, is replaced by addressing the probability conditional on *full adherence* to the assigned treatments.

21.2 The Essentials of the Non-experimental Studies

A study on the prospective effects of an intervention is non-experimental if it lacks the feature that would have made it experimental. Thus, an intervention-prognostic study is *non-experimental* if the interventions in it are not assigned for the purposes of the study (for learning about their effects) but take place independently of the study (to achieve their intended effects). For the term 'non-experimental' here, a commonly-used synonym is 'observational'; but: experimental studies also are observational, observations-deploying.

The *study population* of non-experimental studies on the effects of interventions, different from their experimental counterparts, *is not inherently of the cohort type.* While the experimental assignments of treatments are tantamount to study subjects' enrolments into the study cohort, the absence of these assignments in the non-experimental studies leaves open the possibility of studying the effects in the framework of a *dynamic* study-population. As such a study-population is an inherent feature of the other, etiognostic species of causal studies for clinicians' gnoses (Sect. 15.6), studies which generally are non-experimental (Chap. 17), the question arises, whether at least some of non-experimental intervention-prognostic studies could be *patterned after etiognostic studies.*

The concept of a study of the etiognostic type actually serving an intervention-prognostic purpose gains impetus from the prevailing essence of experimental studies to this end. For, *the paradigmatic experimental studies on the now well-established level (Level 1,* Sect. 21.1, *above) is about a causal incidence-density ratio, which etiognostic research generally is about* (Sect. 15.6).

Thus, the non-experimental counterpart of its *Level 1* experimental intervention-prognostic cohort study paradigm (Sect. 21.1, above) can be taken to be *a set of non-cohort studies of the etiogenetic/etiognostic type*, each of them specific to one of the outcomes addressed in the experiment paradigmatic to this set of studies. The essence of any given one of these studies is that of etiogenetic/etiognostic studies in general (Sect. 15.6). In the (retrospective) studies at issue here, the *causal histories are about the intervention at issue*, classified as index and reference (and 'other') histories. Different from the Level 1 experimental studies with their 'intention-to-treat' comparisons, the comparisons of the index and reference segments of the non-experimental study base address the *actual treatments* of comparative interest.

A note on the validity of such non-experimental studies relative to the corresponding (Level 1) experimental studies is in order. *By no means is it the case that a non-experimental study is, inherently, less valid than its experimental counterpart.* It is true, of course, that the experimental prevention of confounding (by random assignments of the interventions) prevents even undocumented confounding (at prognostic T_0), different from non-experimental control of confounding; but a countervailing fact is the experimental bias due to non-adherence to the assigned treatments (cf. Chap. 20) as well as losses to follow-up, with no counterpart of either one of these in the non-experimental study. Besides, the confounders that need to be controlled – bearing on the medications' use – are not secrets of Nature but matters of purposive human behavior and, thus, subject to specification, documentation, and control.

Important to note also is that *this etiologic-type study serving an intervention-prognostic purpose actually corresponds to its Level 2 experimental counterpart* (above). For, this non-experimental study inherently has the case-base (case-referent) structure which, in the synthesis of the data assembled in an intervention-prognostic trial, raises the trial from Level 1 to Level 2 – at which the (prospective) incidence-density ratio (causal) no longer is treated as though inherently constant over the attained duration of the treatment, but is studied as a function of this time (in the framework of logistic, rather than Cox, regression).

A *non-experimental intervention-prognostic study can be quasi-experimental* (i.e., like an experiment without actually being one). In such a study, the study population is a cohort, with the divergence in treatment taking place at cohort T_0, not by experimental arrangement but by suitable selection of the study subjects. This study need not and therefore does not emulate the major source of bias in its experimental paradigm, the generally unavoidable non-adherence to the assigned treatments: the study cohort's members can be taken to contribute to the study base only as long as they adhere to the (algorithm of) treatment adopted at entry into the cohort, and they also can be chosen on the basis of following the treatment algorithms throughout the time horizon of the prognoses at issue.

This quasi-experimental intervention-prognostic cohort study is, of course, much more demanding to implement than is its dynamic-population alternative. It therefore is *truly justifiable only insofar as it represents the non-experimental counterpart of Level 3 experimental intervention-prognostic study*; that is, insofar as it addresses all the outcomes of concern in the context of the choice between the options for treatment and, for each of these outcomes, the probability of its occurrence as a function of all three types of its determinants (prognostic indicators, choice of treatment, and prognostic time; cf. Sect. 20.3.3).

21.3 Examples: Studies on 'Hormone Replacement Therapy'

21.3.1 Selection of the Example Studies

In the report on the trial we've been using as an instructive example [1], the background research on the topic – all of it non-experimental – was addressed, very casually, in only one sentence in the first paragraph. But right before the appearance of the report on that trial, an inclusive "*scientific review*" of its background studies was reported [3].

Among all the thus-identified prior studies, we focus on the ones that addressed the illness whose prevention – by postmenopausal use exogenous estrogens

(Premarin) – has been identified [1] as the main purpose of the treatment. This target of the treatment (prophylactic) was, as we've made plain, CHD (coronary heart disease). The "good- or fair-quality studies" included in the report on the review encompassed "11 case-control [refs.] and 10 cohort studies [refs.]."

Among these studies, we narrowed down to the ones that addressed *"current" treatment relative to never having been treated*, as this is what a case-base synthesis of the data from an experimental intervention-prognostic study would address in the context of full adherence to the assigned treatments. And finally, among these studies we chose to focus on the most recent ones, limiting the inclusions (arbitrarily) to the most recent four identified in that review. As it happened, two of these the reviewers classified as "case-control" studies, and the other two as "cohort" studies (while we do not recognize that duality in etiogenetic research; Sect. 15.6).

Our reason for choosing the example studies this way was that 'the state of the art' in the non-experimental intervention-prognostic research is best manifest in the most recent studies addressing the most relevant types of treatment histories (leaving out studies addressing only discontinued treatment). And in the presentation of these examples, the best – most instructive – sequence we took to be the chronologic one of their respective publications.

21.3.2 Some Particulars of the Studies

Of those four studies we chose to address as examples, the earliest two were published almost simultaneously, in 1997. One of these two was by Sidney *et alii* [4].

According to the report's *"abstract,"* the *"Design"* of this study was said to be one of "Retrospective case-control study." The intended meaning of this is, however, quite a mystery. For, at issue is terminology of etiologic/etiogenetic studies, and the characterization of some of these studies as 'retrospective' arose once the 'prospective' alternative to this was introduced (in the early 1950s, without any express rationale); and subsequently, the term 'retrospective study' has been replaced (with questionable rationale) by 'case-control study' (Cf. Sect. 15.6). So the original term is not an apt modifier of the current one.

Despite this curious specification of its "design," this study can be seen to have been a *non-experimental intervention-prognostic study of the etiogenetic/etiognostic rather than quasi-experimental type*, about the effects of postmenopausal use of (exogenous) hormones on the occurrence of MI (myocardial infarction) – one corresponding to Level 1 or 2 of its experimental counterparts (Sect. 21.1). It was a *non-cohort* intervention-prognostic study (Sect. 18.6.2).

The report's abstract specifies the study's *"Objective"* as having been "To estimate the relative risk [*sic*] for incident acute [*sic*] myocardial infarction in relation to the current [*sic*] use of estrogen and [*sic*] estrogen-progestogen." But one of the two *"Results"* in the abstract is about the magnitude of "odds ratio" in reference to "current" use of estrogen or [*sic*] estrogen-progestogen, and the other is about "past" [*sic*] use of one "or" the other of those two types of medication. (An MI is inherently an acute illness).

So, from the Objectives and Results sections of the report's abstract, the reader does not learn whether addressed in a segment of this study was the treatment that was the focus in the trial [1], namely the use of estrogens alone. For clarity on this, the reader naturally turns to the section of the report's abstract that is devoted to (succinct) specification of the interventions that were addressed, recognizing that various interventions' effects (on a single outcome) can be addressed in an etiogenetic-type intervention-prognostic study (while the effects of only a single intervention, on various outcomes, can be addressed in an intervention-prognostic experiment and in its quasi-experimental counterpart).

In this pursuit of the (centrally important) clarification of what interventions were studied, the reader is taken aback, in two stages. First, the title for the relevant section in the abstract is "*Intervention*," this singular form implying (the falsehood) that only a single type of intervention could be addressed in an etiognostic-type intervention-prognostic study of Level 1 or 2. But downright jolting to the reader is the actual content of this section: the specification of the "intervention" (singular) was constituted, solely, by *the questions that were included in "an in-person interview."*

With such questions as the stated "intervention" at issue, the "*Main outcome measures*" (concerning its effects) are said to be these: "Odds ratios for myocardial infarction associated with use of estrogen and [*sic*] estrogen-progestogen." But, as we noted above, reported in the Results section of the abstract is one "odds ratio" (rather than "relative risk") for "current" use and another for "past" use of estrogen or [*sic*] estrogen-progestogen, and nothing for the two of these together.

As the *abstract* of the report proper on this study, *more meaningful,* we suggest, would have been this:

Objects of study: The efficacy of hormonal prophylaxes of MI (myocardial infarction) in postmenopausal women.

Interventions: Use of unopposed or opposed estrogens, according as the woman has or has not undergone hysterectomy.

Type of study: Non-experimental, of the etiologic (case-referent) type.

Measure of effect: Incidence-density ratio of the occurrence of MI, contrasting the medication's still-continuing use with never having used it, adjusted for various potential confounders.

Result: For the measure of effect, the value 0.96, with its 95% imprecision interval ranging from 0.66 to 1.40.

With this substitute abstract giving the reader an orientational understanding of the objects and methodology (and results) of this study, we proceed to present a review – descriptive-cum-critical – of this study, with a view to the reader's learning about the theory – concepts and principles (and terminology too) – of Level 1–2 etiologic-type intervention-prognostic research. (Cf. "Type of study" in that substitute abstract).

The *source population* for this (etiologic-type/non-cohort) study – misrepresented as a case-control study (cf. Sect. 15.6.2) – was the client population of the Kaiser Permanente Medical Care Program for Northern California, and the study's *source base* was the population-time of this population's course over the period of its deployment for the study's data-collection (from November 1991 to November 1994). Within that source base, the actual *study base* was the population-time within it that was formed by the corresponding course of the actual study population – the source population's sub-population (dynamic) whose membership criteria (apart from being alive) were the states of: female gender, age 45–74 years, post-menopausal, either index or reference history of the intervention; no prior MI or angina pectoris, and English- and/or Spanish-speaking.

The *identification of cases* of non-fatal MI occurring in this this source base was a serious effort to be both timely and thorough in this. Strict criteria were applied to verification of the MI diagnoses of clinical practice, and included in the case series from the actual study base were only "definite" and "probable" cases of MI (non-fatal).

For the thus-obtained case series, a corresponding *base (referent) series* was selected with the aim of obtaining, for each "case-patient," "one control, matched for year of birth and facility of usual care." No rationale for that matching is given in the report, nor can any tenable rationale be given to it (Sect. 17.2.2). In the table entitled "Summary of exclusion criteria," given are *numbers of exclusions* from the case and base series from the source base, numbers specific to select criteria for it (e.g., "Used progestogen only"), but included are not criteria of non-representation of the actual study base in terms of positive history for coronary heart disease or risk factors for it. The CHD exclusions were initially made on the basis of hospital records in the case series alone (rather than in both series) and then by means of an interview in both the case and base series. According to another table, these exclusions actually remained incomplete in both series.

Against the backdrop of the serious effort to assure correctness of the (rule-in) diagnoses in the case series, it is curious that the *information on the intervention* was based on interviews – misconstrued as intervention (cf. abstract) – and not on abstraction of the Program's pharmacy records. Evidently, no effort was made to verify – on a sampling basis, even – the information on the presence/absence of "current" treatment, most notably.

The meaning of the use (current) of "estrogen or estrogen-progestogen" in the report's abstract becomes clear from the Results section of the report proper: addressed were not two types of treatment, each of them relative to no treatment, but *a single treatment, the nature of which depends on whether hysterectomy had been performed*. No rationale for this was given, nor can a tenable rationale be given, for this amalgamation of the two types of intervention addressed in the two separate (and parallel) WHI trials [1, 2], with different indications.

Various possible *confounders* were controlled in the logistic regression "if an appreciable change was seen in the exposure coefficients with the addition of that variable." On the basis of this common but untenable principle, "only body mass index was added to the final model." Controlled in that model were "hypertension, diabetes, body mass index, smoking, race or ethnicity, level of education, and history of coronary heart disease." The extent to which this represents under- or over-inclusiveness of potential confounders is a matter of judgement; but notable is the sketchiness with which the elements in this were documented – with age conspicuous by its absence from this set, presumably for the untenable reason that it was a matching factor in the selection of the base series.

"Duration (in years) of hormone replacement therapy [prophylaxis] in current hormone users was examined by replacing the main hormone replacement treatment variable (estrogen for women who had had hysterectomy; estrogen-progestogen for women who had not) with years of use of either therapy." The proper minimalist modelling would have been addition of this duration variate to the indicator of the treatment (as the product of these two). But the results presented on *duration* of the medication's use (in Table 3) evidently were not derived by any regression modelling. And curiously, the rate-ratio's potential modification by age (at the time of the involvement in the study series) was not explored.

At the end of the Results section is this little paragraph:

> Table 4 shows data [statistics from the data] stratified by [specific according to] hysterectomy status. The odds ratios [incidence-density ratios] for women who had had hysterectomy (odds ratio, 0.95 [CI, 0.50–1.80]) and current use of estrogen-progestogen in women who had not had hysterectomy (odds ratio, 0.89 [CI, 0.52–1.53]) were consistent with the results of the main analysis [synthesis of the data].

So, insofar as this study provided a non-experimental counterpart of the result from the estrogen trial [1] for coronary heart disease, it was that "0.95 [CI, 0.50–1.80]" corresponding to the "0.91 (0.75 1.12)" from that trial.

In the report's opening paragraph, the investigators comment on the "numerous" already-published non-experimental studies on the CHD effects of women's use of "estrogen replacement therapy," saying that "the lack of experimental studies of estrogen use limits the ability to draw definitive conclusions about cause and effect." We say that conclusions shouldn't be drawn from those trials either (Sect. 19.2.2). And to this we add that to us it is unclear which one of those two results, the non-experimental 0.95 or the experimental 0.91, is more valid. In this comparison, the clearest factual element is the upward bias in the experimental result on account of the quite incomplete adherence to the assigned treatments.

***

The other of the two reports in 1997 was by Heckbert *et alii* [5].

According to the *"Abstract"* in this report, the *"Background"* of this study was that "There is little information about whether an increasing duration of estrogen replacement therapy is associated with a decreasing risk for myocardial infarction in postmenopausal women." The (consequent) *"Objective"* of the study is said to have been "To conduct a population-based case-control study among enrollees of the Group Health Cooperative (GHC) of Puget Sound, Seattle, Wash." The ensuing section, on *"Subjects and methods,"* is a delineation of who the "case subjects" were and how the "controls" were selected, as well as of how the data were collected.

Next, in the "*Results*" section are presented "odds ratios" describing how "Among women who were currently using estrogen, the duration of estrogen use was inversely associated with a risk for myocardial infarction after adjustment for age, year of identification, diabetes mellitus, angina, and smoking." This is supplemented by a remark on the corresponding pattern "Among women who had used estrogen in the past." Finally, presented as "*Conclusion*" is a restatement of the main result.

Different from the abstract in the study report addressed above [4], this one may be seen to be quite comprehensible, and agreeable too. Nevertheless, rather extensive *annotations on this abstract*, both explanatory and critical, we deem to be in order:

1. In that *Background* statement, the expression of the form of something being (or not being) "*associated with*" something else, while ingrained in the jargon of etiologic (etiogenetic) research, is a less-than-apt expression of the idea that something is causing (or being caused by) something else. Explicitly stated, the background was that there was a paucity of information about whether the efficacy – momentary – of the treatment (prophylactic rather than therapeutic) increases with increasing duration of it.
2. That statement about the "*Objective*" of the study prompts us to say, again, something that *should go without saying*: that the objective of any gnostic clinical study (in scientific rather than careerist or other non-scientific terms) is to produce evidence about the magnitudes of its object parameter(s), and that, therefore, the now-common statement of the objective of such a study should be replaced by one of the *object(s)* of it.
3. The *object of the study* should have been addressed as a topic unto itself. It could have been specified, for instance, this way: 'In postmenopausal women, the duration of the use of hormonal prophylaxis against myocardial infarction as a determinant of its efficacy' (Cf. # 1, above).
4. As for the "*Subjects and methods*" topic in this abstract, a bit of history is of note for a start. A precursor of this phrase, now routinely used in clinical research, was "Materials and methods." Then, an aversion justifiably developed to the related phrase 'patient material,' and this therefore got to be replaced 'study subjects' or 'study participants.' But a conceptual point about that "Subjects and methods" phrase is of much greater note: that term implies a need to distinguish between the subjects involved and the methods used in a gnostic clinical study; but this distinction-making is untenable. For, *the definition/selection of the persons contributing to the study base is an aspect – an eminent one – of the methodology of such a study (*rather than distinct from this*)*. Instead, a salient (and very propitious) feature of the methods (*sic*) of the study at issue here was the way in which the study 'subjects'/'participants' were defined (as the contributors to the study base, secondary to the selection of the source population-time, the source base).
5. With the "Subjects and methods" phrase reduced to *Methods* (à la # 4, above), the first, most broadly orientational point to be made about this study (under Methods rather than "Objectives") would have been that *the study was non-*

experimental, of the etiogenetic/etiognostic, case-referent type (rather than quasi-experimental). To say that it was a "case-control" study is to perpetuate the 'trohoc' fallacy (Sect. 15.3). The elements in this should not have been misrepresented as though ones in a case-control study (cf. Sects. 15.6.1 and 15.6.2).

6. Given the de-facto case-base (case-referent) structure of the study at issue here, the *subjects* in it were not the persons on whom data were collected, the "case subjects" together with the "controls." As in these studies in general, *the subjects of this study were those who contributed to the population-time of the study base* (cf. above). The case and base series are involved in the documentation of the study result for its referent, which is the study base rather than the union of those two series. (The case-control study has no study base as the referent of the result).
7. To say that this study was "*population-based*" is meaningless. For, all *theoretically sound etiologic/etiogenetic studies – case-referent (case-base) studies, different from case-control studies – are population-based* (in the meaning of # 6 above), 'nested' in the study population-time. The point about this study that could have been made is that the study's *source population was defined directly* (as the enrollees of the GHC) rather than indirectly (as the 'catchment population' of the way in which cases of the illness were identified) (Sect. 17.3.2).
8. As for the "Results" section, writing about "*odds ratios*" is one more perpetuation of the case-control fallacy, going back to comparisons of 'exposure odds' between 'cases' and 'controls.' In a case-referent study, the first-order results are the index and reference quasi-rates in reference to the study base, and the ratio of these is, inherently, the result for the corresponding *incidence-density ratio.* Logistic modelling of the duality constituted by the case and base series in a study of the etiogenetic (case-referent) type – whether for etiognosis or intervention-prognosis – is modelling for the logarithm of the quasi-rate as such, and thereby for the logarithm of the incidence-density ratio – rather than the logarithm of any "odds ratio" (Sects. 7.4.4 and 20.1.2).
9. The summary of the results presented in the report's abstract was not an actual "*Conclusion*," nor should any conclusion be drawn from the results obtained in a gnostic clinical study (original or, even, derivative). The heading for this section in the abstract could have been that for the last section in the report proper, namely *Comment.* And the content of this could have been that, 'The evidence from this study is reasonably persuasive about a trend of appreciable increase in the momentary efficacy at issue with increasing duration of the intervention.'

With these understandings of the Abstract of the report on the study at issue here [5] – in terms of the teachings in this book – the principal questions about the study's *report proper* naturally have to do with the specific meaning and basis of the above-suggested substitute for the investigators' "Conclusion." The first of these questions is this qualitative one: *In what sense and on what basis is the evidence from this study reasonably persuasive* about the existence of the trend which the study directly addressed, namely the postulated increase in the proportional reduction in the incidence-density of MI with increasing duration of the hormone's past use among its still-continuing users, relative to those who never used it, in the domain of the study? And a related other question is this: Insofar as the study indeed provided reasonably persuasive evidence about the magnitude of this trend, *what does it indicate as being that "appreciable" magnitude of the intervention's prognostic implication?* Our answers follow.

The reported pattern of the incidence-density ratio in relation to the duration of the medication's past use in this result's referent (the study base of still-continuing users and never-users) is obviously consistent with the postulated pattern in reference to the study object's domain (abstract); but the empirical pattern is *reasonably persuasive* about the existence and causal interpretability of this pattern in the abstract only *if two conditions obtain:* the trend in the result is reasonably significant statistically, and reasonably valid besides (so that the statistical significance would remain even upon the result's 'adjustment' – correction – for its bias).

Regarding the *statistical significance* of the trend in the study base, the report gives for it P = 0.05, "2-tailed." With focus on the postulated increase in the treatment's efficacy (implying decrease in the causal incidence-density ratio over increasing duration of the treatment's use), the P-value (suitably one-sided) actually was half of this: P = 0.025. This statistical significance of the trend in this study is at variance with the essential absence of such a trend in the results of the study by Sidney *et alii* [4]; and it challenges the aprioristic premise of no such trend in the WHI trial [1] and in the derivative study by Nelson *et alii* [3], in both of which it was incorporated in the "proportional hazards" model deployed in the syntheses of the data.

The *validity* of this study was superior to that of the study by Sidney *et alii* [4], and it was, arguably at least, reasonably good as such. In both of these studies, *the source population had a direct definition* (cf. above), and it was, very propitiously, the participants in a system of prepaid healthcare. But only Heckbert *et alii* made full use of the potential for validity-assurance afforded by such a source population for a study of the case-referent type. While in both of these studies this type of setting was used to good advantage in validity-assurance of the *identification of the cases of MI* that occurred in the source base, and also as the source for a suitable sampling frame for *valid selection of the corresponding base series*, only Heckbert *et alii* abstracted most of the information needed on these two series from the system's database, most notably the *information on the use of the medications at issue* (estrogen alone and estrogen together with progestin, which were addressed, as is necessary, separately in this report).

In judging the extent of *residual confounding* in the results of Heckbert *et alii*, the place to start is the comparison between the unadjusted and adjusted ratios of incidence density contrasting still-continuing users of estrogen with its never-users, considering these ratios for the shortest, intermediate, and longest duration of the use. The *unadjusted ratios* for these three durations can be calculated from the statistics in the report's Table 5, and they are, respectively, 0.81, 0.61, and 0.48. The *adjusted ratios* are given in that Table as 0.91 for the shortest duration of use and as 0.55 for the longest, while for the two durations here combined as intermediate they are given as 0.70 and 0.65 for the shorter and longer one of these, respectively. So, the adjustments for confounding – inherently incomplete – shifted the ratios toward their null value (of 1.00), reducing the differences among them; and *the question is, whether complete adjustment would have eliminated the trend pattern in the results.*

The characteristics on which the adjustments (for potential confounding) were made (jointly, in the model for logistic regression) were "age, year of identification, diabetes mellitus, angina, and current smoking," after having excluded from the study series, most notably, the instances that were associated with a prior MI. "Data were complete for the variables defining duration of hormone use, and information on medical conditions, such as angina, diabetes mellitus, and hypertension, was uniformly available from the review of the medical record." But as for whether this set of potential confounders was reasonably complete, one may wonder about *inattention to SES* (socioeconomic status) in particular, given that the report by Sidney *et alii* [4] gives evidence of decrease in the incidence of MI with increasing levels of education and income. Presuming this negative association between SES and the incidence of MI to be true in general, and presuming also that postmenopausal estrogen use was positively associated with SES in the study base of Heckbert *et alii*, one can conclude that the pattern reported from the latter study was *exaggerated by lack of adjustment for SES*. That this residual confounding together with other biases completely explains the pattern reported by Heckbert *et alii* is of course possible in principle, but it may be judged to be dubitable in the light of the extent to which those empirical ratios fall below unity.

"Overall," the authors say, "current use [of estrogen] was associated with a 30% decrease in risk [of MI] (OR, 0.70; 95% CI, 0.55–0.89)." But *this 30%, even if taken at face value, is quantitatively meaningless in respect to the "risk of MI,"* insofar as the magnitude of the reduction depends on the duration of the hormone's use (sustained, prophylactic) by postmenopausal women. From the vantage of this study, quantitatively meaningful (even on the face-value premise of the results' complete validity and precision) are only the (apparent) reductions (in incidence-density of MI) specific to the four durations of the hormone's past use (among those who still use it), the percentages for the successively increasing durations of the medication's use (9%, 30%, 35%, and 45%; cf. above).

The question arises, In what sense, if any, would these retrospectively caused reductions, if taken at face value, represent attainable proportional reductions in the "risk" – inherently prospective – of MI over various durations of the hormone's prospective use (by postmenopausal women who have not previously used it). The beginning of the answer is that, *according to the results of this study*, a first use of estrogen for 1.8 years produces a 9% reduction in the incidence density of MI that determines the cumulative incidence of MI from time 0 to 1.8 years; and that, in the periods from 1.8 to 4.2 years, 4.2–8.2 years, and 8.2–10.0 years, say, the corresponding reductions are those 30%, 35%, 45%, respectively. To derive the proportional reduction in, say, the 10-year risk, needed added inputs are the values of the incidence density in each of those periods of prognostic time conditional on no use of the hormone. Then the computations proceed as outlined in Sect. 20.2. The point here is that *results on interventions-contrasting ratios of incidence density are not, in themselves, results on "relative risk" for the outcome at issue*, contrary to the implication in this report and in those of etiogenetic-type (case-referent) studies quite generally.

***

The third of the four most-recent non-experimental studies on estrogen prophylaxis of MI included in the 2002 review by Nelson *et alii* [3] was published in 1998, by Sourander *et alii* [6]. Its title is a bit eyebrow-raising by its implication that "cardiovascular mortality" does not cover cases of "sudden cardiac death."

In the report's "*Summary,*" under "*Background,*" the authors say that "We aimed to analyse the relation between postmenopausal oestrogen replacement therapy (ERT), cardiovascular disease, and cancer." In the next section, on "*Methods,*" they imply that this study was appended to a program of screening for breast cancer. They give the number of women they "examined" and the numbers of "current" and "former" users of "ERT" but without indicating whether at issue is use as of the time of the outcome event at issue (as in the two studies addressed above) or as of some other time; and nothing is said about never-users. This section closes with, "We used proportional-hazards models to calculate risk ratios and 95% CIs, adjusted for eight confounding variables." Then, the section on "*Results*" opens with the point that "Current HRT was associated with decreased cardiovascular mortality and a decrease in sudden cardiac death" (cf. note on this duality above), still with no indication of the meaning of "current" nor of the alternative to it. The particulars that follow address the magnitudes (empirical) of "absolute risk per 1000 person-years," inter alia. "*Interpretation*" of the evidence includes the idea that "Current ERT predicted [*sic*] reduced cardiovascular mortality."

The report's Summary aside, orientational information on the *background* and *object(s)* of the study should be found in the "Introduction" section of the report proper, notably since there is no section for either one of these before the one on "Methods." In the first of the Introduction's two paragraphs the opening two sentences are these: "Observational studies have shown a reduction in cardiovascular-disease risk and mortality in postmenopausal women on oestrogen replacement therapy (ERT), but to what extent this reduction results from selection bias is contested [refs.]. Weaknesses in the studies have been insufficient recording of cardiovascular disease, and lack of information on sudden cardiac death." In the second paragraph the salient point is this: "We report results from a community-based prospective cohort study."

Our understanding of the essence of this study – on the effects of the use of "ERT" by postmenopausal women – is this: The entire *cohort* of women who elected to avail themselves of a 1987–1988 municipal offering of screening for breast cancer were adopted, right away, as *the study (rather than source) population* for the purpose at issue here. The women were interviewed about matters relevant to this study at the baseline screening and also at its three biennial repetitions, regarding "ERT" use, occupation, etc.; and information on *health outcomes in the 8-year period of follow-up* was obtained by the use of various routine registries.

Very notable about the particulars of this study were the definitions of the *compared treatments:*

> Women who did not report ERT before 1987 or during follow-up were classified as never users. Those who reported that they had used ERT before 1987 but not in 1987 or during follow-up were deemed former users. Current users were those who used oestrogen at baseline of the study.

The cohort entering the screening program should not have been treated as the study population. It should have been treated as the study's *source-population*, with its follow-up producing the study's *source-base*. This source-base (in the course of the cohort over cohort time) should have been deployed the same way the source-base (in the course of a dynamic population over calendar time) was deployed in the two studies addressed above – including, very importantly, the definition of the treatment's *current use* and *never-use* as of the person-moments in the case and base series (initially from the source base but then reduced to instances from the actual study base within the source base).

That extraordinary way the temporal aspects of the compared interventions were defined is not consistent with the authors' characterization this study as a "cohort study" – not in the meaning of the term in the 'cohort fallacy' of etiologic/etiogenetic studies (Sect. 15.6.3) nor in reference to the intervention-prognostic cohort study (Sect. 18.6.1). Nor does this study represent a defensible conceptual innovation in the intervention-prognostic class of clinical studies. The structure of this study was seriously malformed.

It is instructive to note that Nelson *et alii* in their review [3] classified this study as being of the "*case-control*" type, and as being of "good" or "fair" quality, 1 of the 11 of these at the time. So, not only is that duality a fallacy (Sect. 15.6.3); there is common confusion about the nature of its constituent fallacies.

***

The last of the latest four non-experimental ('observational') studies contributing to the derivative study ("scientific review") by Nelson *et alii* [3] was by Grodstein *et alii* [7].

In the "*Abstract*" of the report, following the "Background" section, the section on "*Objective*" specifies it thus: "To investigate duration, dose, and type of post-menopausal hormone therapy and primary prevention of cardiovascular disease," presumably meaning of the *objects* of the study had to do with the CVD effects of such treatment (prophylactic rather than "therapeutic") in women with no prior CVD, with special reference to the particulars of the treatment. Then come four sections on *methods* (without the Methods heading), with the successive headings of "Design," "Setting," "Patients," and "Measurements." Under "*Results*," the first item is this: "When all cardiovascular risk factors were considered, the risk for major coronary events was lower among current users of hormone therapy, including short-term users, compared with never-users (relative risk 0.61 [95% CI, 0.52–0.71])." A number of other results, all of this form, follow. Finally, under "*Conclusions*," the first is that "Postmenopausal hormone use appears to reduce risk for major coronary events in women without previous heart disease."

In the Abstract, the "*Design*" of this study is specified as "Prospective, observational cohort study"; its "*Setting*" as "Nurses' Health Study, with follow-up from 1976 to 1996"; the "*Patients*" in it as "70 533 postmenopausal women, in whom 1258 major coronary events (nonfatal myocardial infarction or fatal coronary disease) and 767 strokes were identified"; and the "Measurements" in it are specified as having involved questionnaires, medical record reviews, and logistic regression models "to calculate relative risks and 95% CIs, adjusted for confounders." That so-called Nurses' Health Study (misnomer) is a program of routine data-collection, biennial, on a cohort (of nurses) for whatever studies on human (rather than specifically nurses') health can be based on those data.

The question arises, Why was the "design" of this study specified as "prospective, observational cohort study" while that of Sidney *et alii* was said to be a "retrospective case-control study" and that of Heckbert *et alii* a "population-based, case-control study? The beginning of the answer is that neither one of those other two studies actually was a "case-control" study, as a case series in each of them was coupled with a base (referent) series, instead of involving a 'case group' together with a 'control group' (Sect. 15.6.3); they both had the structure – singular – of genuine etiologic (etiogenetic) studies (Sects. 7.4.4 and 15.6.2). Accordingly, both of these studies were retrospective (Sect. 15.2), in the meaning of involving causal contrasts of etiogenetic histories as of the person-moments in the case and base series; and both of them were population-based, based on their respective study populations (dynamic; Sect. 17.3.1). As a lege-artis etiologic (etiogenetic) study has its particular, singular structure a priori, it is unnecessary and only confusing to write about these studies as "case-control" studies with some of those features specified.

The orientational point here is that *Grodstein et alii definitely had the option of doing what was done in those etiognostic-type – non-cohort – intervention-prognostic studies,* different only in terms of the type of *source population*: Focusing on a chosen segment of the cohort's course from 1976 to 1996, Grodstein *et alii* could have identified the series of cases of the CVD at issue that had been documented as having occurred in this source base; they could have drawn a sample of the person-moments (infinite in number) constituting that source base; they could have abstracted the relevant data on the instances constituting these two series and reduced them to the actual study series (from the actual study base); etc. So, *What did they do instead of this, and what, if anything, justified it?*

The 20-year follow-up of the source cohort was divided into ten successive 2-year periods within it, corresponding to the biennial updates of the information (on the cohort's members still alive and available to fill out the questionnaire). At the beginning of each of these periods, included in the sub-cohort for the ensuing 2-year follow-up were only those satisfying, at that time, the criteria for the domain of the study (freedom from prior CVD, etc.). "To maintain the prospective nature of the study, hormone use (including duration) during the [prior] 2-year period was established from women's reports at the start of the [next] period." And, "We used pooled logistic regression across the ten 2-year periods to adjust simultaneously for potential confounding factors [ref.]. In this approach, independent blocks of person-time are pooled … Simulation studies have established the asymptomatic equivalence of pooled logistic regression to Cox regression with time-dependent covariates [ref.]."

Nothing is said in justification of the concern "to maintain the prospective nature of the study." If this had merit, Heckbert *et alii*, for example, could have formed such blocks from their non-cohort, dynamic-population source-base. But *it has no justification* as an alternative to the case-referent structuring of the study; and addressing "time-dependent covariates" is not only feasible but actually quite routine in (inherently retrospective) etiognostic-type (non-cohort) intervention-prognostic studies. In the various tables in the Grodstein *et alii* report, shown is the distribution of the case series according to the determinant at issue, but the reader is left missing the corresponding distribution of the study's base series – because the selection of such a supplement to the cases series, one can presume, would not have served the (unjustifiable) concern "to maintain the prospective nature of the study" (Cf. Sects. 15.6.2, 15.6.3, and 20.1.2).

Insofar as the meaning of the study's "prospective nature" is taken to be the recording of the determinant information (here on the medication use) prior to the outcome events (here cases of CHD), with this considered relevant for validity, there would have been no problem in drawing the determinant information from the beginning of the intervals in which the events occurred. (Ditto for the person-moments in the base series).

21.3.3 Some General Notes on the Studies

The four studies addressed in Sect. 21.3.2 above [4–7] illustrate the point that non-experimental intervention-prognostic studies are *not necessarily patterned after their experimental counterparts* (clinical trials); that they are not inherently, or even typically, of the quasi-experimental type (Sect. 21.2): they are, commonly, of the type familiar from epidemiological research on the etiology/etiogenesis of illness, addressing treatment in the etiogenesis of illness. While all four studies addressed in the Section above were about the prognostic topic of 'HRT' prophylaxis of acute CHD, they thereby were about the 'etiognostic' topic of 'HRT' in the etiogenesis (negative) of acute CHD outcome in those so treated. This is a way – a very useful way – of viewing the objects of the corresponding experimental study [1] as well, as for each of the outcome events addressed in it (Sect. 21.1, above). It thereby should have been the outlook, also, in the study by Grodstein *et alii*.

Those studies illustrate, also, the *confusion* about the theory of etiogenetic research in contemporary epidemiologic academia [8]. Thus, as for what these studies were about – in the background of the ensuing experimental study [1] reporting on the "hazard ratio" of CHD (i.a.) – the *object of study* (implicit in the reported result) was "odds ratio" (causal) in two of them, "risk ratio" in another, and "relative risk" in yet another. In point of fact, though, all five of these studies were about incidence density ratio of the occurrence of the outcome in question, contrasting history of 'HRT' use with absence of this. In the trial the histories were about what they were supposed to be, per their experimental assignments, rather than what they should have been, namely histories of continuing adherence to the assignments. In the non-experimental studies, the histories actually were about continuing (current at outcome) use/non-use of the medication in question.

The confusion extended to the *methodology* of these studies. The first two of them were said to be "case-control" studies, one of them specifically a "retrospective" study of this type, the other as "population-based." But the structure of these two studies was identical, that of *the* etiogenetic study – the case-base/case-referent study – which inherently is retrospective (in its etiogenetic histories) and also population-based (per its study base, absent from the case-control study). The third study was unclassifiable as to type, very confusing about this. The remaining, fourth study was characterized as "prospective." In it, there was a rather complex effort "to maintain the prospective nature of the study," a quality that commonly is held as superior to the 'retrospective nature' of other etiogenetic studies. But conducting a case-base study – retrospective – in the framework of that study's pre-existing database (on a cohort) would have been preferable. All of these distinctions are vacuous in the conceptual framework of *the* etiogenetic study, the structure of which is very usefully involved in intervention-prognostic cohort studies as well as in their non-cohort alternatives.

In the midst of this confusion, the investigators conducting the "scientific review" of – the *derivative study* based on – all the original non-experimental studies on "postmenopausal hormone replacement therapy" [3] obviously faced quite a challenge in grasping what each of these 'HRT'-CHD studies was about, and what their respective methodological types were. For this was the necessary framework for their complete identification – as studies with the same object in reference to the same domain as was the case in the trial [1] – for potential inclusion in the synthesis of the evidence. And even more importantly, this understanding was a prerequisite for identification of the "good-or fair-quality studies" for the inclusion.

References

1. The Women's Health Initiative steering committee (2004) Effects of conjugated equine estrogen in postmenopausal women with hysterectomy. JAMA 291:1701–1712
2. Writing group for the Women's Health Initiative investigators (2002) Risks and benefits of estrogen plus progestin in healthy postmenopausal women: principal results from the Women's Health Initiative randomized controlled trial. JAMA 288:321–333
3. Nelson HD, Humphrey LL, Nygren P *et alii* (2002) Postmenopausal hormone replacement therapy: scientific review. JAMA 288:872–888
4. Sidney S, Petitti DB, Quesenberry CP (1997) Myocardial infarction and the use of estrogen and estrogen-progestogen in postmenopausal women. Ann Intern Med 127:501–508

5. Heckbert SR, Weiss NS, Koepsell TD *et alii* (1997) Duration of estrogen replacement therapy in relation to the risk of incident myocardial infarction in postmenopausal women. Arch Intern Med 157:1330–1336
6. Sourander L, Rajala T, Räihä I, Mäkinen J *et alii* (1998) Cardiovascular and cancer morbidity and mortality and sudden cardiac death in postmenopausal women on oestrogen replacement therapy (ERT). Lancet 352:1965–1969
7. Grodstein F, Manson JE, Colditz GA *et alii* (2000) A prospective, observational study of postmenopausal hormone therapy and primary prevention of cardiovascular disease. Ann Intern Med 133:933–941
8. Miettinen OS (2017) On progress in epidemiologic academia. Eur J Epidemiol 32:173–179

Chapter 22
Intervention-Prognostic Derivative Research

Contents

Abstract The enormous rate with which original studies for the advancement of the knowledge-base of clinicians' intervention-prognoses are now being published, creates both an opportunity and a need for its corresponding *derivative research*; and this derivative research, too, has become dauntingly voluminous, even on closely-demarcated topics. As this is research that draws from original research with critical selectivity, it *requires understanding of the quality-assurance of the original studies on a level higher than is characteristic of the 'peer reviews' of the reports on these*. And it requires a keen sense not only of the *generic mission* in it but also of its requisite *quality-assurance*. Eminent examples indicate that the quality of derivative intervention-prognostic studies, even ones commissioned for authoritative promulgation of recommendations for clinicians' practices, remains quite wanting.

Keywords Mission · Quality assurance · Examples · Overview of the examples

22.1 The Mission in Derivative Gnostic Research

In teachings about clinical research, the mission – purpose or objective – of conducting a study is commonly said to be that of 'answering the research question.' But: *the study report generally does not specify a question that was going to be answered by means of the study, nor does the report present a meaningful answer to an unspecified question*. Instead of an answer to a specified question, the report's abstract, already, commonly culminates in at least one 'conclusion' – as though it

O. S. Miettinen et al., *Clinical Research Transformed*,
https://doi.org/10.1007/978-3-030-06176-0_22

were feasible to logically deduce abstract truths from the data assembled in a piece of clinical research. In the eminent study we extensively addressed in Chaps. 19 and 20 [1], the "objective" was "to assess" the effects of the treatment at issue, and the assessment was reported to have culminated, inter alia, in the "conclusion" that Premarin treatment for status post menopause "does not affect [coronary heart disease] incidence" among the treated. (Abstract knowledge is expressed in present tense, study results in past tense).

We have repeatedly asserted our conception of the *mission in a piece of original gnostic research as that of producing evidence* – new evidence – about the parameters in a gnostic probability function. At issue inherently are the *magnitudes* of those parameters. In gnostic clinical research, the magnitude of a given parameter – an effect parameter in particular – may be addressed in merely *qualitative* terms, focusing on its possible deviation from its null value; but practice-relevant generally is only *quantitative* knowledge about the magnitudes of the parameters in a gnostic probability function.

In respect to any given parameter, *the result of a gnostic study inherently is, as we've illustrated, quantitative:* it is the parameter's empirical value (descriptive of its referent, the study base), even if at issue is, merely, testing of the tenability of the parameter's null value. And we've illustrated how, in the report from a gnostic clinical study, associated with the empirical value of a parameter routinely is a *measure of its imprecision* – usually the 95% 'confidence interval.' The imprecision of the result on any given parameter is, as is well understood, the inescapable consequence of the necessarily finite size of the study. By the same token, the imprecision of a parameter's empirical value from a given study, while unavoidable, could have been reduced in magnitude by increasing the size of the study, if that was possible.

When the initial study on a given gnostic probability function (in reference to a given domain) has been replicated with the same object and also with the same validity (freedom from bias), *the results' variation among those original studies reflects nothing but their respective imprecisions* – their *irreproducibility* on account of their imprecision, due to the limited amounts of information in them. This represents an opportunity for *a meaningful derivative study*, the mission in which is to produce, on the basis the original studies (and thus without any original data), a *more precise result* than that of any of the original studies.

The opportunity for a derivative study is well worth exploiting, provided also that the shared objects design for the original studies – inherently shared also by their derivative study – satisfies the relevance-to-practice requirement that is ubiquitous in gnostic clinical studies, and that the original studies are, uniformly, of sufficiently high quality. On the other hand, *deriving a relatively precise result from original studies with heterogeneous objects and/or varying levels of validity is an unworthy, counterproductive mission* – though, alas, a common one.

22.2 Quality Assurance in Derivative Gnostic Research

When a derivative gnostic clinical study has a *justification for its mission* (Sect. 22.1, above), the research nevertheless is justified only if, in addition, its methodology conforms to the cardinal principles of validity assurance in it. The process of a derivative gnostic study is bi-phasic, and so accordingly is the necessary *validity-assurance* in it. A derivative gnostic study is to be valid, first, in respect to what original studies are included in the study base for it; and second, in respect to how the results of the derivative study, and the measures of the imprecisions of these, are derived from the statistics reported on the included original studies.

The cardinal principle that should govern the *inclusion of original studies* into the study base of a derivative gnostic study is not that to be included are all of the valid studies on the object(s) of study at issue in reference to the domain in question. Rather, it is that the inclusions of original studies are to be independent of their respective results. Thus, *the included studies (valid) must have been completed – including the publication phase that completes the process – independently of their results* (i.e., free of 'publication bias'), and *the set of the included studies must be chosen from such (valid) studies independently of their respective results.* On the other hand, selectivity on the basis of the results' *precision*, notably with natural preference for more precise – larger – studies is consistent with validity of a derivative gnostic study.

Valid synthesis of the various results on a given parameter from the included original studies into the corresponding derivative result is a matter of suitable averaging of those original results. Suitable for this in respect to each of the parameters in a logistic (or Cox) regression-model is information-weighted averaging of the original results, the weights being the inverses of the squares of their respective 'standard errors.'

When the results of the original studies are the study-specific values for a *rate ratio* and reported on each of these is its 95% 'confidence' (imprecision) interval (cf. Chaps. 19 and 20), the weighted averaging is to be carried out in respect to their *logarithms*, with the 'standard errors' of these derived from the logarithms of the interval's boundaries. The derivative result on any given ratio-type parameter is the antilog (exponential) of the logarithms' information-weighted average. For the derivative result's logarithm, the 'standard error' is based on the study-specific amounts of information, as the square root of the inverse of their sum. The examples in Sect. 22.3.1 below illustrate all of this.

22.3 Examples: Studies on 'Hormone Replacement Therapy'

22.3.1 The Study Reported in 2002

In 2002, when the report on the original experimental study on the effects of the 'unopposed' use of Premarin (extensively addressed in Chaps. 19 and 20) appeared [1], published also was a major derivative study on the effects of postmenopausal use of "hormone replacement therapy" at large [2] – that is, of hormonal prophylaxis in postmenopausal women, directed mainly to acute CHD (coronary heart disease). Addressed in this derivative study, just as in that original one, were the treatment's effects not only on the occurrence of CHD but on that of various other illnesses as well. We've touched upon this derivative study in Sects. 19.3 and 21.3.1.

We here focus on this derivative study to the extent that addressed in it was *the effect of Premarin use on the occurrence of CHD*. In the report on that original study [1], prior research on this effect was covered by saying, merely, that "Observational [i.e., non-experimental] studies primarily examining unopposed estrogen preparations [i.e., Premarin alone] have suggested a 30–50% reduction in coronary events [refs.]." In the derivative study [2] this literature was addressed in full, "by reviewing the literature, conducting meta-analyses, and calculating outcome rates" (Cf. Sect. 21.3.1).

Just as in that new original study, the mission in this derivative study on its background studies was that of service to clinical-level preventive medicine, specifically *primary prevention* (directed to the events' first occurrence rather than recurrence). Accordingly, in line with that original study, the *domain* of this derivative study was restricted to persons who had not experienced the outcome events before. A further, somewhat related restriction was that the persons were to be free of "conditions associated with higher risks for targeted outcomes." And whereas in that trial [1] the *object* in respect to any given illness was a single parameter, namely the incidence-density ratio contrasting use of Premarin with non-use of it, this was the object in this derivative study as well. We've seen this in the four examples of these studies in Sect. 21.3.2, though with the term for it varying.

"Our review [concerning CHD]," the investigators say, "focuses on the good- and fair-quality studies, including 11 case-control [refs.] and 10 cohort studies [refs.] and 1 small trial [ref,]." *Emblematic of the quality of the included etiogenetic-type intervention-prognostic studies* is the nature of the temporal aspect of the histories of the use of the hormones. The included studies were classified into these three "mutually exclusive" types in this (very important) respect: addressed in any given study was either "current" use, "ever" use, or "past" use; but among these, only studies addressing *"current" use* – meaning past use that has not been discontinued – should have been included. (Cf. non-adherence bias in experimental intervention-prognostic studies in Sect. 20.3.3, and the respective meanings of 'current use' in "case-control" and "cohort" studies in Sect. 21.3).

The results of the original studies on CHD "incidence" (distinct from "mortality") were first synthesized within those three "mutually exclusive" types of study (based on the temporal aspect of the medications' use), leaving unspecified whether progestin was involved, and the dosage(s) as well. The temporal vantage of that classification is not specified in the report, but it is fair to presume that in the "case-control" studies it was the time of the CHD event, while in the "cohort" studies it likely was different: the time of entry into the cohort in a "cohort study" on the 'HRT' etiogenesis of acute CHD. These syntheses were supplemented by one across all three of these subsets of the studies. For each of the syntheses, "Relative risk (95% confidence interval)" is given (in the report's Table 1).

Potentially *meaningful* among the reported derivative results were ones that synthesized original results varying only on account of their respective imprecisions. This means that the focus should have been on the "case control" studies' results in reference to "current" use in these. What is reported is less than meaningful – per inadmissible pooling of the results of "case control" studies with those of "cohort" studies on "current" use and even pooling with these the results on "past" use.

Critical examination of a reported derivative, synthetic result on an ostensibly meaningful rate ratio and its associated 'confidence' (imprecision) limits might well begin with checking the mutual consistency of these numbers. In respect to each of these triads of values the question is, Are the interval's limits on the logarithmic scale symmetrical around the result's logarithm (as generally is the intent)?; that is, Is the reported ratio proper the geometric mean of its reported 'confidence limits' (i.e., the square root of the product of the limits)? Unfortunately, the meaningful synthesis (about) was not among the three that were reported. What is reported regarding "current" and "past" use is consistent in this sense. But as for "ever" use, the square root of the reported limits' product (of 0.67×1.33) is 0.94, not the reported 0.91.

Checked next might well be *whether the reported precision of the ostensibly meaningful derivative/synthetic result indeed is, as it should be, greater than that of the most precise result involved in the synthesis.* For the original studies addressing "current," "ever," and "past" use, the 'standard errors' of the ratio's logarithm – derived here as one-quarter of the difference between the logarithms of the reported 95% limits – are 0.08, 0.017, and 0.08, respectively. Thus, the 'standard error' of their synthetic result's logarithm is expected to be smaller than the smallest one of those three, smaller than 0.08; but in the reported synthetic result it actually is – based on "0.88 (0.64–1.21)" –0.16, twice as large (*sic*) as that 0.08.

Correct synthesis of the three input ratios –0.80, 0.94 (replacing 0.91; cf. above), and 0.89 – is based on their logarithms: –0.22, –0.06, and –0.12, respectively. The logarithm of the synthetic result is the weighted average of those logarithms, with their respective amounts of 'information' (statistical) the weights. The weights are the inverses of the squares of the respective 'standard errors' (above). Thus the logarithm of the synthetic rate-ratio is:

$$\log(\text{RR}) = -\left[156(0.22) + 35(0.06) + 156(0.12)\right]/347 = -0.16,$$

implying RR = 0.85, different from the reported 0.88. The discrepancy would be even greater if 0.91 were used in lieu of 0.94; cf. above.

The *'standard error'* of the synthetic overall result's logarithm (that −0.16) is the square root of the inverse of the total information about it (that 347), which is 0.054, indeed smaller than the smallest one among the inputs (cf. above). This implies the 95% interval from −0.27 to −0.052 on the logarithmic level and the *correct overall synthetic result, corresponding to the reported "0.88 (0.64–1.21)," thus would have been 0.85 (0.77–0.94).*

The main point of note about this synthesis is that *a cardinal principle was violated:* Insofar as the distinctions among those three types of history are to be made – as indeed obviously is the case – the synthesis of the results across them is inadmissible!

From the synthesis of the results of the studies addressing the relevant, *"current" use*, the reported result (on the incidence of CHD) was "0.80 (0.68–0.95)." As the inputs to this are not shown in the report, these numbers cannot be readily verified. But, in the face of the discrepancies that were identifiable, the question is, Would the derivative result and its imprecision interval specific to the relevant studies, if correctly derived from the statistics from these studies, have been even more compelling than these (just as identifiably is the case in respect to the statistics on the inadmissible synthesis of the results across the different definitions of the medication use).

In the report's final, "*Comment*" section, the investigators say this: "Prevention of CHD, previously believed to be an important indication for long-term HRT [hormone replacement therapy], is not supported by our analysis of observational studies." *This evidence-summarizing comment is correct, but only because of the mistaken "analysis."* As we imply above, that "previous" belief is *supported* by the "analysis" specific to the studies that addressed the relevant histories (those of "current" use of the hormones); and it would have been supported even by the result drawing from all of the included studies – the *relevant and irrelevant studies combined* – had the synthetic result from these and its imprecision interval been correctly derived.

Among the aberrations of note in this "scientific review" is the investigators' treatment of the *cardinal validity-issue in the original studies* that were included. Said in the report's Results section is this:

> When [the studies addressing current use with control for socioeconomic status] were combined, the summary RR became nonsignificant (RR, 0.97; 95% CI, 0.82–1.16), suggesting confounding. Further sensitivity analysis evaluating only studies that adjusted for alcohol use, exercise, or major cardiovascular risk factors confirmed this finding [refs.].

Among the implications of this is, that *included in the synthesis of the original results were those of studies – non-experimental – in which a notable confounder was not controlled.*

Concerning the genesis of this "scientific review" [2], the investigators say that "This review was initiated to aid the current USPSTF [U.S. Preventive Services Task Force] in making new recommendations that will be released this fall. The focus of the USPSTF is to develop recommendations on screening, counseling, and chemoprophylaxis for asymptomatic populations." Two of the five investigators were among the 14 members of that Task Force. The *Task Force* indeed made its recommendations [3]: "The USPSTF found fair to good evidence that" the harms of "the combination of estrogen and progestin ... include increased risk for ... coronary heart disease," and that "Evidence is insufficient to determine the effects of unopposed estrogens on the risks for ... CHD, ..." As the basis for these, *it repeated, quite verbatim, the derivative results addressed above, with no criticism about the way they were derived* (including without that distinction between 'opposed' and 'unopposed' estrogens.; cf. above). In its own collective voice, and apparently in reference to the original studies, it posited the impression that "selection bias (the tendency of healthier women to use HRT) appears to explain the apparent protective effect of estrogen on CHD seen in observational studies."

That perceived explanation is, however, not one of selection bias but confounding; and at issue in this is confounding by level of cardiovascular health. In the review, "Studies were excluded if the population was selected according to prior events or presence of conditions associated with higher risks for targeted outcomes."

In the face of all of this, the Task Force did not conclude that the original research, and especially its review, provides inadequate basis for any recommendation. Instead, it found it feasible to be quite categorical: "The USPSTF has concluded that HRT does not decrease, and may in fact increase, the incidence of CHD." And, very notably, this was the TF's conclusion when the only relevant derivative result – presumably diluted by the inclusion of results of "cohort" studies – was, as noted above, "0.80 (0.68–0.95)."

22.3.2 The Study Reported in 2012

The 2002 Task Force [3] set the direction for an update of the then review [2]:

> Better data on benefits and harms are expected from ongoing randomized trials, including from the Women's Health Initiative (WHI) of unopposed estrogen in women who have had hysterectomy [ref.].

Accordingly, in the "systematic review to update the U.S. Preventive Services Task Force recommendations" published *in 2012* [4], the focus was on "randomized, double-blind trials" on the subject, "published in English since 2002," and "The Women's Health Initiative reported most of the results." "We did not include observational studies because of the existence of published randomized trials ..."

"We used results from the WHI trials as the main estimates for each outcome rather than perform meta-analysis of all trials because the trials were heterogeneous, they were most applicable to the key questions, and their results would dominate the meta-analysis because of their large enrollment."

Thus, *this "systematic review" to update the inputs to the Task Force did not amount to an updated derivative study on the effects of the treatments at issue*. It reflected full-on devotion to the commonly-held doctrine that the results of randomized trials are, inherently, of superior validity relative to those from any non-experimental studies; that in the face of such experimental results their non-experimental counterparts can be ignored.

The Task Force, in its report published in 2013 [5], payed heed to that "systematic review." In respect to the effect we've been focusing on, it noted that the WHI trial on estrogen alone, after 8 years of follow-up, produced for CHD "(HR, 0.95 [CI, 0.78–1.15])." This the TF took to mean that "For the overall enrolled population, there was no reduction in the risk for CHD with estrogen alone." And it noted, too, that "Subgroup analysis did reveal a potential reduction in women aged 50–59 years (HR, 0.59 [CI, 0.38–0.90]." *There was no allusion to the 'dilution' of the reported "reduction" in CHD incidence on account of the poor adherence to the assigned treatments, even before the experimental treatment's termination in the trial* (Sect. 20.3.3).

Nevertheless, elsewhere in the report the TF drew a *categorical, nihilistic conclusion, from the trial alone*: "There is convincing evidence that estrogen does not have a beneficial effect on CHD" – without specification of that "convincing evidence."

22.3.3 The Burden of These Examples

Given the importance of the topic (Sect. 19.1) and the eminent-and-instructive original research on it (Sects. 19.2 and 21.3), derivative research on it also is instructive to examine, notably research commissioned by the USPSTF (U.S. Preventive Services Task Force) for the purposes of its promulgation of "recommendations" about prophylactic use of 'HRT.'

As the example in Sect. 22.3.2 above illustrates, derivative gnostic studies are now termed systematic reviews. The general denotation of *'systematic'* is, according to our Oxford American Writer's Thesaurus, "structured, methodical, organized, orderly, planned, systematized, regular, routine, standardized, standard; logical, coherent, consistent; efficient, businesslike, practical," with "disorganized" given as the word's antonym. We suggest that it would go without saying that any appropriate derivative gnostic study, like any appropriate original one, is systematic, and this in the particular meaning that it is *protocol-driven* (rather than haphazard).

In dealing with those example reviews [2, 4] we did not address the principal sense in which the first on of these [2], like derivative clinical studies in general, was protocol-driven, namely in their *mission to identify every original study of the targeted type* as to objects and methods (at least the ones published in English). The main reason why we did not cover this aspect of those derivative-study reports is that *we don't regard it as very important* for the study's validity (Sect. 22.2). Indeed, in the first one of those studies (Sect. 22.3.1) the main (efficacy) result was derived by synthesizing too many original results; and in the second one of those two examples (Sect. 22.3.2) the findings of the derivative study were drawn solely from the dominant one among the identified original studies of the targeted type (without any "meta-analysis").

As the example in Sect. 22.3.1 illustrates, *even a very high-profile derivative clinical study, very rigorous in its systematic identification of all of the potentially admissible studies, can be quite untidy in its protocol concerning the actual admissibility* of original studies into the synthesis of the results. Examples of this in the synthesis of non-experimental results (Sect. 22.3.1) were, for one, the inclusion of studies in which a positive history of the medication's use was its having been used "ever," and without regard for its type or dosage; and for another, the untidy way the eminently-important topic of potential confounding was dealt with. We here add the feature that, "In general, studies were included if they included a comparison group of HRT nonusers and reported data relating to HRT and clinical outcomes of interest." Yet in none of the 11 "case-control" studies on the etiogenesis of CHD could there have been a "comparison group of HRT nonusers."

And as for the derivative studies themselves in respect to the included original studies, *the original results' "meta-analysis" (synthesis) can be downright antithetical to the study's purported systematic nature*, as we made plain in Sect. 22.3.1.

The second one of those two examples reflects the generally strong tendency in derivative intervention-prognostic studies to accent the evidence from *randomized trials*, if available. And notable in this is that, even when the concern expressly is to provide for evidence-based recommendations for practitioners, the evidence drawn from the thus-revered trials is *not about prognostic probabilities* but about the magnitudes of "hazard ratios" (incidence-density ratios) presumed to be constant over prognostic time (cf. Sect. 19.2); and this empirical ratio is taken at its face value, notably in disregard of even very major *non-adherence* to the assigned treatments.

In addition to illustrating the level of systematicity commonly involved in 'systematic' derivative studies for intervention-prognosis, the two examples in the Sections above illustrate the tendency in these studies to focus on the production of *synthetic study results* – for each of the effects at issue a single-valued measure of it, together with an imprecision interval for this – rather than results in the sense of *justified beliefs* about the magnitudes of the parameters at issue. This is most eminently illustrated by the focus, in that second example, on long-term results in a trial without any concern to adjust these numerics – judgementally at least – for the major non-adherence to the assigned treatments, even in the period when the assignments were in force (Cf. Sect. 20.3.3).

And in the end, in this vein, the basis of authoritative "recommendations" gets to be, in essence, those numerics alone – less than tidy, synthesized from original studies with heterogeneous and poorly thought-out objects of study and with wanting validity of methods. They leave practicing doctors without critically-updated knowledge as to the basis for the intervention-prognosis at issue, even in such superficial terms as are characteristic of these studies.

References

1. The Women's Health Initiative Steering Committee (2004) Effects of conjugated equine estrogen in postmenopausal women with hysterectomy. The Women's Health Initiative randomized trial. JAMA 291:1701–1712
2. Nelson HD, Humphrey LL, Nygren P *et alii* (2002) Postmenopausal hormone replacement therapy: scientific review. JAMA 288:872–888
3. U.S. Preventive Services Task Force (2002) Postmenopausal hormone replacement therapy for primary prevention of chronic conditions: recommendations and rationale. Ann Intern Med 137:834–839
4. Nelson HD, Walker M, Zakher B, Mitchell J (2012) Menopausal hormone therapy for the primary prevention of chronic conditions: a systematic review to update the U.S. Preventive Services Task Force recommendations. Ann Intern Med 157:104–113
5. Moyer AV (2013) Menopausal hormone therapy for the primary prevention of chronic conditions: U.S. Preventive Services Task Force recommendation statement. Ann Intern Med 158:47–54

Part VII
Retrospective Overview of the Precepts in This Book

Chapter 23
Theory of Medicine Defining the Essential Missions for Clinical Research

Contents

Abstract In this book on clinical research, the first – most broadly introductory – part (Part I) includes a delineation of our critically-adopted conception of *the essence of clinical medicine* and, related to this, that of the essence of *scientific medicine*. And in the framework of these most fundamental concepts, then, we present our answer to the most fundamentally-orientational question about clinical research, namely: *What is clinical research for scientific medicine in principle about?* We here present an overview of these fundamentally-orientational tenets in our general theory-framework for clinical medicine and clinical research.

Keywords Theory of medicine · Essence of clinical medicine · Requisite knowledgebase of clinical medicine · Core missions for clinical research

23.1 Esoteric Ad-hoc Knowing – Gnosis – in the Essence of Clinical Medicine

We see clinical doctors' work centering on their *pursuit (and attainment) of first-hand knowing about hidden-but-relevant truths* concerning the health of their clients. For, such knowing is needed as the basis for clinical doctors' *teaching* – L. doctor, teacher – their clients about their own health (in those hidden-but-relevant respects; Sect. 1.2.1).

We distinguish among three species of such knowing in clinical medicine: *diagnosis*, which concerns the client's health at present; *etiognosis*, which is about the causal origin – etiology/etiogenesis – of the client's illness (or sickness not due to

O. S. Miettinen et al., *Clinical Research Transformed*,
https://doi.org/10.1007/978-3-030-06176-0_23

illness); and *prognosis*, or knowing about the future course of the client's health, especially about the ways in which this would depend on the choice of treatment. Our omnibus term for this esoteric ad-hoc knowing is '*gnosis.*'

Pursuit of gnoses about their clients' health and teaching the clients about the thus-attained insights we see as both universal in and unique to doctors' work in clinical healthcare, and we hence deem these two, closely interrelated, functions to constitute *the essence of clinical medicine* (Sect. 1.2.2). This essence of it we see as the 'specific difference' distinguishing clinical medicine from clinical nursing and other 'paramedical' disciplines of clinical healthcare. (As a separate topic, we distinguish clinical medicine from community medicine – from epidemiology, that is; Sect. 1.5).

That conception of the essence of clinical medicine presupposes clinical doctors' active possession of, or else ready access to, the general – abstract (placeless and timeless) – *medical knowledge* that constitutes the basis of the gnoses at the core of the practice of clinical medicine (Sect. 1.2.3). That knowledge can only derive from medical science, from the quintessentially-applied branch of it.

From these premises we've deduced our conception of the essence of *scientific medicine* as a core element in our theory-framework of medicine: To us, medicine is scientific to the extent that its theoretical framework is rational (logical) and its knowledge-base derives from science (Sect. 2.4) – from gnostic clinical research, that is.

23.2 The Requisite Knowledge-Base – Probabilistic – for Clinicians' Gnoses

As the available facts on the case at issue generally underdetermine the truths (hidden) that a clinical doctor's gnoses are about, gnostic clinical knowledge can generally be only about the *probability* of the truth in question (Sect. 1.2.3).

And by the same token, the knowledge (probabilistic) relevant to any given case is predicated by the set of available, gnostically relevant (but inconclusive) set of facts on it – the *gnostic profile* of the case (Sect. 1.2.3).

While attainment of knowledge of this critically-relevant type – gnostic – has not been the consequence of the already-ample gnostic clinical research (Sect. 3.3), the fundamental reason for this has been a lack of appreciation of the nature of the requisite knowledge.

23.3 The Essential Missions – Gnostic – for Clinical Research

Clinical research, in our conception of it, encompasses laboratory-level, biological-type research in addition to human-level, statistical-type research (Sect. 2.3). The former, even though commonly termed 'basic' medical research, also is *applied* research (Sect. 3.2.1), as it in medical contexts generally is motivated by hope for results that would provide for the development of new products and processes for potential deployment in clinical medicine.

But *essential* in all of clinical medicine is the appropriate *knowledge-base* for the deployment of that which already is available to consider; and thus, *quintessentially applied* (Sect. 3.2.1) is clinical research that serves advancement of the knowledge-base of clinical medicine, of knowing, in it, about the magnitudes of the gnostic probabilities of concern in it (Sect. 23.2, above).

This implies that the *essential missions* in clinical research are ones in the realm of gnostic clinical research, ones of serving advancement of the knowledge-base of clinicians' gnoses – of probability estimation in clinicians' diagnoses, etiognoses, and prognoses (Sect. 23.1, above). The essential missions in clinical research thus are those of diagnostic, etiognostic, and prognostic clinical research.

The direct contributions from clinical studies to the advancement of clinicians' gnoses are ones of new *evidence* about the objects of gnosis-relevant knowledge (Sect. 19.1.3) rather than actual new knowledge of that type. The new evidence is for the relevant scientific communities to consider, in their updating of the knowledge.

Chapter 24
Theory of Clinical Research for its Gnosis-Serving Missions

Contents

Abstract After Parts I, II, and III – constituting a general introduction to clinical research and then presentations of select epidemiological and statistical propedeutics of specifically gnostic clinical research – the bulk of this book on transformed (and thereby practice-transformative) clinical research naturally is devoted to critical theory of quintessentially-applied – gnostic – clinical research. In the present overview of that theory, we first reassert *the requisite form of the objects* of that research, and then highlight some *key principles* of objects and methods design for, and of the *reporting* on, the three species of such research.

Keywords Theory of essential clinical research · Generic objects of the studies · Objects design for the studies · Methods design for the studies · Reporting on the new evidence

24.1 Generic Objects of the Studies

In the coverage of the theory of quintessentially-applied – gnostic – clinical research in this book, our focus is on the studies' objects design before their methods design, as we placed great emphasis on the former as a necessary predicate for the latter. And indeed, as for the already-ample gnostic clinical research, its failure to have provided for material advancement of the requisite knowledge-base of scientific medicine we attribute to it not having addressed the critically-relevant objects of study, namely the gnostic probabilities of clinicians' concern (Preface).

A salient challenge in the objects design for gnostic clinical studies we understand to be the *complexity* of the requisite knowledge-base of the gnoses, even in

O. S. Miettinen et al., *Clinical Research Transformed*,
https://doi.org/10.1007/978-3-030-06176-0_24

quite narrowly-defined disciplines of clinical medicine, the complexity arising from the great multiplicity of gnostic profiles of cases from whichever domain of their presentation for gnoses. But we invoke a ready solution to this ubiquitous, serious problem, namely *statistical modelling* – thereby treating the magnitude of any *gnostic probability as a function of the gnostic indicators* involved in the gnostic profiles of cases from whatever defined *domain* of their presentation for gnosis.

Now, insofar as there is a *singular idea transformative of clinical research* such that the research, in turn, serves to transform today's clinical medicine – essentially opinion-based – into genuinely scientific medicine, this idea is the invocation of such statistical modelling of the profile-specificity of gnostic probabilities (Sect. 4.1).

In these terms, for any given truth (hidden) of gnostic concern in a defined domain of case presentations, the *overall object of study* – addressing the great multitude of case profiles from the domain – is the designed *Gnostic Probability Function, GPF*. And the corresponding *component objects* of study are (the magnitudes of) the parameters in such a function, the manageably small number of these (Sect. 7.4).

24.2 Objects Design for the Studies

Those objects of a gnostic clinical study (above) we present as resulting from an express, principles-guided *objects design*, for the referent *domain* of the objects. The designed object function we present as always being a regression model and, more specifically, always a model of *logistic regression* (Sect. 7.4).

We repeatedly emphasize that design of the objects (statistical in form) for a gnostic clinical study is tantamount to designing, secondarily, *the form, and type of referent, for the study's result*. The actual study – following its objects design – will thus be tantamount to a project to obtain empirical content of the designed object-function's form, from the designed domain of the case-presentations and gnoses at issue. This brings to focus the primacy of these studies' objects design over their methods design.

Objects design for a gnostic clinical study, we explain, is the context in which assurance of the study's *relevance* for the development of the knowledge-base of clinical practice – this principal quality-desideratum of a human-level clinical study (Sect. 23.3, above) – comes to focus. The overarching principle to this end we noted above, namely the attainment of *specificity* to the great multitude of gnostic profiles from a given domain of case presentations in the framework of a *statistical model* for the probabilities in the multifarious cases from the domain in question (Sect. 24.1, above).

We do, however, caution against excessive provision for profile-specificity in the overall object of a gnostic clinical study, as this conduces to 'overparametrization bias' in the study's result (Sect. 8.3).

Among the other desiderata for a gnostic study's objects design, preeminent we present to be definition of the study objects' *domain* with a view to the degree of need for development or advancement of the knowledge-base of the gnoses in it (Sects. 2.2 and 19.1.1, i.a.) – implied by the commonality of case presentations from it, the importance of well-informed gnoses in those cases, and the state of the existing knowledge-base of the gnoses.

Appreciation of the generic nature of the truly practice-relevant objects of gnostic clinical research (Sect. 24.1, above), and then of the need for express, principles-guided design of these in the framework of statistical modelling of gnostic probabilities, has remained seriously wanting, we hold, due to a still-prevalent *research-cultural aberration* in medical academia. In epidemiologic academia, a distinction is still being made between 'epidemiologists' in the meaning of epidemiological researchers and 'biostatisticians' focusing on epidemiological research; and there is a counterpart of this in clinical academia. This runs counter to our teaching that, in statistical science such as gnostic clinical research, the purely medical and purely statistical aspects should be suitably integrated in the mind of the Principal Investigator at least (Sects. 4.2 and 19.2, i.a.).

24.3 Methods Design for the Studies

In regard to methods design for a gnostic clinical study, our cardinal principle is viewing this – the design of the study proper – as *subordinate to the study's objects design*. From this vantage, the mission in a gnostic clinical study is to produce empirical content of the form of the study's overall object from the referent domain of this (cf. Sect. 24.2, above).

The first-order upshot of that cardinal principle is, to us, the need to deduce the essence of a gnostic clinical study from its objects design. In these terms, *the essence of a gnostic study on a given type of object of study* – one on a diagnostic probability, for instance (Sect. 12.1) – *we regard as an aprioristic given*, singular in type and hence not the result of the study's methods design. Whereas the generic type of a first-principles gnostic clinical study is dictated (logically) by the design of its objects (and domain), actual method design defines only the *ad-hoc particulars of the study*.

Instructive examples of this cardinal principle of study design in gnostic clinical research are the logic-dictated *structural essence* – aprioristic, singular – of studies on *diagnostic* probability functions (Sect. 12.1) and, especially, the case-base/case-referent structure of *etiognostic* studies in the context of an event-type health outcome (Sect. 15.6.2). As these examples illustrate, the essentials of the structure of any first-principles gnostic clinical study include, first, its particular *study base*, representing the designed GPF's (gnostic probability function's) domain (abstract); and second, the study's result in reference to the study base. The essence of the study process in reference to the study base is the production of the study result – by *documentation* of the designed GPF's empirical counterpart in reference to the study base.

From the reports on a number of *intervention-prognostic studies* we closely examined (Chaps. 19, 20, 21, and 22), it is evident that for none of them was the methods design governed by its antecedent objects design; to it there was no allusion, even. And hence, the form and referent of each of the results was determined by the study's methods design, "statistical methods" included, rather than by the study's objects design – statistical – for a defined domain. The study result is, consistently, a single number, in total disregard of the variation in the prognostic profiles of the persons. (Instead, the term for what result was generically about, even in a synthesis of these, varied from one study to another). Among the non-experimental studies there are "case-control studies" and "cohort studies" without appreciation of the case-base or case-referent structure of etiologic-type intervention-prognostic studies (cf. above). And more than anything else, on display was, unwittingly, *confusion* about the theory – concepts and principles – of these studies.

24.4 Reporting on the New Evidence

An integral part of any piece of gnostic clinical research is the *published report* on it. And just as the other parts of any gnostic clinical study, the report on it is to be *designed,* and specifically in the framework of tenable principles specific to it.

As we, for the purposes of concrete instruction late in this book (Chaps. 19, 20, 21, and 22), extensively describe recent reports on some very high-profile gnostic clinical studies, salient is the *confusion* at the root of the failure that has thus-far marked this research for the scientific knowledge-base for clinical medicine (Chap. 23, above). And very notably, while the objects and methods of those studies are wanting, particularly flaring we find to be the flaws in their respective reports.

In that context we posit some utterly elementary – and, we think, obviously incontrovertible – propositions concerning the design of the report on an intervention-prognostic study – or, for that matter, on any study, original or derivative, intended to contribute to the evidence-base of the knowledge-base of clinical medicine. Among these are propositions concerning the structuring ('architecture') of the report:

1. The title of the report should be simple, merely giving an indication of what the study was about.
2. The structure should be the same for the Abstract/Summary of the report and the report proper.
3. Objective is unworthy as element in those structures.
4. Conclusion(s) is absolutely unjustifiable as an element in those structures.
5. Extensive presentation of the study's results in its Abstract/Summary is unjustifiable.
6. The main sections in the report's Abstract/Summary and the report proper might best be these: Background, Objects, Methods, Results, and Comments.

We also give some advice about the appropriate contents under these headings.

The *Background* section, we say, is meaningless if it merely states the obvious: that the evidence on that which the study is about is insufficient. It should specify the gnostic concerns that are at issue in the study. To be meaningful, it would give a sense of the state of the available evidence for the knowledge-base of those gnoses.

The *Objects* section naturally would sketch the domain of the case presentations addressed in the study and the gnostic probability function(s) in reference to the domain that the study addresses.

The *Methods* section would cover everything that in that part of the report (the Abstract, say) is said as specification of the study's methodology, without delegating some of the specifics to contents under the Results heading. And correspondingly, the *Results* section would address the study results alone, without involving content that belongs in the Methods section of the report – most notably features of the *actual methods* as distinct from the designed ones.

Comprehensibility – to the members of the relevant scientific community – is not merely a desideratum in the design of the study report. It is a scientific imperative. While the intended readers are a community of gnostic researchers, they are not a community of statisticians. Yet, the examples we cover illustrate that the statistical aspects of the reports presumably are, quite commonly, incomprehensible to statisticians, even.

Effective reporting on a gnostic clinical study is orderly in its structuring, suitably focused under its topic headings, cohesive in is flow across and also within those topics and, above all, comprehensible in its contents. The imperative of comprehensibility of the study report translates to the desideratum of *simplicity* in it – echoing the call for simplicity in the formulation of complex knowledge needed in clinical gnoses (Sect. 24.1) and, correspondingly, in the objects of gnostic clinical studies (Sect. 24.2).

The *Comments* section, conveying the authors' closing points on the study to the report's readers, would be relevant only if it brought forth something that is relevant about the study but does not really fit under the other headings in the report. For instance, the authors might apologize for the illogical structure of and elements in the report which the journal's *editorial policy* imposed. This might be specific in reference to the mutually incoherent structurings of the Abstract (or Summary) section vis-à-vis the body of the report, and/or the purported Conclusions, and/or reporting on the so-called sample size determination, among other editorial impositions.

Progress in research for the knowledge-base of clinical medicine does not optimally flourish under editorial constraints on researchers' expression of their ideas about the research, their own studies or those of others. It would flourish best if the editors of all medical journals would provide for, and otherwise cultivate, free exchange of ideas about this eminently important research. The ideal we outline in the Section below (Sect. 25.3.2).

Chapter 25
Toward Worldwide Scientific Medicine

Contents

Abstract While this book is about the radical transformation that is urgently needed in the vast enterprise of clinical research – in order that it provide for the development of the requisite knowledge-base for genuinely-scientific clinical medicine – our presentation of the theory of the suitably-transformed research we here supplement by a sketch of the way in which we see the needed transformation of the research, and then of the practice of clinical medicine, to come about, without undue delay. So we here sketch the way we see the *sequentially-evolving developments* – the educating of the researchers, the designing of a *global program* of the research, the implementing of that program, the translating of the accrued evidence into knowledge, and ultimately: bringing the critically-relevant knowledge to guide the practices of clinicians everywhere.

Keywords Arranging for the education · Designing the requisite program · Implementing the research · Translating the evidence into knowledge · Making the knowledge accessible in practice

O. S. Miettinen et al., *Clinical Research Transformed*,
https://doi.org/10.1007/978-3-030-06176-0_25

25.1 Educating the Researchers

For clinical research to undergo the needed transformation that this book is about, clinical researchers need to be educated in the transformed statistical-type medical research (Sect. 4.2). In this, the top priority is high-quality education for the *vanguard* of these researchers. For, their transformed research, once commonly accepted as paradigmatic, will be the essence of the needed "paradigm shift" (à la Thomas Kuhn) in the research.

We envision this education to be introduced, for global purposes, in the epidemiologic segment of a leading faculty of medicine (App. 2). This vision focuses on *epidemiologic* academia because the theory at issue is an extension of the theory of epidemiological research to (meta-epidemiological) clinical research (Sect. 6.4); and it focuses on a *leading* faculty of medicine, as the needed major transformation in clinical research is primarily a concern for faculties with an engrained culture of global leadership in medical research. In fact, we've identified a faculty that is particularly well-suited for this pioneering role (App. 2).

Our vision of the pioneering education being *centered* in a leading faculty for global purposes reflects our vision of the education being closely connected to global leadership in the research proper (Sect. 25.2.1, below), and to the development of a global community-cum-fellowship of these researchers.

25.2 Designing the Global Program

25.2.1 Forming the Leadership Group

A program of pioneering, *globally-oriented education* in the transformed clinical research naturally spawns, in the same faculty, the concern to develop, collaboratively between the epidemiologic and clinical segments of it (Sect. 6.5), an actual, *globally coordinated program of research* – a program of the human-level, statistical-type clinical research that, in its eminence and significance, is the equivalent of the two parallel programs of laboratory-level, biological-type clinical research that accomplished the feat of decoding of the human genome.

The requisite *leadership* for such a program can only be provided by a suitably-educated *Leadership Group* involving epidemiologic and clinical members of that leading faculty of medicine. Needed is a group that represents the requisite expertise in the epidemiologic and clinical segments of the faculty and is, also, multidisciplinary in its clinical subject-matter. The members all master the key aspects of the theory of gnostic clinical research, and they all are dedicated to expeditious advancement of the research and, thereby, the development of scientific medicine, on a global basis.

25.2.2 Designing Example Informatics

The Leadership Group of the Program will understand that the Program will only thrive in the context of digital systems of clinical informatics in teaching facilities of clinical care, systems designed to serve not only the documentation and teaching needs in these facilities, but secondarily, also those of gnostic clinical research (Sect. 17.4).

Such an all-purpose system of clinical informatics needs to be organized, most broadly, according *the three generic types of case presentation for gnosis* in clinical medicine: there needs be a well-designed structure for the clinical data on cases in which the presentation calls for the pursuit of diagnosis; another for cases that prompt etiognostic concerns; and finally, a structure for cases in which the doctor needs to document the prognostic profile of the case and invoke prognostic knowledge specific to the profile.

The Leadership Group needs to illustrate each of these three types of data structure by suitable examples, to thereby clarify the respective missions for the three main types of *informatics working groups,* each of them *subdivided* according to suitably-grouped types of case presentation for the species of gnosis at issue. Those sub-groups, when rationally defined, will represent rational sub-disciplines of clinical medicine.

25.2.3 Designing Example Protocols

The natural next phase in the Leadership Group's exercise of leadership we take to be its design of suitably-illustrative example protocols for possible actual studies for the three species of gnosis, for implementation in the framework of the to-be-developed all-purpose clinical informatics system.

The objects designs in these, in particular, serve to make concrete what the Program will be about, in its comprehensive way, and how the research will be implemented in the framework of the informatics system expressly designed for it (together with the needs of clinical practice itself).

25.2.4 Designing the Gestalt of the Program

Once the Leadership Group has gained a concrete sense of the nature of the informatics system that needs to be developed for the operation of the Program, and how this system indeed provides the requisite database for comprehensive conduct of the research that is needed for the development of the requisite knowledge-base for scientific clinical medicine, they are ready to design the main features of the Program's structure and functioning in that context.

As we see it, the principal features of the Program's *structure* are that *Leadership Group* in a leading faculty of medicine (Sect. 25.2.1) together with a set of participating *Investigator Groups* in medical faculties around the world, chosen (critically) by the Leadership Group. And the principal features of the program's *functioning* are the studies' initiations by Principal investigators in the participating faculties and their quality-assurance by the Leadership Group. Only thus-sanctioned studies, with reports of them approved by the Leadership Group, can be attributed to the Program.

25.3 Implementing the Global Program

25.3.1 Securing Financing for the Program

The Leadership Group, with its ambitious planning for the Program – of clinical research that will serve to transform clinical medicine from its prevailing, essentially opinion-based practices to genuinely knowledge-based, scientific medicine – is in a situation that in its practicability is fundamentally different from its counterparts in 'basic' medical research. The knowledge-base of clinical medicine is not proprietary, subject to patenting and commercial exploitation. Thus, its financing by venture capital is not an option. The Program needs to be financed by a non-commercial source, whether some major foundation engaging in support of health research or, perhaps, the World Health Organization.

At issue in this is, first-off, funding of the central functions of the Program, enabling the investigator education and the functions of the Leadership Group of the research. The funding should cover, also, the design and implementation of the all-purpose clinical informatics system, designed under guidance of the Leadership Group for its home university but thereby also serving as the model to the other participating universities. The informatics systems and actual research by the participating other Investigator Groups would be need to be locally financed.

25.3.2 Effecting Operation of the Program

Once the Leadership Group has secured long-term financing for the Program, it can initiate its operation, with appointment of its *Director* the first task in this. Presumably, this will be the chairperson, or some other member, of that the Leadership Group. That Group's own role will change from the Program's planning to functioning, very actively, as its *Board of Directors.*

The *top priority* in the Program's operation will be the development of its clinical informatics infrastructure for the teaching hospitals (and other clinical care facilities) of the Leadership Group's own university (cf. Sect. 25.2.2), for implementation in all of the participating universities. In this task, the Director will depend heavily on experts in the various disciplines of clinical medicine, disciplines defined for this purpose according to types of case presentation for gnosis (cf. Sect. 25.2.2). To this end, the Director needs to form a thus-defined set of *Discipline-specific Expert Panels,* supplemented by one of experts representing the discipline of the theory of gnostic clinical research.

While the informatics infrastructure of the Program is being developed and the education of the investigators (Sect. 25.1) continues, the Program naturally prepares for its work in its framework and in matters closely related to this (Sect. 23.3, below).

25.4 Translating the Evidence into Knowledge

25.4.1 The Work of the Discipline-Specific Expert Panels

The Expert Panels that have a critical role in the development of the Program's informatics infrastructure (Sect. 25.2.6, above), have a new, related and equally critical role subsequent to this initial function. It focuses on gnostic the research proper.

In its initial phase, this work by each of the clinical Expert Panels is a direct extension of their planning for their presentation-specific segments of the Program's informatics infrastructure. For, in each Panel the work naturally focuses on provisional *objects design* for the requisite knowledge-base of the clinical discipline represented by it. After all, a sense of these objects of study was already needed and deployed in the design of the discipline-specific structures for the Program's informatics system.

The second phase is the obvious extension of this to provisional *methods design* for studying those GPFs (Gnostic Probability Functions).

The remaining, equally critical process-type function of those Expert Panels is *quality-assurance* of all of the scientific work in their respective segments of the Program. In this, their main role is not peer review of manuscripts; it is their *expert review.* This work can be directed, also, to manuscripts from outside the Program, notably when its database still is prohibitively sparse.

Finally, those Expert Panels – including, inter alia, one (diagnostic) on preclinical detection of breast cancer, one (etiognostic) on gastro-intestinal bleeding, and one (prognostic) on status post menopause – have the task of defining, for their respective segments of gnostic challenges in clinical medicine, *the state of the knowledge-base for the gnoses,* with updating of this as new evidence or something else warrants.

25.4.2 *The Public Forum for Use by the Expert Panels*

Scientific *research* inherently being a public enterprise, the Program's work needs a public forum, one that is truly suitable for this role in the Program.

This forum – in cyberspace – needs to provide for *public discourse* about the development and continual improvement of the Program's database; and about its studies' objects design methods design. And it needs to serve as the setting for *publication* of reports on gnostic clinical studies, derivative studies included, upon their expert (*sic*!) approval (cf. above) – this together with practically unlimited and free critical discussion of them. The reported studies need not be endogenous to the Program.

This forum for the Expert Panels naturally also is the forum for their specifications of the *state of the knowledge-base of gnoses* in their respective domains of types of case presentation for gnosis – their expert, maximally evidence-based knowledge about the magnitudes of the parameters in particular GPFs (gnostic probability functions) for defined domains.

25.5 Making the Knowledge Available in Practice

Once there is actual knowledge (rather than mere evidence; Sect. 23.3.2, above) about the gnostic probabilities relevant in the context of cases from a given domain of their presentations for gnosis, there generally can be no reasonable expectation that a doctor possesses this knowledge in terms of having stored the GPF in his/her neural memory-space and can quickly evaluate this function at the gnostic profile of the case at hand. It is, as we've said, an aprioristic given about the requisite knowledge-base of clinical medicine in this Information Age, that it resides, in the form of GPFs, in cyberspace, in an electronic 'expert system,' and that it is there automatically applied to the gnostic profile of the case at hand to produce state-of-the-art-knowledge about the gnostic probability in question, together with relevant collateral knowledge.

It follows that development of gnostic 'expert systems,' founded on the knowledge formulated by the Program's Expert Panels, is an integral part – and indeed the ever-evolving end product – of the Program.

Glossary

Abstract (as a quality of the referent of gnostic probabilities and of the objects of gnostic clinical studies): General in the meaning of not being specific to any place or time; that is, being abstract-general. See Particularistic.

Acausal (as a quality of a relation): Viewed without regard for causality (or lack thereof). See Causal.

Acute (as a quality in medicine): 1. Concerning the onset of an illness: Abrupt (rather than insidious). 2. Concerning the course of an illness: Short (episodic, rather than long, chronic).

Analysis (statistical, of data, into a result and its related other statistics): Misnomer (common) for Synthesis. See Synthesis.

Assessment (in clinical medicine and in gnostic clinical research): Facts-based estimation of the magnitude of something unmeasurable (such as the severity of a symptom). See Evaluation.

Base (of a gnostic clinical study): See Study base.

Baseline (of a cohort): Time of entry into the cohort, in cohort time (at time zero of this).

Basic medical research: See Medical research.

Note: Basic research, different from applied research, is driven by investigators' interest/curiosity rather than by their concern to provide for useful applications of the resulting knowledge; and as medical research is (medicine-serving) applied research, 'basic medical research' is a *contradiction in terms*. It generally denotes laboratory-level biological research, as distinct from its patient-level, statistical-type counterpart.

Bayesian statistics: Statistics involving subjective probabilities; that is, probabilities as matters of subjective belief.

Note: Scientific knowledge (about a gnostic probability, say) is a matter of subjective beliefs, notably when they are reasonably convergent rather than widely dispersed.

O. S. Miettinen et al., *Clinical Research Transformed*,
https://doi.org/10.1007/978-3-030-06176-0

Bernoulli distribution (in statistics): Distribution of a binary random variate (Y) taking on realizations 0 and 1. A particular Bernoulli distribution is defined by its mean, the probability of Y = 1.

Bias (in a gnostic study and, hence, in its result): Lack of validity, notably in terms of the extent of systematic error. See Systematic error.

Biostatistics: Statistics relevant to scholarly and professional work on particular aspects of the biosphere – from biology to demography (incl. of non-human species) to medicine and medical research. See Statistics.

Note: Most notably relevant to gnostic clinical research is statistics in the sense in which it bears on the *objects design* of the studies. The inferential statistics and statistical software packages used in the synthesis of data in this research are not peculiar to this context of their use.

Case (of a particular type of presentation for gnosis, or of a particular type of health outcome): An instance (of it).

Note: A *person* with a case of something *is not a case* over that something.

Case-base/case-referent study (in etiogenetic/etiognostic research): Study in which the outcome's incidence-density ratio, conditional on potential confounders, is documented for a defined *study base* in terms of (suitably-derived) case series and base/referent series. See Study base.

Case-control/retrospective study (in etiogenetic/etiognostic research): Study in which a group of persons with the illness at issue ('case group') is compared with a group of persons without the illness ('control group') as to their distributions by histories in respect to the etiogenetic determinant at issue. See Cohort study and Etiogenetic/etiognostic study.

Note: This concept is *malformed*, representing the original understanding – misconception – of the requisite nature – essence – of etiogenetic studies. At present, this type of study is commonly viewed as one of the two principal types of etiogenetic study (the other one being cohort study).

Case-fatality rate (of an illness): Of the cases (of an illness in a particular experience or in general), the proportion having a fatal outcome.

Note: For any subacute or chronic illness, this rate has scientific meaning only if it is made conditional on not succumbing to some other, 'competing' cause of death. In these (counterfactual) terms it is the asymptote of the fatalities' rate of cumulative incidence.

Catchment population (of a specified means of case identification): The population (dynamic) whose members satisfy the 'were-would' state of: Were a case of the event at issue now to occur, it would be caught (by the specified means of case identification).

Causal, as a quality of a determinant of *prospective* occurrence on an outcome: The outcome's occurrence/non-occurrence may depend crucially (i.e., causally) on its background in respect to this factor. See Acausal.

Note 1: In clinical medicine, this is the quality of prognostic concern in respect to the options for *intervention*.

Note 2: Interventive causation in prognosis is either *negative* or *positive* according as it decreases or increases the outcomes' probability.

Causal, as a quality of an outcomes' relation to an antecedent: The outcome would not have occurred but for the presence of the *antecedent*, ceteris paribus. See Acausal.

Note: In clinical medicine, this is the causal concern in *etiognosis.*

Ceteris paribus (in definitions of causality): All else being the same.

Clinical (as a quality of a datum or a process): Having to do with doctor-client interaction directly (in contrast to activities in laboratories or those of paramedical clinical personnel).

Clinical epidemiology: Misnomer (a contradiction in terms) in reference to 'evidence-based' clinical practice and/or to research producing the (purportedly) requisite evidence for the practice of clinical medicine. See Evidence-based medicine.

Clinical medicine: The species of medicine in which a doctor serves individual clients, individually. See Medicine.

Note: Clinical medicine is distinct from community medicine, in which a doctor serves a population, as a population (as distinct from its members individually).

Clinical research: See Clinical medicine and Medical research.

Closed population: Population whose membership is closed for exit; that is, once a member, always a member. See Open population and Cohort.

Cohort (in a gnostic study, clinical or epidemiological): Population whose membership is clinched by an event and lasts forever (including post mortem). See Closed population.

Cohort/prospective study in etiogenetic/etiognostic research: Study in which cohorts representing the compared (index and reference) categories of the etiogenetic determinant are compared in terms of the respective rates of occurrence of the illness at issue (in cohort/prospective time). See Case-control/retrospective study and Etiogenetic/etiognostic study.

Note 1: Like its case-control/retrospective precursor, this concept too is *malformed*. The cohort in it should be construed as the *source* population for an actual, first-principles etiogenetic study, whose *study* population is dynamic.

Note 2: In proper usage, 'cohort study' denotes a study with a cohort-type *study* population (distinct from a dynamic one).

Cohort/prospective study in intervention-prognostic research: Study in which the study population is a cohort. See Cohort study in etiogenetic/etiognostic research and Non-cohort intervention-prognostic study.

Cohort time: For each member of a cohort, the time since his/her entry into the cohort; and for a cohort at large, the time since the notionally synchronous entries into the cohort.

Note: Entries into a cohort, while synchronous in cohort time (by definition), are generally asynchronous in calendar time and study time.

Complication (of an illness or a treatment): Illness caused by it.

Confidence interval (for the value of a parameter in statistics): Interval so derived that with a given probability it covers the value (abstract) of the parameter – on the premise that the data are valid.

Note 1: This term is a *misnomer* for the statistic in question. For, confidence is a state of the mind of the interval's interpreter (in respect to the parameter's value), and not a feature of this statistic. This statistic actually is a measure of a result's imprecision; it is the result's *imprecision interval.*

Note 2: Any X% imprecision interval for the result on a parameter in statistical science (such as gnostic clinical research) serves as an X% confidence interval for the parameters' value if, and only if, two conditions obtain: the interval was validly derived from valid data, and these data are the only basis for the interpreter having any idea about the value in question.

Confounder (in an etiogenetic/etiognostic or intervention-prognostic study): Extraneous causal determinant of (the rate of) the outcome's occurrence with imbalanced distribution between the index and reference segments of the study base (thereby requiring control of it to prevent confounding bias from this imbalance), or a proxy for such a determinant.

Control group (in an intervention-prognostic cohort study): Sub-cohort representing the index treatment's alternative.

Counterfactual (in an etiognostic or intervention-prognostic study): The alternative to the causal category (factual) characterizing the index segment of the study base.

Cumulative incidence of a non-fatal event: See Note 2 under Cumulative incidence of death from a particular cause.

Cumulative incidence of death from a particular cause (in a cohort's course over cohort time), in reference to a particular point in cohort time: 1. The proportion of the cohort's members who died from the cause at issue before that point in cohort time. 2. The proportion – counterfactual – of the cohort's members who would have died from the cause at issue before that point in cohort time had there been no other, 'competing' causes of death.

Note 1: Only the latter type of cumulative incidence of death (from a particular cause) is meaningful in clinical research (for prognosis about fatal outcome of an illness or a treatment).

Note 2: That meaningful cumulative incidence (of death, cause-specific) can be quantified on the basis of the *incidence density* of death from the cause at issue as a function of cohort time. This conception of cumulative incidence applies to *non-fatal events* as well.

Cumulative incidence of death from any cause (in a cohort's course over cohort time): In reference to any particular point in cohort time, the proportion of the cohort's members who died before that point in cohort time.

Note: This rate – a simple proportion – is, due to its lack of specificity to any particular cause of death, quite empty of relevance in epidemiology and, especially, in medical research (epidemiological or clinical); but it is a useful point of departure in seeking to understand cumulative incidence of death from a particular cause and, finally, that of various non-fatal events.

Data: The plural of datum.

Note: It has become commonplace, in loose locution in particular, to treat the word 'data' as a singular (à la "The data is …").

Datum: Documented fact or factoid, especially when expressed in numerical code.

Defect: A state-type illness.

Note: A defect is either congenital or acquired (later); and an acquired defect is either a status post a disease or a status post injury – with the disease or injury the pathogenesis of the defect.

Derivative study (gnostic): Study in which the results of some original studies on a given object of study are synthesized into their corresponding meta-result.

Note 1: The result of a derivative study has the virtue of being more precise (re each of the parameters) than that of any of the original studies contributing to it. In principle, thus, a derivative study supplants the set of original studies it draws from.

Note 2: Quality assurance in gnosis-serving derivative clinical studies is more demanding of the investigators' competence than is its counterpart in the original studies on which these studies are based. For, derivative studies commonly involve the need to override the judgements of the original studies' investigators and their peer reviewers.

Design (of a gnostic study's objects or methods): Development of the specifics of the study plan, or these specifics as such.

Note: When the objects of study call for a singular type of study, this is the type of study a-priori and not by design; only the particulars in this framework are subject to design.

Determinant (of the level of a quantity): Something on which the level at issue depends.

Note 1: A determinant in the meaning of a *gnostic indicator* is an aspect (operational) of the cases from the domain at issue – a dimension of their characterization – and not the (set of) statistical variate (s) representing it in the probability function designed for the domain (as to its form).

Note 2: Such a determinant is either *acausal* or *causal* in its intended role in a gnostic probability function.

Development (research-based, for medicine): The process of by which knowledge ('biomedical') from 'basic' medical research can become consequential to medicine – in terms of a new product or process.

Note: Research can be an element in, and not merely the background of, such development. A prime example of this is 'drug development' in its three Phases.

Diagnosis (in clinical medicine): A doctor's first-hand knowing (esoteric) about possible hidden presence of a particular illness in the client.

Note: Commonly, only uncertain knowing of this type is possible, even in principle; and hence, diagnosis about a particular illness is, specifically, knowing about the *probability* of its presence (with certainty a special case of this).

Diagnostic (as an entity in clinical medicine): Test producing diagnostically-relevant information; that is, diagnostic test (in a clinical doctor's pursuit of diagnosis).

Diagnostic probability: The probability – theoretical/abstract – with which the illness in question is present, given the diagnostic profile of the case.

Note: Diagnostic probability of the presence (hidden) of the illness in question is (numerically) the proportion of cases of the profile in general – in the abstract – such that it actually is present.

Diagnostic profile (of a case presenting for diagnosis): The set of available, diagnostically- relevant facts (on the case).

Diagnostic study: Study producing evidence about the probabilities of the presence – hidden – of a particular illness, probabilities specific to the diagnostic profiles of the cases. See Diagnostic probability, Etiognostic study and Intervention-prognostic study.

Note: A diagnostic study addresses a (designed) diagnostic probability function for a particular (selected/designed) domain of case presentations for diagnosis.

Diagnostic test (in clinical medicine): Procedure revealing a (set of) hidden diagnostically-relevant fact(s) on the client (for incorporation into the diagnostic profile).

Discipline of medicine: Segment of medicine constituting the focus of practice for a segment of doctors.

Note. The common term for this still is '*specialty*' (of medicine), with the implication that there is modern medicine without such a focus. But this implication is untenable; for, no one can competently practice all, or even several, well-construed disciplines of modern medicine.

Disease: Process-type illness with natural (non-traumatic) pathogenesis. See Injury.

Doctor (medical): Practitioner of medicine. See Medicine and Clinical medicine.

Domain (of the object function of a gnostic clinical study): The type of situation – defined in abstract terms – in reference to which the probability function is, or was, designed (as to its form).

Dynamic population: Population with turnover of membership. See Open population.

Effect: Change in an outcome caused by an antecedent of it, present in lieu of the defined alternative of it.

Efficiency (of a gnostic clinical study): Information yield (about the magnitudes of the object parameters) in relation to the size or cost of the study.

Empirical value (of a parameter, from a study): Result of study. See Estimate.

Note: In statistics, such a statistic is termed estimate, or point estimate (of a parameter's value).

Entity: Thing (an illness, say) that has an existence in itself, rather than merely as a quality (severity, say) of such a thing or as a relation (causal, say) between such things.

Epidemiologic (as used in this book): Having to do with epidemiology.

Epidemiological (as used in this book): Being inherent in epidemiology or consistent with the essence of epidemiology.

Epidemiological research: Research (scientific) for the advancement of epidemiology. See Clinical research.

Note: In epidemiological research, analogously with clinical research, a salient duality is constituted by 'basic' epidemiological research versus gnostic epidemiological research.

Epidemiology: Community medicine. See Medicine.

Note: Community medicine is medicine in which a doctor cares for the population of a community, as a population (rather than for its members individually).

Epistemology (of gnostic clinical research): Theory of methodology. See Ontology.

Note: Epistemological (epistemic) theory is subordinate to ontological (ontal) theory.

Estimate (of a parameter's value): 1. In statistical science (such as gnostic clinical research), the value in question in the judgement of a particular expert on the matter, or typically among such experts. 2. In statistics, an empirical value (of the parameter at issue). See Empirical value.

Etiogenesis/etiology (of an illness, or a sickness not due to illness): Causal origin. See Pathogenesis.

Note 1: Etiogenesis is explanatory (causally) of pathogenesis.

Note 2: In etiogenesis a distinction can be made between producing – *positive* – causation and preventing – *negative* – causation. Etiognosis generally is about the former.

Etiogenetic/etiognostic study: Study producing evidence about etiognostic probabilities for an antecedent of cases of an illness (or sickness not due to illness), specific to the etiognostic profiles of the cases. See Etiognostic probability, Diagnostic study, and Intervention-prognostic study.

Note: A first-principles etiogenetic/etiognostic study has a singular essence, that of the *case-base/case-referent* study. See Case-base/case-referent study.

Etiognosis (in clinical medicine): A doctor's first-hand knowing (esoteric) about whether a particular antecedent of the case (of illness, or sickness not due to illness), known to have been present, actually was causal – etiogenetic/etiologic – to the case.

Note: Commonly, only uncertain knowing of this type is possible, even in principle; and hence, etiognosis about a particular antecedent (known) of the case is, specifically, knowing about the *probability* of its etiogenetic role (with certainty a special case of this).

Etiognostic probability: The probability – theoretical, abstract – with which an antecedent (actual) of a health outcome was etiogenetic to the outcome, given the etiognostic profile of the case.

Note: Etiognostic probability is (numerically) the proportion of cases of the profile (of the antecedent-outcome-host complex) in general – in the abstract – such that the antecedent of the outcome was causal (etiogenetic) to it.

Etiology: See Etiogenesis.

Evaluation (in clinical medicine and in gnostic clinical research): Facts-based judgement of the quality of something (such as a patient's 'health-related quality of life' or the validity of a study), on a scale of preference. See Assessment.

Note. The term is, unjustifiably, in very wide use in medicine and in clinical-level/('patient'-level) clinical research, in the meaning of assessment.

Event-type illness: Illness which, distinct from state-type illnesses, is of a duration so short that what really matters is its happening per se, without regard for the duration of its course.

Note 1: Examples of event-type illnesses are myocardial infarction and pulmonary embolism, but not the *states* of cardiac or pulmonary fibrosis.

Note 2: This distinction/duality is eminently manifest in the way population-level (epidemiological) rates of occurrence of particular illnesses are formulated and termed: Rates of event-type illnesses are, inherently, ones of incidence, while those of state-type illnesses ones of the incidence of (the event of) their inception or detection and/or ones of the prevalence of (the state of) their being present, prevailing.

Evidence (about the objects of a gnostic study): The result of the study together with the referent and genesis of it, as documented in the study's published report. See Result, Method, and Methodology.

Note: The genesis of the study result is the methodology of the study. It needs to be documented on two levels: first, as to what it was designed to be; and then, as to what it actually got to be.

Evidence-based medicine: Doctrine recently introduced by 'clinical epidemiologists' at McMaster University. The core idea in it is that practitioners of clinical medicine need to comprehensively follow research relevant to their work – critically, as instructed by those 'clinical epidemiologists.'

Note: Practitioners of clinical medicine do not have the time to do the reading, nor does mastery of the precepts of 'clinical epidemiology' constitute the requisite competence for doing it critically.

Experimental (as a quality of a gnostic clinical study): Involving a study base in which some determinant(s) of the gnostic probabilities at issue are 'manipulated' in the interest of learning about their implications (gnostic).

Note: Experimental gnostic studies are not all intervention-prognostic trials. For, notably, a diagnostic study is experimental if it involves diagnostic testing done for the purposes of the study (in cases without such testing in actual practice).

Factor (gnostic): Causal determinant of the rate/probability of occurrence of the health outcome at issue, or a category of this.

Fatal outcome (of the course of an illness): Death from (caused by) the illness at issue.

Finding (in clinical medicine): A sign pointing to a hidden anomaly.

Note: While a finding clinical medicine inherently is an abnormality, in clinical research any result is referred to as a finding.

General linear model (in statistics): Model in which the mean of a Gaussian ('normal') random variate of interest is formulated as a linear compound of a set of parameters. See Linear compound.

Note: The GLM is general in the sense of encompassing the models for each of 'analysis of variance,' 'analysis of covariance,' and 'regression analysis.'

Generalized linear model (in statistics): Model in which a transform of the mean or the random variate of interest – non-Gaussian, perhaps – is formulated as a linear compound of a set of parameters.

Note: A salient example of generalized linear models is that for *logistic regression*.

Gnosis (in clinical medicine): A doctor's first-hand knowing (esoteric) about some hidden truth(s) concerning the health of the client. See Diagnosis, Etiognosis, and Prognosis.

Gnostic probability (in clinical medicine): See Diagnosis, Etiognosis, and Prognosis.

Hazard (in the jargon of statistics): Incidence density (in the jargon of epidemiology and gnostic clinical research).

Health (in clinical medicine): 1. Absence of particular illness(es) (in a client). 2. Status regarding the presence/absence of particular illness(es) (of a client).

Hypothesis: 1. In science, a conjecture about a truth (abstract) of scientific concern. 2. In statistics, any value or range of values entertained for a parameter.

Note 1: In reference to a particular probability function in gnostic clinical research, any hypothesis is a conjecture positing that a particular parameter in the function (designed as to its form for a particular domain) has a *non-null value*, one that deviates from the null value in a *particular direction.*

Note 2: In statistics – in statistical hypothesis-testing – actually tested is the tenability of the parameter's null value, termed the *null hypothesis.* Its 'rejection,' in the light of the P-value from the test, is tantamount to 'acceptance' of the non-null, *alternative hypothesis.*

Iatrogenic (as a quality of case of illness or of sickness not due to illness): Having etiogenesis from a medical action (such as recommending a particular treatment).

Illness: Somatic anomaly, either hidden but causing sickness (at least potentially) or one that inherently is overt.

Note: Illness encompasses three species of it: disease, defect, and injury.

Impact of a piece of gnostic clinical research: The extent to which the study provides for advancement of (the practice of) clinical medicine.

Note. This concept bears no relation to the now ubiquitously-deployed 'impact factor' of the journal in which the study's report is published.

Imprecision (of a parameter's empirical magnitude/value): The extent of the lack of reproducibility (in hypothetical replications of the study with the same methodology in all result-relevant respects, including the size of the study).

Imprecision interval: See Note 1 under Confidence interval.

Incidence (as a property of an event-type entity of health): Frequency of occurrence in a population over time. See Prevalence.

Incidence density: Number of cases (of an event-type entity, such as death) divided by the amount of population-time of opportunity for the cases' occurrence. See Incidence and Cumulative Incidence.

Note: An incidence density is generally expressed in the form of the number of cases per a given unit-amount of population-time (e.g., 100,000 person-years).

Index category (of a causal determinant): The category representing the cause in question. See Reference category.

Indication (gnostic)*:* The realization of an indicator (gnostic). See Indicator.

Indicator (gnostic, in a gnostic clinical study): An aspect of characterization of cases from the domain of the study, involved in the profiles of the cases and, hence, in the definition of the (independent) variates (Xs) in the designed gnostic probability function. See Indication.

Indicator variate (in statistical science, such as gnostic clinical research): Variate that is binary in in its realizations: the realization is 1 for the category the variate is designed to indicate, 0 otherwise.

Information (from a gnostic clinical study on a parameter's value): The inverse of the square of the standard error of the empirical value. See Standard error.

Injury/trauma: Process-type illness whose pathogenesis is unnatural (traumatic). See Disease.

Note: The outcome of the non-fatal course of an injury commonly is a defect – with the course of the injury the pathogenesis of the defect.

Interaction (between two entities): Mutual action; that is, acting on – and influencing – each other.

Note: The word is *commonly misused* in medicine, as in 'drug interaction' and 'gene- environment interaction.' In statistics, similarly, a product terms in a regression model is mischaracterized as an 'interaction term.' If the effect of one determinant (causal) depends on another one, at issue is not interaction (involving, say, the influence of the genome on the environment) but *modification* of the effect of one of the factors by the other.

Interval estimate (of a parameter in statistics): Confidence interval.

Intervention (on the course of an individual's health): Action on the person's soma with the aim of changing the course of his/her health (for the better).

Note: Doctoring (teaching) a client about their future health (incl. as to how it could be changed for the better) is not intervention, nor is referral for treatment or writing a prescription.

Intervention-prognostic study (clinical): Prognostic study addressing one or more effects of an intervention, ideally in the framework of a designed prognostic probability function, for the designed/defined domain of this.

Laboratory (clinical): Setting other than that of the doctor-client interaction, for the conduct of a gnostic test (radiologic, say).

Latent (*as* a quality of a case of illness): Not manifest in sickness. See Sickness and Overt.

Level of significance (in statistics): 1. Concerning the deviation of a parameter's empirical value from its null value, the extent of this in terms of the P-value it implies. 2. The adopted maximum for this deviation's P-value, α, for classification of the deviation as statistically significant.

Likelihood ratio (for a particular result of a diagnostic test for a particular illness): The probability that the test would/will produce that result in the presence of the illness at issue divided by the probability of this result in the absence of that illness. See Note 1 under Properties of diagnostic tests.

Linear compound (of a set of quantities, in mathematics): The sum of the quantities at issue upon them having been multiplied by their respective coefficients (definitional to the formation of the compound).

Note: Definitional to 'linear' regression models is the formulation of the dependent parameter – the mean of Y or a transform of this – as a linear compound of the independent parameters B_0, B_1, etc., the respective coefficients being 1, X_1, X_2, etc.

Logistic model (in statistics and, centrally, in gnostic clinical research): Formulation of the logit of the mean of a Bernoulli distribution as a linear compound of a set of parameters (with $X_0 = 1$). That is, a logistic model is of the form of:

Log [P/(1 – P)] = B0 + B1X1 + B2X2 + … ;
P = Pr (Y = 1).

Logit (transform of the Bernoulli parameter): The logarithm of the odds of Pr (Y = 1). See Logistic model.

Medical research: Research (scientific) for the advancement of medicine.

Note: The principal species of medical research are its 'basic' and gnostic branches. '*Basic*' medical research – biological in nature – produces knowledge relevant to the development of new tools (products and processes) for deployment in (the practice of) medicine, while *gnostic* medical research – statistical in nature – produces evidence for the development of the knowledge-base (gnostic, of the practice) of medicine.

Medicine (in the professional meaning of the term): Professional healthcare by a (medical) doctor; that is, professional healthcare in which central is the provider's first-hand esoteric knowing – gnosis – about the client's (person's or population's) health. See Clinical medicine and Community medicine.

Note 1: The essence of medical healthcare (by a doctor) is gnosis-based teaching of the client about their own health. Everything else in medicine is incidental yet also predicated on gnosis.

Note 2: The genus medicine subsumes (only) two species: clinical medicine and community medicine. These, in turn, subsume differentiated sub-species – differentiated disciplines such as 'general practice' (misnomer) and communicative-disease epidemiology.

Note 3: The term 'medicine' is much overused: 'Experimental medicine' and 'laboratory medicine,' for instance, are contradictions in terms, and 'translational medicine' is a misnomer for an (inchoate) amalgam of laboratory-level research and clinical-level research and practice. By contrast, the now-fashionable terms 'personalized medicine' and 'precision medicine' do denote medicine, but the they falsely imply that medicine without a role for genomics (in its gnoses) is not personalized, while whatever involvement of genomics makes clinicians' gnoses precise – even in the absence of suitable gnostic probability functions (involving genomic indicators).

Meta-analysis (in statistical science, such as gnostic clinical research): Misnomer for synthesis, in a derivative study, of the results of a set of original studies into their corresponding synthetic result.

Meta-result: Result of a derivative study.

Method: Means to a pre-set end.

Methodology (in a gnostic clinical study): The aggregate of methods (in the production of evidence about the magnitudes of the parameters in the designed gnostic probability function).

Model (statistical, in gnostic clinical research): The designed-and-adopted way of thinking about the rate of occurrence, in a particular domain, of the entity of health addressed in the gnoses the study is to serve.

Note 1: In its fully-developed form, this model involves statistical formulation of the determinants of the rate (in terms of statistical variates, Xs).

Note 2: The objects of study are the parameters in the model.

Morbidity (from an illness): The 'emergent property' of illness on the population level: the frequency of its occurrence. See Rate of morbidity.

Note: On the individual level, the occurrence of an illness is a qualitative matter: in a given individual at any given point in time (i.e., at any given person-moment), the illness either is, or is not, present. But in a population, the occurrence – morbidity – is quantitative, characterized by the (pattern of the) frequency – *rate* – of it.

Mortality (from an illness): The 'emergent property' of death on the population level: the frequency of its occurrence.

Note: Like morbidity, mortality (from an illness) is characterized by the (pattern of the) frequency – *rate* – of it.

Multiple regression model (in statistics): Regression model involving multiple (more than one) independent (non-random) variates (Xs).

Multivariate regression model (in statistics): Regression model involving more than one dependent (random) variates; that is, a vector-valued dependent variate.

Natural experiment (in gnostic clinical research): Malformed concept, as any experimental study on gnostic probabilities involves, by definition, some unnatural determinant(s) of the probability at issue, either acausal one(s) whose very existence in the study base is an artifact of, and for, the study, or causal one(s) whose realizations in the study base are unnatural in this sense. The 'natural experiment' term is self-contradictory, a contradiction in terms. See Experimental study.

Note: While an intervention-prognostic trial – with or without randomization of the experimental (and in this sense unnatural, alien-to-practice) allocations of the treatments – obviously is an experimental study, its quasi-experimental facsimile – involving naturally-occurring choices of the treatments – is not a natural experiment; for, even though such a study has the structure of the corresponding experimental study, the choices of the treatments in its study base are not experimental. The trial involves simulated practice, while its facsimile involves (selections from) actual practice.

Non-cohort study in intervention-prognostic research: Study in which the study population is an open, dynamic one. See Cohort/prospective study in intervention-prognostic research.

Note: When addressing treatments-comparing incidence-density *ratio,* this study can be construed, also, as an etiogenetic/etiognostic study (for etiognosis about iatrogenesis of the outcome in question).

Null hypothesis (about a parameter): 1. In statistical science (such as gnostic clinical research), the conjecture that the parameter in question has its null value. 2. In statistics, any value entertained in testing its tenability as the true value.

Null value (of a parameter in a gnostic probability function): The value representing the simplest possible conception of the relation at issue; that is, the value 0 for the parameter at issue.

Object of study (gnostic): The gnostic probability function addressed in the study – designed (as to its form) for a defined/designed domain of case presentations for gnosis.

Objective of study (gnostic): To produce evidence about the magnitudes of the parameters in the object of the study. See Object of study.

Objects of study (gnostic): The parameters in the object of study. See Object of study.

Observational (as a quality of a gnostic clinical study): Non-experimental.

Note: The word 'observational' is very commonly used as the antonym of 'experimental.' But: observations are just as germane to experimental gnostic studies as they are to non-experimental ones, and it thus would be preferable to use the word 'non-experimental.'

Occurrence (of an entity of health): Happening (i.e., taking place) or being present.

Note: The happening and being present have to do with event- and state-type entities, respectively.

Odds (of Bernoulli realization Y = 1): The probability of the realization divided by its complement; that is, the odds of Y = 1 is $P/(1 - P)$, where $P = \Pr(Y = 1)$.

Note: It is a common misapprehension that deployment of a logistic model for the occurrence of an event-type outcome in an etiogenetic study, or in a non-cohort intervention-prognostic study, inherently produces a result on an odds ratio (rather than an incidence-density ratio).

Ontology (of gnostic clinical research): Theory of admissible concepts. See Epistemology.

Note: In this book, the principal ontological (ontal) precept is that the requisite *knowledge-base* of clinical medicine is of the form of *gnostic probability functions* for defined domains of case presentation for gnosis.

Open population: Population open for exit. See Closed population and Dynamic population.

Note: Membership in an open population is based on a *state* of being (transient, à la being alive). An open population generally is a *dynamic* population.

Original study (gnostic): Study producing new evidence (about the magnitudes of the parameters in the object of study). See Objects of study and Derivative study.

Outcome (in clinical medicine and in gnostic clinical research): 1. Concerning the course of a case of an illness, the way in which it ends, if not terminated by death from an intercurrent extraneous cause; that is: full recovery, survival with some sequela(e), or death from it. 2. Concerning an adopted treatment, any entity of health whose occurrence may be a result of the treatment. See Effect.

Note: Outcome of a treatment is an *acausal* concept: it is merely descriptive of what may happen or has happened under the treatment; for, even though any outcome's possible causal connection to the treatment is of interest, this is not observable.

Overfitting/overparametrization bias (in a result on a gnostic probability function): Bias in the meaning of excessive discrimination (among different gnostic profiles) in the probabilities from the empirical function, due to the number of parameters being too large in relation to the amount of information in the data (or, conversely, the information in the data being insufficient in the face of the number of parameters in the model).

Note: The result can be corrected for this bias by 'shrinkage' of it; but the bias is, without any correction, lesser in the result of a derivative study on the function at issue than in any of the original results contributing to it (due to the larger amount of information deployed in the derivative study).

Overt (as a quality of a case of illness): Manifest in sickness. See Sickness and Latent.

Palliation: Treatment of sickness (rather than its underlying illness). See Therapy.

Parameter: 1. In clinical medicine, any quantitative measure of the state of the client's soma (such as heart rate and systolic blood-pressure). 2. In science (such as gnostic clinical research), any (presumed) constant of Nature (such as a coefficient of an independent variate in an object function for gnostic clinical research). 3. In statistics, a quantity definitional, wholly or in part, of a particular distribution in a family of these (Bernoulli, Gaussian, Poisson, …) or a constant in a function-type model (logistic, say).

Particularistic (as a quality of the referent of gnosis and of the result of a gnostic study): Having a particular case, or a particular study base, as its referent. See Referent and Abstract.

Pathogenesis (of an illness): The process of transition from a normal somatic state to the anomaly definitional to the illness in question. See Etiogenesis.

Note: Pathogenesis is the genesis of an illness in *acausal*, descriptive terms, distinct from the causal counterpart of this, etiogenesis.

Pathognomonic (as a quality of an element in a diagnostic profile, or of the profile as a whole): Practically conclusive about the presence, or absence, of the illness at issue.

Patient (of a clinical doctor): 1. Client being cared for on account of existing illness (or sickness not due to illness). 2. In common usage, client (even if presenting no illness or complaint).

Point estimate (of a parameter in statistics): Empirical value. See Empirical value and Estimate.

Population-based (as a quality of a gnostic clinical study): Involving a study base of (an aggregate of) population-time (as distinct from a series of person-moments).

Note: The term is now commonly used to underscore that the study involves the use in a defined population (as distinct from a 'case-control' study not 'nested' in such a population). Once it gets to be commonly understood that properly-construed etiogenetic/etiognostic and non-cohort intervention-prognostic studies inherently are population-based (while diagnostic studies are not), there will be little use for this term (except in making this orientational point).

Population-time (for quantification of an empirical incidence density): The average size of the rate's (incidence density's) referent population over a particular span of time multiplied by the duration of that time.

Note: Conceptually, this quantity is the integral of the population's size (time-specific) over the span of time involved. It therefore is time-dimensioned; it is a given amount of time, of so-called population-time.

Power of a study (as a concept in statistics): The probability with which a study, as designed (incl. as to its size), will reject the null value of the perimeter under study – with the rejection based on the study producing, for the parameter, an empirical value whose deviation from the null value is statistically significant on the specified level of this, conditionally on the parameter actually having a particular non-null value.

Power of a test (gnostic): The probability with which the test completes a practically conclusive gnostic profile conditionally on a particular inconclusive pre-test profile.

Prediction (in medicine as in general): Foretelling something about the future.

Note 1: Prognostic probability-setting is prediction (of the outcome at issue) only when the probability is set very high (as though having foreknowledge about the outcome).

Note 2: Diagnosis, even with very high probability, is not prediction, as at issue is something about the present (or the past). Yet, all diagnostic probability-setting is prediction in the jargon of 'clinical epidemiologists.'

Prevalence (as a property of a state-type entity of health): Frequency of occurrence (presence) in a population cross-section (at a point in time) or in some other series of person-moments (such as the study base of a diagnostic probability study). See Prevalence rate.

Prevalence rate (of a state of health): The proportion of the person-moments in question such that the state is present (prevails at that moment). See Prevalence.

Probability (gnostic): The proportion of instances like the one at hand in general (i.e., in the abstract) such that the hidden truth being considered actually is, was, or will be the truth (according as at issue is diagnosis, etiognosis, or prognosis).

Prognosis (in clinical medicine): A doctor's first-hand knowing (esoteric) about the future health of the client, specifically about whether a particular entity of health will occur.

Note: Commonly, only uncertain knowing of this type is possible, even in principle; and hence, prognosis about a particular entity of health is, specifically, knowing about the *probability* of its (future) occurrence (with certainty a special case of this).

Precision (of a parameter's empirical value): The extent of freedom from imprecision. See Imprecision.

Properties of diagnostic tests (in 'clinical epidemiology'): 'Sensitivity' and 'specificity' (together with certain derivatives of these, incl. 'likelihood ratio'). See Power of a test.

Note 1: All of these are *malformed* concepts – ontologically inadmissible – as they are, or are based on, conditional probabilities with the respective conditions generally quite non-singular. They have no place in a tenable theory of medicine.

Note 2: A soundly-construed, real property of a diagnostic test, or of a particular set of these, is its 'power' to provide provide for a sufficiently conclusive post-test probability (diagnostic), conditionally on a particular pre-test profile (inconclusive, but singular in its meaning).

Prophylaxis (of illness): Treatment aimed at prevention.

Prospective study (in etiogenetic/etiognostic research): See Cohort/prospective study in etiogenetic/etiognostic research.

Public health: 1. The health of a community (the population of a municipality, say). 2. The field of community-level healthcare.

Note: Different from epidemiology, *clinical medicine* is commonly viewed as not being a public-health field. However, clinical medicine is a very major determinant of public health in meaning # 1 above; and clinical medicine increasingly is a governmental concern – as to the education of clinical doctors as well as the organization, regulation, and even providing of the care, in the context of national health insurance in particular.

P-value (in testing the tenability a statistical null hypothesis): Statistic so constructed that on the null hypothesis its distribution is uniform in the range from 0 to 1, while on the alternative hypothesis the distribution, still in this range, is shifted toward the lower end of it. See Hypothesis.

Note 1: This formulation of the essence of the P-value statistic is exceptional. It has the virtues of being analogous to the common definition of confidence interval and serving to prevent its common, serious misinterpretation as the probability that the null hypothesis (in the statistical meaning of this) is true.
Note 2: With α a value in that range, $\Pr(P < \alpha) = \alpha$ on the null hypothesis, and $\Pr(P < \alpha) > \alpha$ on the alternative hypothesis. By no means is the P-value the probability that the null hypothesis is true.

Quasi-experimental (as a quality of a gnostic clinical study, specifically an intervention-prognostic study): Having the structure of the corresponding experimental study, without actually being experimental.

Note: The experiment-emulating structure of a quasi-experimental intervention-prognostic trial arises from selective enrolments into the compared sub-cohorts, the actual-practice treatments in these corresponding to the experimentally-assigned ones the trial serving as the paradigm for the study.

Rate of morbidity (from an illness in a population): Number of cases of the illness divided by the amount of opportunity for the cases' occurrence.

Note: A rate of morbidity is either *empirical* (with a particular documented experience as its referent) or *theoretical* (with an abstract domain as its referent).

Reference category (of a causal determinant): The defined alternative of the index category of a causal determinant, representing absence of the cause at issue (in the causal contrast). See Index category.
Referent (of a piece of gnostic knowledge or of the result of a gnostic study): That to which it refers.

Note: The referent of knowledge about a gnostic probability is an abstract domain of case presentations, while that of the result of a gnostic study is the study base.

Rehabilitation (for sequelae of an illness): Treatment to restore lost functionality.
Research (scientific, gnostic or other): The aggregate of studies on a given class of objects of study.

Result (of a gnostic study): Empirical values (from the study) of the objects of the study. See Object of study and Objects of study.

Retrospective study (in etiogenetic/etiognostic research): See Case-control study.

Risk (in medicine as in general): The possibility, or probability, of an adverse outcome (prospective).

Risk factor (for an adverse outcome): Causal determinant of the rate/probability of the outcome's occurrence. See Risk indicator.

Note 1: In this meaning of the term, everyone has, at all times, particular realizations for all risk factors for the outcome at issue.

Note 2: In another meaning of it, the term denotes a particular category of the determinant at issue, specifically an/the index category of it (representing higher risk of the outcome relative to that represented by the reference category). In these terms, a person at a particular time may not have the factor at issue.

Risk indicator (for an adverse outcome): Acausal determinant of the rate/probability of the outcome's occurrence; that is, a prognostic indicator for an adverse outcome. See Risk factor.

Sample-size determination (statistical, for a study on the value of a parameter): Calculation of the size of the study (otherwise fully designed) which implies a given level of power for the study. See Power of a study.

Note: In gnostic clinical research, truly-relevant studies are not ones of hypothesis-testing. Rather, in each of these studies the overall objective is one of quantification: the production of evidence about the magnitudes of the parameters in a pre-specified gnostic probability function. This 'sample-size determination' therefore has *no justifiable place* in the design of these studies – nor, actually, in any others. The calculated study size is not the optimal size of the study, nor does it have any bearing on the synthesis of the study data into the result of the study and the inferential statistics on this, or the interpretation of these.

Scientific medicine: Medicine with a rational theoretical framework and knowledge-base (for gnoses) from science (gnostic research).

Screening (in clinical medicine): Preliminary testing for the presence of a latent case of a particular illness, with the result bearing on the decision to more seriously pursue rule-in diagnosis about the illness.

Sensitivity (of a diagnostic test with binary or dichotomized results, to the presence of a particular illness): The probability that the test would/will produce its positive result, conditionally on the illness at issue being present. See Note 1 under Properties of diagnostic tests. See Specificity and Properties of diagnostic tests.

Sequela (of an illness): Defect as an outcome. See Outcome and Complication.

Setting (for a gnostic clinical study): The framework for the definition/formation of the study base (such as the practices of a particular discipline of medicine in a particular set of institutions).

Shrinkage (of the empirical values of multiple-regression parameters): Adjustment of the empirical values toward their respective null values. See Overfitting/over-parametrization bias.
Sickness: Symptom(s) and/or overt sign(s) of an illness (hidden) or from a non-somatic direct cause (behavioral or environmental).
Sign (in clinical medicine): An objective manifestation of a hidden anomaly of the patient's soma, detected by the doctor. See Finding.

Note. A sign is a finding in the person's physical examination or from a laboratory test.

Specialty (in medicine): See Discipline.
Specificity (of a diagnostic test with binary or dichotomized results, to the absence of a particular illness): The probability that the test would/will produce its negative result, conditionally on the illness at issue being absent. See Sensitivity and Note 1 under Properties of diagnostic tests.
Standard deviation (as a descriptor of a distribution): Square root of variance.

Note: This measure, like variance, is a meaningful descriptor of Gaussian ('Normal') distributions alone. Very commonly, this measure is used inappropriately.

Standard error (of a parameter's empirical value): Empirical value (from the study data) of the standard deviation of a result's distribution (asymptotically Gaussian) in hypothetical replications of the study. See Standard deviation.
State-type illness: See Event-type illness.
Statistic: 1. Datum. 2. Number derived, in a particular way, from a body of data.
Statistical significance (of the extent to which a parameter's empirical value deviates from its null value): 1. The amount of the deviation as measured by its P-value, by how small the value of this statistic is. 2. The deviation's extent being statistically significant. See Statistically significant.
Statistically significant (as a quality of the extent to which a parameter's empirical value deviates from its null value): The amount of deviation being sufficiently large to translate into a P-value smaller than the cut-off level α chosen for statistical significance. See Statistical significance.
Statistics (as a scholarly and professional field): 1. The field concerned with documentation of numerical information (à la, e.g., 'vital statistics'). 2. The branch of mathematics that treats of distribution theory, including in its relation to probability theory. See Biostatistics.

Note: Highly relevant to gnostic clinical research is statistics in meaning # 2 above.

Stochastic (as a quality of a fact or a set of facts): Involving a role for chance in its genesis.
Study (gnostic): Piece of research, original or derivative, on the magnitudes of the parameters constituting the objects of it. See Original study, Derivative study, and Objects of study.

Note: The process of a gnostic (or any other scientific) study is completed only by the publication of the *report* on it. For, scientific research is a public enterprise.

Study base (of a gnostic clinical study): The series of instances (person-moments) or the aggregate of population-time representing the domain of the object of the study and documented in the study (in terms of empirical values for the parameters constituting the objects of the study). See Referent.

Symptom (in clinical medicine): A subjective manifestation of an anomalous state of the patient's soma, reported by the patient. See Sign.

Note. The *anomalous state need not be an unhealthy one*; it can be a state – transient – of a healthy soma under abnormal stress (iatrogenic, say).

Synthesis (of study data): Derivation of a/the study result (original of synthetic) from the study data (the 'raw' data of an original study or the results of a set of these). See Analysis.

Systematic error (in an empirical value of a parameter): The extent to which a parameter's empirical value (from a study with its methodological particulars) would deviate from the corresponding theoretical value, if that result were free of its imprecision.

Systematic review (in statistical science, such as gnostic clinical research): See Derivative study.

Test (in clinical medicine and in gnostic clinical research): Procedure – generally on the laboratory level – to obtain some gnostically relevant indication on the state of the client's soma supplementary to that from history and physical examination. See Indication and Diagnostic test.

Note: According to teachings about '*clinical epidemiology*,' even symptoms (from history-taking) and overt signs (from physical examination) are results of tests (diagnostic). This allows diagnostic probability-setting in the context of the full diagnostic profile of the case at hand on the basis of knowledge about certain properties of diagnostic tests, *misguided* though this idea is (as an alternative to understanding the relevant knowledge to be about diagnostic probability functions).

Theoretical: Based on, or having to do with, or being in the nature of theory (reasoning-based, rather than empirical).

Theoretical value (of a parameter in a gnostic study's object function): The value in the function's referent domain (abstract). See Empirical value.

Theory (of medicine, or of medical research): Concepts and principles of the field in question, notably when in accord with facts about that field and also rational (i.e., in accord with the imperatives of logic).

Therapy: Treatment directed to amelioration, or cure, of an illness (of the anomaly in its essence). See Palliation and Prophylaxis.

Transformed/transformative clinical research: Patient-level clinical research transformed to production of the critically-relevant knowledge-base (gnostic) of (the practice of) clinical medicine; that is, clinical research transformative of clinical medicine, in its gnostic probability-setting, from pre-scientific (opinion-based) to scientific (scientifically knowledge-based).

Trauma: Injury. See Illness.

Treatment (in clinical medicine): See Prophylaxis, Therapy, Palliation, and Rehabilitation.

Validity (of the methodology of a gnostic clinical study, original or derivative, and hence of the result produced by it): The extent to which the empirical magnitudes of the object parameters (in the result of the study) are free of 'systematic' errors. See Systematic error and Bias.

Variable/variate (in statistics): Numerical entity that has random (chance) variation of its realizations.

Note 1: While 'variable' now is (by far) the more commonly-used term for this concept, 'variate' is preferable; for, an apposite term for this (and any other) entity is not an adjectival one but a noun, as in saying that one of the defining qualities of variates (noun) is that they are variable (adjective) in their realizations.

Note 2: The term 'variable' is, at present, in common usage, also, in reference to various non-statistical entities (such as a person's age and gender), even in statisticians' scholarly writings. In this book, however, a sharp distinction is made between gnostic indicators and the variates representing them in gnostic probability functions.

Variance (as a descriptor of a distribution): Average of the squares of the variate's realizations' deviations from the mean.

Appendices

Abstract Some experts on 'artificial intelligence' are very sanguine about the potential of 'machine learning' as the source of the knowledge-base of clinical medicine, one of them saying, "Take any old classification problem where you have a lot of data, and it's going to be solved by deep learning" (i.e., by machine learning). We therefore needed to consider the question, Is machine learning a realistic alternative to the gnostic clinical research we're outlining and advocating, making this research superfluous? Even though we have no expertise on machine learning, it is evident to us that this technology can serve clinical gnosis and gnostic clinical research in the production of inputs to gnostic profiles by means of high-quality reading of electronic images and tracings; and equally clear to us is, that even with access to lots of high-quality data on clinical practices, machine learning cannot produce valid estimates of profile-specific causal probabilities, whether etiognostic or prognostic. We thus believe that the correct answer to that overall question is No.

Appendix 1: What About 'Machine Learning'?

A1.1 Expert Introduction to Machine Learning for Medicine

For this book of ours we developed, with careful deliberation, our vision of clinical research so transformed that it, in turn, would transform clinical medicine from its status quo of still being largely opinion-based, pre-scientific to becoming generally knowledge-based, genuinely scientific medicine (cf. Preface).

In the presentation of all of this, we made no reference to *machine learning* as a source of the knowledge-base of clinicians' gnoses. But we're filling that void here, prompted by the great expectations that some in the vanguard of health-related information technology now exhibit about this species of 'artificial intelligence' as

O. S. Miettinen et al., *Clinical Research Transformed*,
https://doi.org/10.1007/978-3-030-06176-0

a contributor to doctors' esoteric knowing (gnosis) about hidden truths concerning their patients' health, to doctors' diagnoses in particular.

This vision about AI in relation to doctors' practices came to focus in a recent (April 3, 2017) issue of The New Yorker. In it was an article by *Siddhartha Mukherjee*, this author of the celebrated books "The Emperor of All Maladies" and "The Gene: An Intimate History." In that recent article he addressed the question, *"When it comes to diagnosis, will A.I. replace the M.D.?"* The title of that piece was as telling as it was witty: "The Algorithm Will See You Now."

Mukherjee attributed a good part of the ideas – about the principles and prospects of machine learning in the advancement of the knowledge-base of medicine – to two experts on the subject.

One of those two experts is *Sebastian Thrun.* He had become "convinced that he could do better than [the] first-generation diagnostic devices" that performed pattern-recognition in the meaning of rule-based mapping from digital electrocardiograms and mammograms into diagnostic categories such as 'atrial fibrillation' or 'breast cancer.' Different from these rule-implementing algorithms, "learning algorithms of the kind that Thrun works with involve [emulation of] how the brain functions. … The more powerful [digital systems] have something akin to layers of neurons, each processing the input data and sending the results up to the next layer. Hence, 'deep learning.'"

In his studies on deep learning for diagnoses, "Thrun began [with the question,] Could a machine be taught to distinguish skin cancer from a benign skin condition by scanning a photograph? 'If a dermatologist can do it, then a machine should be able to do it as well,' Thrun reasoned. 'Perhaps a machine could do it even better.'"

The mathematical foundations of the approach aside, Thrun's deep-learning scheme is this: "The machine learning algorithm … pulls information from a training set that has been classified." The thus-developed system classifies any given image into one of a pre-specified set of diagnostic categories; it translates the image into ostensible rule-in diagnosis about one of these possibilities; but this actually is the category of the highest probability, which may be quite low. "(The actual output of the algorithm is not 'yes' or 'no' but a probability that a given lesion belongs to a category of interest.)" How the machine arrived at its diagnosis "it can't tell us."

"Thrun insists that these deep-learning devices will not replace dermatologists and radiologists. They will *augment* the professionals, offering them expertise and assistance."

The other expert Mukherjee interviewed is *Geoffrey Hinton.* He is more sanguine than Thrun about the prospects of machine learning for applications in medicine. For, Mukherjee quotes Hinton as saying that, "It's just completely obvious that in 5 years deep learning is going to do better than radiologists. It *might* be ten years. … They should stop training radiologists now."

Hinton's "prognosis for the future of automated medicine," says Mukherjee, "is based on a simple principle: *Take any old classification problem where you have a lot of data, and it's going to be solved by deep learning* [italics ours]. He wants to use learning algorithms to read X-rays, CT scans, and MRIs of every variety – and that's just what he considers the near-term projects. In the future, … learning algorithms will make pathological diagnoses," presumably meaning diagnoses on the basis of digital images of tissues.

Very notable to us is those experts' evident agreement on two other things: for one, that at issue is, initially at least, the knowledge-base of *only diagnosis,* exclusive of etiognosis and prognosis (intervention-prognosis in particular); and for another, that needed for machine learning relevant to diagnosis is *"a vast trove" of data – "a lot of data" (commonly called big data) – on, specifically, clinicians' actual in-practice classifications (diagnostic) together with whatever data of whatever quality happen to be associated with the classifications in the practice records constituting the learning's source base.*

Mukherjee makes a passing allusion to some of "the most ambitious versions of diagnostic machine-learning," ones that "seek to integrate natural-language processing (permitting them to read medical records) and an encyclopedic knowledge of medical conditions gleaned from textbooks, journals, and medical databases." As examples of this he mentions IBM's Watson Health and Google's DeepMind.

A1.2 Our Non-expert Thoughts on Those Expert Precepts

In our conception of it, *scientific dermatology* of the future is driven by its 'expert systems,' and those AI devises assist diagnoses by providing the lesion-descriptive inputs into the diagnostic profiles of the cases. This is not machine diagnosis about the nature of skin lesions; it is *machine reading* of images of the lesions, for description of these. This point has its counterpart in the context of radiologic images.

Hinton's prognosis about the development of machine interpretation of radiologic images – about this going to be superior to radiologists' diagnoses – we strongly believe. But to us this is nothing to be sanguine about. For, as we implied above, image-reading machines are not diagnosing devises nor should radiologists presume to be diagnosticians; and even diagnoses based on machine reading of images will be inferior to the scientific diagnoses for which reading of images is but a source of a part of the inputs into the diagnostic profiles.

As *Thrun* and *Hinton* agree that machine learning for medicine will, initially at least, be limited to *diagnosis,* we unhesitatingly agree, though only in the pre-diagnostic, fact-finding meaning of 'diagnosis' (above). As for the possibility of machine learning for *etiognoses*, our position is that – by virtue of the non-phenomenal (noumenal) nature of any causal connection – there can be no body of training data for a machine's learning (etiognostic) in which cases of the outcome are classified according to whether the antecedent caused the outcome.

And any given *prognostic* concern in modern medicine also generally is about a causal connection, about the prospective effects of a particular algorithm of prospective treatment relative to those of a particular alternative algorithm. A machine can learn about associations between treatment and outcome, but it scarcely can *learn not to 'learn,'* for instance, that chemo- and radiotherapy for a cancer are major positive causes of fatal outcomes of its course.

Those experts' agreement about the *diagnostic big-data doctrine* – that a machine can learn diagnostic probabilities from any sufficiently large body of clinical data, without any other requirements on it – is downright astounding to us. And IBM's *Watson Health* and Google's *DeepMind,* as Mukherjee describes them, leave us even more baffled.

A1.3 Will Machine Learning Supplant Gnostic Clinical Research?

Even though we have no expertise in machine learning, we have in the foregoing demarcated the limited, though by no means unimportant, role that we envision for machine learning in the development of the requisite knowledge-base for clinical medicine; and even for this limited role, we question the purported usefulness of 'big data' from clinical records without any constraints on their suitability for the purpose.

Whereas for the development of this view we deployed a single article delineating the views of two experts on the essence and potential of machine learning for diagnoses (Sect. A1.1), and whereas we here criticize some fundamentals of those views, experts on this topic may well have criticisms of what we say here. For presentation of such counterpoints it would not suffice, we suggest, to study this Appendix. Needed is, we believe, study of this book more extensively so as to be clear on what we in this Appendix are saying about gnostic clinical research. For, the topic is quite challenging and generally ill-understood, and in this book we present serious criticisms of the entire enterprise of contemporary research for the knowledge-base of clinical medicine – this as the backdrop for positing what we regard as a tenable theoretical framework for the needed research.

This book is about *human learning* – scientific, about probability functions for all three species of clinicians' gnoses – the directly practice-relevant knowledge-base of clinical medicine, to be codified, explicitly, in *machines of a different kind,* in practice-guiding 'expert systems.' In this, we don't see any 'machine learning' supplanting human learning the theory of this research and, then, humans conducting the requisite research – as a global program of transformative clinical research (Appendix 2, below).

Appendix 2: On Excellence of Epidemiologic Academia

A Lecture by O.S. Miettinen at the Karolinska Institute on 23/02/2018

Thank you Anders for that gracious and generous introduction. And, I wish all of you a good afternoon for the next hour – good in the sense of it leading to further elevations in your already-high cruising altitudes in epidemiologic academia.

As you well know, I am here to talk to you about that very topic – high cruising altitudes in epidemiologic academia, with focus on them here at this KI.

This very advanced topic the organizers of this session – Anders Ahlbom and Anita Berglund – deemed me to be qualified to address. The basis for this judgement of theirs I presume to have been, simply, my status as a very advanced epidemiologist – yes, and this by the well-established criterion of exhibiting a very advanced case of being broken down by age and sex.

From this lofty vantage, *I'll guide you through a dozen displays* of bare-bones text; and, as noted in this procedural one, you'll receive copies of those texts.

This being the Nobel Forum of the KI, I prepared written remarks on the text displays, having never done such a thing before; and I'll make them available to you along with the text displays. For the same reason, I'm wearing a tie for this academic business session, which also is very extraordinary.

1. This lecture's premises and missions

The main *premises* of this lecture are these two:

1. Here at the KI, the general imperative of *academic excellence* presumably is felt with heightened intensity. For this is, after all, the KI.
2. In the *epidemiologic segment* of the medical faculty here, the felt burden of this imperative presumably is heightened further by awareness of the *confusion* that now plagues epidemiologic academia everywhere; and in this segment of the faculty here, there therefore presumably is felt a *burning need to resolve this confusion* – locally for a start, and then, under KI's leadership, globally.

My main missions in this lecture, therefore, are these two:

1. To present *my conception of what excellence of epidemiologic academia consists in.*
2. To advance *my vision of the epidemiologic segment of the KI medical faculty as the prospective pioneer and leader of an exceptionally excellent program, global in scope, of medical research.*

In this first one of those text displays I specify, for your orientation, the predicates of, and missions in, this talk.

The *principal predicate* is, otherwise put, my presumption that you epidemiologic academics here at the KI are – like I also am – imbued with Aristotelian ethics and are, hence, seeking personal happiness by striving for personal excellence, specifically as epidemiologic academics. And an *added predicate* is my presumption that you – different from me – now are frustrated in this pursuit, by confusion about the nature of that aspirational excellence of yours.

My *mission* in this talk therefore will be a dual one: first, to dissipate your confusion about the nature of the excellence you aspire to; and then, to paint a picture of such outstanding excellence as you, quite uniquely, can attain – and by my presumption will attain.

That prospective super-excellence of yours, while making for your full-on happiness, will have the same consequence for me, as I'll be very happy about you effecting the major transformation in medical research that I now am dreaming of. For *at issue ultimately is nothing less than transformation of the prevailing, essentially pre-scientific medicine into genuinely scientific medicine*.

2. The prevailing confusion in epidemiologic academia, fundamentally

The depth of the prevailing confusion in epidemiologic academia comes to view, most notably, in the prevailing conceptions of *the essence of epidemiology* in it:

Some academic 'epidemiologists' now define epidemiology as a *study* or a *science,* while others among them define it as a *method.* Besides, equally ill-defined '*clinical epidemiology*' has arisen in clinical academia and has become an element even in epidemiologic academia, confounding it further as to the essence of epidemiology.

In epidemiologic academia there thus is, at present, no shared conception of the essence of epidemiology, much less a shared-and-tenable conception of this.

Epidemiologic academia thus lacks, at present, the requisite foundation for the development of truly productive programs of education and research.

As you see here, in epidemiologic academia in general there now indeed is *serious confusion, even about the very essence of the field* whose knowledge-base in principle is the object of its teaching, advanced by its research.

I felt this lack of solid foundation for the edifice of epidemiologic academia, keenly, at the beginning of my epidemiologic studies already, in the early 1960s, when the essence of epidemiology was being debated – without any denouement – in the AJPH.

As a follow-up to this, I invited an eminent 'shoe-leather' epidemiologist – Alex Langmuir of the Center for Disease Control in Atlanta – to come and explain to us epidemiologic academics at Harvard what epidemiology – out there in the real world – actually is. His hour-long screed on this converged to the proposition, "Epidemiology is long division." And in accord with this, some define an epidemiologist as a doctor who can count.

But critically weighing and considering this description of epidemiologists' work – counting of cases and noses and then dividing the case count by the nose count – I just couldn't adopt it as my considered conception of the essence of epidemiology.

In this direction, though, I have come to a conception of epidemiology with which I am entirely happy, and have also reached gratifying understandings of various issues subordinate to this – ones of epidemiology proper and epidemiological research for a start; and then, distinctly more importantly, ones of clinical research.

The main ones of these points of happiness I'll briefly address in what follows, ultimately with special reference to this KI – aiming to leave enough time for an initial Q & A exchange, to be supplemented in correspondence.

3. Tenable conception of epidemiology: proposition

In a tenable conception of it, I firmly hold, epidemiology is a species – branch – of *medicine*. Specifically, I define epidemiology as *population medicine,* a.k.a. *community* medicine and *social* medicine, serving its client *populations* re *morbidity* in them.

Explication of the 'notes' in this:

1. *Medicine* has *professional healthcare* (to humans) as its 'proximate genus.' And its 'specific difference' within this genus is the centrality of *first-hand esoteric knowing – gnosis –* about relevant-but- hidden truths concerning the client's health – dia-, etio-, and/or prognosis, that is.
2. *Populations* (humans) are of two generic, logically-defined types: *closed* (cohort-type) and *open* (dynamic). Client populations of epidemiology are all open.
3. *Morbidity* is the population-medicine counterpart of illness in clinical medicine. It is the *frequency* of the occurrence of an illness in the cared-for population. It is quantified in terms of *rates* of it – rates of *incidence* of events of illness, *prevalence* of states of illness.

Like that definition of epidemiology, these related concepts in that definition also are far from ingrained in today's epidemiologic academia.

Medicine, as you see here, I define as a species of professional healthcare, to humans. While the meaning of 'professional healthcare' presumably is quite unambiguous, there is serious confusion about the essence of the medical species of this genus among us medical academics, even.

That which distinguishes medicine from nursing, most notably, is that *medical doctors are supposed to have, uniquely, the capacity to attain first-hand knowing about relevant-but-hidden truths concerning their clients' health.*

This uniquely medical knowing is about the current state of the client's health, the causal origin of that state, and/or the future course of the client's health. These three species of esoteric knowing I term *diagnosis, etiognosis,* and *prognosis*, respectively; and for the three of them, my omnibus term is *gnosis*.

Gnosis, in that meaning of this word, is the basis for what to me is real doctoring, namely medical doctors' teaching their clients about *their* own health, most importantly about the ways in which it could be changed for the better – *doctor* being Latin for 'teacher.'

The *foundation of medicine* I consequently take to be the requisite knowledge-base – abstract – for those ad-hoc gnoses. And definitional to genuine medicine I thus take to be the role in it of suitably knowledge-based gnoses – their lege artis attainment and use.

In sharp contrast to my conception of medicine as such a species of professional healthcare, preeminent *dictionaries of medicine* now specify the proximate genus of medicine as an amalgam of art and science. Yet, Aristotle already made a sharp distinction between 'productive arts' such as medicine and sciences such as biology. And in truth, even *scientific medicine is art*, in the still-apposite, Aristotelian meaning of 'productive arts,' and thus *it definitely is not science*, not even in part.

The modern mischaracterization of medicine as science is codified in the very word for medicine in a language I know – the Finnish word *laaketiede*, which translates into 'medicinal science.' And the category error this misnomer reflects has been embraced en masse by practicing doctors, as they've donned the lab coat of scientists ever since the time – late nineteenth century – when laboratory science first really asserted itself as the basis for the development of new tools – vaccines – for deployment in medicine.

As for human *populations*, early in my career as a teacher of epidemiological research I posited a *logical duality* in the types of them. Memberships in the two types of population I defined by an event and a state, respectively; and consequent to this, the two types of population I understood to be, respectively, closed and open for exits. I characterized those two types of population as being of cohort type and dynamic, respectively.

Soon after this, Alvan Feinstein quipped having heard that I had made cohorts to represent "statistical immortality." And indeed, membership is eternal in thus-defined cohorts, such as that of winners of the Nobel Prize in Physiology or Medicine. By contrast, membership is transient in all inherently live populations. These populations therefore are open for exit and are dynamic in the sense of having turnover of membership.

Epidemiologic academics still are, commonly, confused about this logic-dictated duality of types of population. Emblematic about this confusion is the recent neologism 'dynamic cohort' – a contradiction in terms.

Morbidity in the cared-for population – constituting the object of epidemiology as I define it – is the 'emergent property' of any illness on the population level. It is the frequency of the occurrence of the illness, quantified in terms of rates of its occurrence.

In disregard of this principle of epidemiology, Feinstein in clinical academia – one of the two fathers of so-called 'clinical epidemiology' – introduced the term 'co-morbidity' to denote co-illness in the patient. Consistent with this aberrant use of the 'morbidity' term of epidemiology would have been declaration of 'morbidly' as an all-purpose synonym of 'illness,' and 'mortality' as a synonym of 'death.'

But the confusion about the essence of morbidity is no lesser in epidemiologic academia itself. This is eminently manifest in the IEA dictionary of epidemiology – produced by epidemiologic academics.

4. Direct implications (analytic) of that definition of epidemiology

My definition of epidemiology, above, has direct implications (per 'analytic judgements') which also are not part of the conceptual framework of today's epidemiologic academia:

1. Epidemiology is, inherently, *population-level preventive medicine* (supplementing individual-level – clinical – preventive medicine).
2. Epidemiology is, inherently, a segment of the professional realm of *public health* – of societally-provided healthcare (medical & paramedical).
3. Epidemiology is accompanied by *clinical medicine* – therapeutic and rehabilitative, as well as preventive – in the medical segment of public health wherever clinical medicine has been brought into the public domain (per national health insurance).
4. Epidemiologists are community doctors (practicing community medicine).
5. Epidemiologic *academics* are not epidemiologists (as they don't practice community medicine); nor is epidemiological *research* epidemiology (but science).

Among these direct implications of my definition of epidemiology, I call your attention to the principal one among them – the point that epidemiology, as I define it, is a segment of the larger professional field of *public health.*

To me, the proximate genus of public health is the same as that of medicine, namely professional healthcare. But different from medicine, public health encompasses paramedical as well as medical care; hence the term 'public health' and not 'public medicine.' By analogy, by the way, we should have the term 'clinical health' for clinical healthcare at large, provided by paramedical as well as medical professionals.

The specific difference of the professional healthcare in public health is, in my conception of it, simply that it is provided, as the term indicates, in the public domain.

A very important but commonly overlooked aspect of modern public health, thus construed, is illustrated by the following vignette from the late 1980s: I asked my audience of public-health professionals, What do you regard as the greatest innovation in the public-health field since the Second World War? A variety of answers were presented, but not the one I was looking for. I then posited my answer – namely, the introduction of *national health insurance,* which in many countries had brought *clinical medicine* into the public domain. This answer, while wholly unexpected by those public-health professionals, was unhesitatingly embraced by them!

A related point of note is that the main concern of a modern Minister of Health typically is not any problem in their nation's health – in public health in this morbidity meaning of the term. Rather, their main concern typically is a major problem in the country's health care itself – the high and ever-mounting cost of it. And very notably, the cost of healthcare derives, overwhelmingly, from clinical rather than epidemiological care.

Thus, eminent in our public-health concerns we modern epidemiologic academics need to have *clinical medicine* – notably in terms of cultivating *research* for the advancement of its knowledge-base, as this presumably serves to substantially reduce the cost of the care by enhancing its efficiency and, thereby, its cost-effectiveness.

This was famously understood and advocated by our colleague Archie Cochrane; and we need to build on the foundation he laid, guided by critically-developed theory of directly practice-relevant – gnostic – clinical research.

5. Research implications (synthetic) of that definition of epidemiology
Definition: *Epidemiological research is research for the advancement of epidemiology.*

Research-based advancements of epidemiology involve a *fundamental duality,* corresponding to a fundamental duality in the research:

1. Availability of novel *products and processes* for it – as a result of *development* based on (knowledge from) 'basic,' *biological*-type epidemiological research.
2. Improved *knowledge-base* of it – based on (evidence from) 'gnostic,' *statistical-type* epidemiological research.

Relevant research in epidemiologic academia advances its *knowledge-base* of epidemiology, and it thus *focuses on # 2.* (The biological research is conducted elsewhere in academia, and in industry too.)

Regrettably, this sense of relevance does not animate the research in today's epidemiologic academia, even when etiology/etiogenesis of illness is addressed.

Here you see that, while I define epidemiological research at large in terms of its relevance to advancement of epidemiology, the segment of this research in epidemiologic academia I define in terms of its relevance, specifically, to teaching of epidemiology. At issue in this teaching-serving research is advancement of the *knowledge-base* of epidemiology; it thus is exclusive of laboratory-level epidemiological research.

Those terms 'relevance' and 'knowledge-base' are at the core of my thinking about epidemiological research; but they are, remarkably, essentially absent from the active vocabulary in our contemporary epidemiologic academia and, hence, from justification of the research in it.

Thus the research in our contemporary epidemiologic academia is, quite generally, devoid of any raison d'être better than the pursuit of the funding for the work and producing entries into the researchers' bibliographies – with the knowledge-base of epidemiology remaining uninfluenced by these academic goings-on.

6. The methodology of the research in epidemiologic academia
The *methodology* of etiogenetic studies is now commonly taken to logically involve two main design options: the 'case-control study' and the 'cohort study'; but this is a *fallacy,* a paralogism.

Logically, the structure of etiogenetic studies actually is a singular one, that of the *case-referent study*. This term is, now, commonly presumed to be a synonym for 'case-control study.'

The *case-referent* study is founded on a defined *study base,* constituting the *referent* of the study result. The result is derived from the complete *case series* from the study base together with a suitable *base/referent series* from it – upon these two series having been derived by needed reduction of the initial series from the study's *source base* (source population-time), in which the study base is inseparably imbedded.

While relevance to practice and teaching of epidemiology should be assured in the studies' ontological or objects design, their epistemological or methods design should assure, above all, conformity with the imperatives of logic.

Here you read about the central tenet in the research conducted in our contemporary epidemiologic academia, namely the doctrine that the basic design-options in studies into the etiogenesis of illnesses and morbidity rates are the case-control study and the cohort study; and you also read myself saying that the idea of that duality is a fallacy, a mere paralogism, while the corresponding logical structure of etiogenetic studies is a singular one, specifically that of case-referent studies – which I introduced in the 1970s.

The doctrine of those purported basic 'designs' for etiogenetic studies is a legacy of the statistician A. Bradford Hill, who famously worked with Richard Doll on smoking in the etiogenesis of lung cancer. Critically understood, Hill actually consolidated the fallacies in what used to be the singular type of etiogenetic study, now called the case-control study; and he flippantly introduced an even-more-malformed alternative to it, now called the cohort study. These two types of etiogenetic study he termed 'retrospective study' and 'prospective study,' respectively – consequent to which the duality appears to be rooted in logic.

Other statisticians have subsequently expanded on this aberrant logic, in terms of the duality of options in 'sampling' from the margins of a *two-by-two table*. But, nothing has misled the theory of etiogenetic research as much as has the fascination with the two-by-two table.

And for 'clinical epidemiologists' the two-by-two table has been the framework of their favourite yet equally misguided doctrines about purportedly relevant properties of diagnostic tests.

7. Epidemiological research vis-à-vis clinical research: propositions

1. The *fundamental duality* in epidemiological research obtains, *mutatis mutandis,* in clinical research as well.
2. In statistical-type medical research there is, however, a fundamental difference between the two: While the epidemiological research is about rates, the clinical research is about *probabilities – gnostic,* mainly diagnostic and prognostic but also etiognostic.
3. Gnostic probabilities for clinical medicine need to be studied through rates. In this sense, *statistical-type clinical research is meta-epidemiological* in nature. Its theory thus is an extension of the theory of statistical-type epidemiological research.
4. The requisite theory of gnostic clinical research – meta-epidemiological as it is – has not been understood in clinical academia, in the so-called *clinical epidemiology* there; but tenable theory of this research will be presented in an upcoming book, *Clinical Research Transformed,* developed as an extension of critical theory of research for the knowledge-base of community medicine.

In this juxtaposition of epidemiological research with clinical research, I again wish to emphasize the main point, namely that the requisite knowledge-base of clinical medicine is about gnostic probabilities, which need to be studied through empirical rates.

Hence, the theory of the research for the knowledge-base of clinical medicine is an extension of that for epidemiology – to non-epidemiological domains and purposes. This research is, in this sense, *meta-epidemiological clinical research.* True understanding of it requires critical understanding of epidemiological research on morbidity rates – and of its logical extension to the needs of clinical medicine.

This is another reason why *we in epidemiological [sic]academia need to concern ourselves with the theory, and practice, of research for the knowledge-base of clinical medicine* – more even than for the counterparts of these for community medicine.

Critically-developed theory – concepts and principles – of this meta-epidemiological clinical research is the subject of an upcoming book with a telling title: *Clinical Research Transformed.*

I actually am this book's first author, and the second author is Johann Steurer, the head of the Horten Centre for Patient-oriented Research and Knowledge Transfer at the University of Zurich. He is with us here. Johann: Please give the attendees here a bit of face time, and assure them that you will correct me, as needed, in this session, just as you otherwise always do. – Thank you, Johann.

8. Excellence of education in epidemiology: propositions

1. With epidemiology construed as one of the two branches of medicine, *excellence of education in epidemiology is inherent in excellence of medical education in general* (whether for epidemiology or clinical medicine).
2. Excellent education in medicine is founded on two (post-Flexnerian) *predicates*: first, that education in whichever science is not education in medicine; and second, that substantive education covering all of the disciplines of modern medicine is as impossible as it is uncalled for.
3. Excellent education (and training) in modern medicine – for compe-tence in whichever one of its constituent disciplines – begins with studies on *the medical common*: educational content that truly is relevant in preparation for whichever genuine – rationally-defined – discipline of medicine, such as communicable-disease epidemiology. The medical common is about the general theory of medicine.
4. Genuinely excellent education in communicable-disease epidemiology would be *paradigmatic* about excellent education in whichever well-construed discipline of medicine.

As for excellent education in the epidemiological branch of medicine, I say for a start, emphatically, how it does *not* begin: The requisite preparation for practice in whichever art of community medicine does not begin with extensive studies on various sciences, nor with years of nibbling at a motley of clinical arts of medicine.

Rather, it begins with studies on general theory of medicine, followed by theory specific to community medicine. This is followed by studies specific to one's chosen art of community medicine. Remarkably, none of this is the case in our contemporary medical education.

This is to say that the prevailing pre-med-cum-medschool education is, in all essence, irrelevant as preparation for practice of whichever of the arts of epidemiology – communicable-disease epidemiology, community cardiology, and community psychiatry, inter alia – and each of the arts of clinical medicine just the same.

This tragic but unspoken truth was on my mind when I, for the only time ever, went to a reunion of my medical-school class – as an invited speaker from overseas. And this truth also was the conclusion of my commentary there. Afterwards I was privately told that my classmates agree with me about that sad truth, but elect to not say this in public – for reasons of professional self-preservation!

The obvious need for radical reformation of medical education – and licensing – I wrote about in *The Lancet* two decades ago, but authorities on medical-school curricula still ignore it. Denial of the irrelevance of the prevailing type of medical-school education is self-serving to medical academia itself, and so it also is to most graduates of that education. And, regrettably, the temptation to be self-serving quite generally trumps the academic obligation to be *Veritas*-serving.

While the truth about the irrelevance of the prevailing common education in medicine – based on the 'Flexner report' of 1910 – is kept sub rosa in medical academia, the society sponsoring that education remains unaware of this truth. In consequence, the society unwittingly sponsors education in a very large pseudo-common in the requisite knowledge-base of practice in the multifarious arts of modern medicine.

9. Excellence of education in 'epidemiological' research: propositions

1. In excellent education for 'epidemiological' research, preparation for *meta-epidemiological clinical research* is included. (Hence those quotation marks.)
2. Excellent education for this research is suitably *hierarchical*: Thus, the focus is on original research before its extension to derivative research. And as for study design, very importantly, the studies' *objects design* is addressed prior to addressing their *methods design.*
3. Excellent education for the research begins with suitable *propedeutics.* The first module of these is a scholarly *introduction* to medicine and medical research. The second module covers tenable theory of *epidemiology* relevant to 'epidemiological' research. And the third one covers topics of *statistics* relevant to this research.

These principles (i.a.) are heeded in the upcoming book *Clinical Research Transformed.*

These propositions about excellent research-education in 'epidemiologic' academia you see converging to the point that the essential contents of it are covered in the upcoming oeuvre Clinical Research Transformed.

The *leit motif* throughout that book is, that the requisite knowledge-base of clinical medicine needs to be thought of in terms of *gnostic probability functions for suitably defined domains of case presentation* – not for doctors to learn and know but for codification in cyberspace, in directly practice-guiding 'expert systems.'

Addressing the requisite knowledge-base of clinical medicine in terms of such GPFs is dictated by the need to formulate its great complexity in simplest possible terms, amenable to productive research. And its storage in doctors' neurospace is unnecessary in this Information Age and it also is neurophysiologically impossible.

While that book focuses on meta-epidemiological clinical research, it serves epidemiological research as well. For whoever masters the theory of gnostic clinical research – etiognostic research included – thereby also masters its counterpart for epidemiological research, while the converse is far from true.

10. Excellence of 'epidemiological' research proper: propositions

1. The *knowledge-base of medicine* – gnostic – is a global resource, in principle very precious; but at present it still is severely wanting as the basis for the practice of genuinely *scientific medicine* (whether clinical or epidemiological).
2. Preparatory to the development of this global resource of knowledge is the development of a *global repository of needed evidence* – relevant (gnostically) in its objects and valid in its contents.
3. *Excellence* of research contributing to that resource is an attribute of the epidemiologic segment of a medical faculty, of its *research program*. Excellence of the program consists in its making contributions to the global resource of relevant-and-valid evidence (gnostic) at a high rate (given the size of the unit).
4. Excellence of the global repository of the evidence requires excellence of *leadership* in its development and functioning (notably its relevance- and validity-assurance).

Once the education for epidemiological and, especially, meta-epidemiological clinical research is in good order in a leading unit of epidemiologic academia, the concern of that unit naturally turns to advancement of the research proper.

The grand mission in that research these avant-garde epidemiologic academics – in their capacity as public-health academics – will understand to be the development, with a sense of urgency, of the requisite knowledge-base – gnostic – for *genuinely scientific medicine*, essentially focusing on clinical medicine.

This they will understand to require the development of a *global repository of the needed evidence* – original and derivative – relevant in its objects and valid in its contents.

The initiation and continual development of this repository of ever-accruing relevant-and-valid evidence these pioneers understand to require global coordination under their own, expert leadership.

11. Toward global excellence of 'epidemiological' research: a vision

1. A coterie of epidemiologic academics at the KI reflect on the contents of this lecture and study the manuscript of the book *Clinical Research Transformed*. This results in radical revision of *education* in epidemiology and, especially, in meta-epidemiological clinical research at the KI.

2. The epidemiologic academics at the KI, in collaboration with their clinical colleagues, develop an excellent *design* of a global program of developing the evidentiary base for the knowledge-base of scientific medicine.
3. The KI secures the collaboration of medical faculties throughout Sweden and, ultimately, on a global basis, and also helps secure the funding for the program – to be led by the epidemiologic academics at the KI.
4. The program begins

Here I outline my vision of how such a global program of research for the knowledge-base of scientific medicine will most likely come about.

The seminal work actually is already underway here at this KI, as a coterie of pioneers are studying the manuscript of the afore-mentioned book on transformed-and-transformative clinical research. Upon these studies they presumably will institute the substantially-reformed research education outlined and advocated in that book.

In the second stage, that newly-excellent epidemiologic segment of the medical faculty here presumably will proceed to implementation of the urgently-needed research. Thus, in collaboration with members of the clinical segment of the faculty, these epidemiologic academics presumably will produce an excellent design of the particulars of the program. The medical faculty at large presumably will eagerly buy into such an excellence-exuding interdisciplinary plan of clinical research, and so therefore also will the leaders of the KI.

The Institute will then exert its leadership in securing the cooperation of other medical faculties in Sweden and, ultimately, select ones on a global basis; and it will also assume a role in securing the requisite funding for the program.

Et voila! The epidemiologic segment of the KI medical faculty will thus have assumed the leadership in a global program of expeditiously developing the relevant-and-valid evidentiary base for the development of the requisite knowledge-base for genuinely scientific medicine!

12. Closing note

In that vision, I see the epidemiologic segment of the medical faculty of this august Institute heeding – in its planning ('strategic') for its future excellence – the advise Daniel Burnham gave on urban planning (to the Chicago City Council at the turn of the twentieth century):

Make no little plans; they have no magic to stir men's blood, …
Make big plans; aim high in hope and work, …

This I really expect of the epidemiologic academics here at the KI. For, in the face of what I regard as an unassailable vision of global excellence of directly practice-relevant medical research under their leadership, the alternative to taking on the mission would be philistine indifference to the quest for a scientific knowledge-base for medicine – and this I just don't see to be in the culture of the faculty that awards Nobel Prizes in Physiology or Medicine.

As a penultimate note in this talk, I point out that I see you in the epidemiologic segment of the medical faculty of this august Institute, in your upcoming strategic planning of research, heeding Daniel Bunham's advise on urban planning: Make no little plans; they have no magic to stir men's blood, … Make big plans; aim high in hope and work, …

For now that you've been presented with a vision of urgently-needed major program of medical research, led by a centre of excellence in epidemiologic academia, you – imbued with Aristotelian ethics as you are – naturally will seize the opportunity to aim high in happiness through excellence in executing a big plan for such work.

Besides, in terms of Kantian ethics you have the obligation to aim at such high level of excellence, given your membership in the medical faculty which, as a custodian of the legacy of Alfred Nobel, is uniquely dedicated to promotion of exceptional excellence in medical research.

And my ultimate point in this talk has to do with your post-hoc reading of the text displays in it as well as the write-up of its spoken contents. With a view to these readings I ask you to bear in mind a counsel of Francis Bacon's that has become a central maxim of mine in my teachings: Read not to contradict, nor to believe, but to weigh and consider.

Having thus completed this talk, I thank you Anders and Anita for the honour you accorded me by inviting me to appear at this awe-provoking forum of this august Institute. And I thank all of you for your attention to what I had to say – for you to weigh and consider – about prospective excellence of epidemiologic academia, with special reference to this KI.

Index

O. S. Miettinen et al., *Clinical Research Transformed*,
https://doi.org/10.1007/978-3-030-06176-0

The manufacturer's authorised representative in the EU is Springer Nature Customer Service Centre GmbH, Europaplatz 3, 69115 Heidelberg, Germany. If you have any concerns regarding our products, please contact ProductSafety@springernature.com

Printed and bound by CPI Group (UK) Ltd, Croydon, CR0 4YY

30/09/2026

02225237-0010